IMAGING OF ARTHRITIS AND RELATED CONDITIONS

WITH CLINICAL PERSPECTIVES

IMAGING OF ARTHRITIS AND RELATED CONDITIONS

WITH CLINICAL PERSPECTIVES

Edited by

GEORGE B. GREENFIELD, MD, FACR

Professor of Radiology
Department of Radiology
University of South Florida College of Medicine
Tampa, Florida
Attending Radiologist
Department of Radiology
H. Lee Moffitt Cancer Center and Research Institute
Tampa, Florida
Consultant Radiologist
Shriner's Hospital for Crippled Children
Tampa, Florida

JOHN A. ARRINGTON, MD

Associate Professor of Radiology
Department of Radiology
University of South Florida College of Medicine
Tampa, Florida

FRANK B. VASEY, MD

Professor and Director
Department of Internal Medicine
University of South Florida College of Medicine
Tampa, Florida
Chief of Rheumatology
Department of Internal Medicine,
Tampa General Hospital
Tampa, Florida

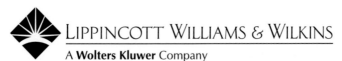

LIPPINCOTT WILLIAMS & WILKINS
A **Wolters Kluwer** Company
Philadelphia • Baltimore • New York • London
Buenos Aires • Hong Kong • Sydney • Tokyo

Acquisitions Editor: Beth Barry
Developmental Editor: Keith Donnellan
Production Editor: Rakesh Rampertab
Manufacturing Manager: Tim Reynolds
Cover Designer: QT Design
Compositor: Maryland Composition Company Inc.
Printer: Maple Press

Library of Congress Cataloging-in-Publication Data

Imaging of arthritis and related conditions: with clinical perspectives/edited by George B. Greenfield, John A. Arrington, Frank B. Vasey.
  p. cm.
  Includes bibliographical references and index.
  ISBN 0-7817-1536-9
  1. Arthritis—Atlases. 2. Arthritis—Diagnosis. 3. Diagnosis, Differential. I. Greenfield, George B., 1928-II. Arrington, John A. III. Vasey, Frank B.

RC933 .I425 2000
616.7′22—dc21   00-041244

Care has been taken to confirm the accuracy of the information presented and to describe generally accepted practices. However, the authors, editors, and publisher are not responsible for errors or omissions or for any consequences from application of the information in this book and make no warranty, expressed or implied, with respect to the currency, completeness, or accuracy of the contents of the publication. Application of this information in a particular situation remains the professional responsibility of the practitioner.

The authors, editors, and publisher have exerted every effort to ensure that drug selection and dosage set forth in this text are in accordance with current recommendations and practice at the time of publication. However, in view of ongoing research, changes in government regulations, and the constant flow of information relating to drug therapy and drug reactions, the reader is urged to check the package insert for each drug for any change in indications and dosage and for added warnings and precautions. This is particularly important when the recommended agent is a new or infrequently employed drug.

Some drugs and medical devices presented in this publication have Food and Drug Administration (FDA) clearance for limited use in restricted research settings. It is the responsibility of the health care provider to ascertain the FDA status of each drug or device planned for use in their clinical practice.

10 9 8 7 6 5 4 3 2 1

CONTENTS

CONTRIBUTING AUTHORS

John A. Arrington, MD   Associate Professor of Radiology, Department of Radiology, University of South Florida College of Medicine, 12901 Bruce B. Downs Boulevard, Tampa, Florida 33612

Gail D. Cawkwell, MD, PhD   Assistant Professor, Department of Pediatrics, P.A.H.O.I, 3920 Southeastern Avenue, Suite 200, Las Vegas, Nevada 89119

George B. Greenfield, MD, FACR   Professor of Radiology, Department of Radiology, University of South Florida College of Medicine; Attending Radiologist, Department of Radiology, H. Lee Moffitt Cancer Center & Research Institute, 12902 Magnolia Drive, Tampa, Florida 33612; and Consultant Radiologist, Department of Radiology, Shriner's Hospital for Crippled Children, Tampa Unit, 12502 North Pine Drive, Tampa, Florida 33612

Keith Kanik, MD, FACP   Assistant Professor, Department of Internal Medicine/Rheumatology, University of South Florida College of Medicine, 12901 Bruce B. Downs Boulevard, Tampa, Florida 33612

G. Douglas Letson, MD   Leader, Sarcoma Program Assistant Professor of Oncology H. Lee Moffitt Cancer Center & Research Institute University of South Florida College of Medicine, 12902 Magnolia Drive, Tampa, Florida 33612

Carlos A. Muro-Cacho, MD, PhD   Associate Professor, Department of Pathology, H. Lee Moffitt Cancer Center & Research Institute, University of South Florida College of Medicine, 12902 Magnolia Drive, Tampa, Florida 33612

Michael D. Neel, MD   Department of Orthopaedics, St. Jude's Children's Research Hospital, 332 North Lauderdale Street, Memphis, Tennessee 38119

Joanne Valeriano-Marcet, MD   Assistant Professor, Department of Internal Medicine, University of South Florida College of Medicine, 12901 Bruce D. Downs Boulevard, Tampa, Florida 33612; and Active Staff Member, Department of Internal Medicine, Tampa General Hospital, Davis Island, Tampa, Florida 33629

Frank B. Vasey, MD   Professor and Director, Department of Internal Medicne, University of South Florida College of Medicine, 12901 Bruce B. Downs Boulevard, Tampa, Florida 33612; and Chief of Rheumatology, Department of Internal Medicine, Tampa General Hospital, Davis Island, Tampa, Florida 33629

PREFACE

The management of the various conditions that can affect joints is often a multidisciplinary endeavor dependent on the skill and expertise of an array of clinical specialists. At the outset and often at later critical points, an accurate radiologic diagnosis is the crucial element for determining the course of treatment and for estimating prognosis. This book provides a comprehensive, extensively illustrated description of the imaging features of arthritis and related conditions.

Imaging of Arthritis and Related Conditions begins with descriptions of the radiologic features of joint disease and illustrations of their differential diagnosis, and concludes with chapters on surgery and pathology related to joint disease. Within these end points are chapters detailing each major entity, along with reports of typical cases as described by expert clinicians. The entities are not limited to the arthritides, but cover other conditions, including tumors, which have overlapping clinical symptoms and imaging features with arthritis. Conventional radiography is stressed, as this modality is most commonly used. Computed tomography and magnetic resonance imaging are also described in detail.

It is my hope that this book will be of assistance to radiologists as well as clinicians who deal with joint diseases.

George B. Greenfield, M.D., F.A.C.R.

ACKNOWLEDGMENTS

We would like to thank Ms. Sally Hammer for her assistance in typing, and Mr. Rick Rouge and Mr. Don Pillae for photography.

IMAGING OF ARTHRITIS AND RELATED CONDITIONS

WITH CLINICAL PERSPECTIVES

RADIOLOGIC FEATURES AND DIFFERENTIAL DIAGNOSIS OF JOINT DISEASE

GEORGE B. GREENFIELD

The conventional radiograph remains the primary modality of diagnosis and follow-up of joint diseases in the peripheral skeleton. Computed tomography (CT) can show greater detail in the central skeleton, and is useful in the periphery. Magnetic resonance imaging (MRI) can show soft-tissue detail and effusions, and demonstrate vascularity as well as the effect of arthritis on the spinal cord and nerve roots. Radionuclide bone scans and ultrasound are helpful also.

The structure of the various joints determines their reaction to disease processes. There are three types of joints: fibrous, cartilaginous, and synovial. *Fibrous joints* (e.g., the cranial sutures) are immobile. These are called *synarthroses*. *Cartilaginous joints,* also called *amphiarthroses* (e.g., the intervertebral discs and the symphysis pubis), contain hyaline cartilage or fibrocartilage. A limited amount of motion is possible.

Most joints are *synovial* or *diarthroses*. The articular surfaces, which are freely movable, are covered with hyaline cartilage, and a capsule surrounds the joint. The outer layer of the joint capsule is fibrous. The inner layer is composed of vascularized connective tissue called the synovium. The synovium does not cover the articular cartilage. It merges with the periosteum, covering the intracapsular portions of bone, except for marginal bare areas. The synovium secretes synovial fluid, which lubricates the joint and nourishes the articular cartilage. Fibrocartilage is present in some joints (e.g., the menisci of the knee). The joints of the extremities and the apophyseal joints of the spine are diarthrodial.

This classification is important because only synovial joints are primarily affected in inflammatory arthritides with generalized synovial involvement.

The spine has two types: the amphiarthrodial intervertebral discs and the diarthrodial apophyseal joints.

The sacroiliac joint is synovial only in its lower two-thirds.

The basic parameters described and illustrated in the following are of importance in interpreting images of arthritis:

1. Patterns of osteopenia
2. Joint effusion and joint space narrowing
3. Erosions, cysts, geodes, and bone resorption
4. Changes in the ossification centers and small bones
5. Subchondral sclerosis and osteophytes
6. Periosteal new bone formation
7. Malalignment, subluxation, dislocation, and fusion
8. Disorganization
9. Ankylosis
10. The distribution and sequence of changes
11. Soft-tissue swelling, atrophy, and calcification
12. The vertebral body
13. The intervertebral disc
14. The apophyseal joints
15. The atlantoaxial articulation
16. The paravertebral area

Osteopenia is associated with several of the arthritides. In inflammatory arthritis, synovial hyperemia leads to early periarticular osteoporosis (Fig. 1.1). Other conditions, such as neurotrophic arthropathy and dialysis arthritis (Fig. 1.2) can also lead to osteoporosis. In chronic arthritis, osteoporosis proceeds to uniform regional bone atrophy, with a thin and sharp cortex (Fig. 1.3). Subchondral osteoporosis occurs in rapidly developing processes such as septic arthritis. Some arthritides, including gout, neurotrophic arthropathy, psoriatic arthritis, Reiter's syndrome, and pigmented villonodular synovitis, are characterized by a relative lack of osteoporosis.

Joint effusion occurs early in synovial disease. Small effusions can be demonstrated earliest by MRI (Fig. 1.4). Large effusions usually can be seen well on conventional radiographs.

Effusions of the proximal interphalangeal (Fig. 1.5) and metacarpophalangeal joints are typical of rheumatoid arthritis (RA) in the hands.

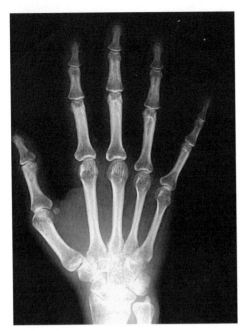

FIGURE 1.1. Periarticular osteoporosis in early rheumatoid arthritis. Hand. No erosions are evident.

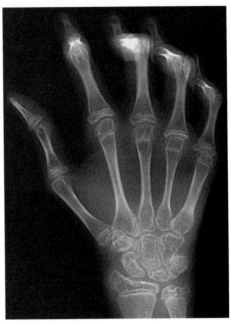

FIGURE 1.3. Juvenile rheumatoid arthritis. Hand. Uniform osteoporosis is noted with a thin, sharp cortex and overtubulation of bones.

The signs of knee effusion are fullness of the suprapatellar pouch seen on lateral view, and curved, displaced radiolucent fat planes medial and lateral to the distal femur in the suprapatellar region, seen on anteroposterior (AP) radiographs (Fig. 1.6).[1] Posterior displacement of the fabella also indicates an effusion. In the elbow, effusion or hemorrhage is indicated by displacement of fat lines, particularly posteriorly. This is called the "fat pad sign" (Fig. 1.7). Haziness is another characteristic of joint effusion, causing a loss of the sharp, white, subchondral cortical line.

Hip effusion in an inflammatory process in children may be detected by displacement of the fat line at the obturator

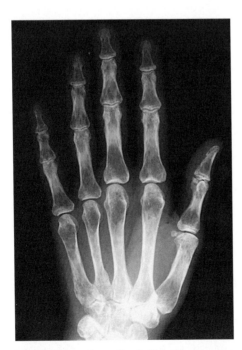

FIGURE 1.2. Dialysis patient. Hand. Periarticular osteoporosis is noted.

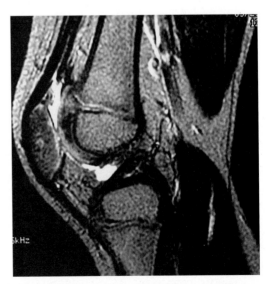

FIGURE 1.4. Hemophilia. Knee. MRI. T2-weighted image. A small effusion is seen as high signal intensity.

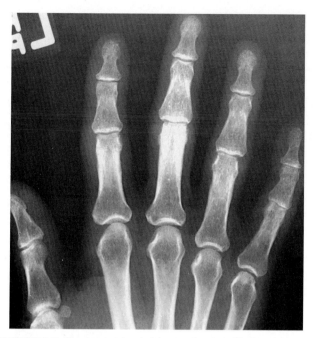

FIGURE 1.5. Rheumatoid arthritis. Hand. Joint effusion and soft-tissue swelling at the proximal interphalangeal joints are noted. Periarticular osteoporosis is also seen.

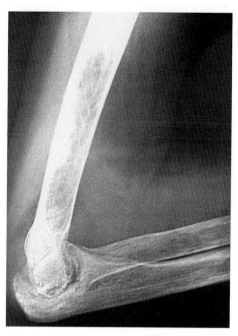

FIGURE 1.7. Rheumatoid arthritis. Lateral view of the elbow. Displacement of fat planes anteriorly and posteriorly at the distal humerus is noted. This is the positive "fat pad" sign.

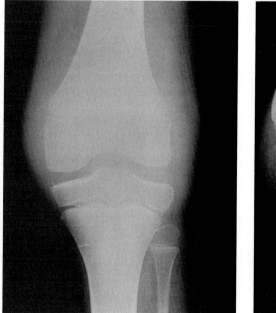

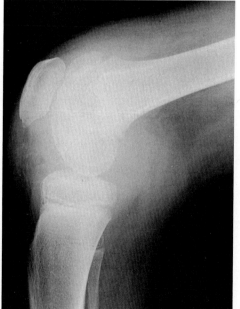

A   B

FIGURE 1.6. **A:** AP view. **B:** Lateral view of the knee shows a large joint effusion.

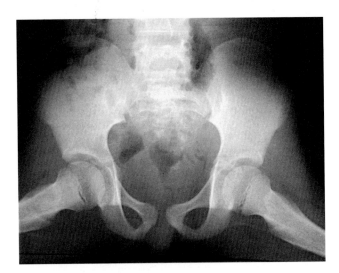

FIGURE 1.8. Early septic arthritis of the left hip. A thin fat line is seen displaced medially owing to edema of the obturator internus muscle. This is called the "obturator sign."

internus muscle medially (Fig. 1.8). This is owing to adjacent muscular edema.

If the amount of fluid increases, joint space widening will occur. If further fluid accumulates, particularly in the hip and shoulder in children, dislocation will follow.

Joint space narrowing may be caused by cartilage atrophy or destruction. Cartilage atrophy may result from disuse. Normal cartilage nutrition is by diffusion of synovial fluid driven by pressure from joint motion. Atrophy may also fol-

low surgical procedures (Fig. 1.9). Rheumatoid arthritis typically results in uniform joint space narrowing, whereas osteoarthritis shows narrowing that is most marked in the weight-bearing areas, which is the medial compartment in the knee, and superiorly in the hip. All three joint compartments are uniformly narrowed in rheumatoid arthritis of the knee (Fig. 1.10). Usually the medial joint compartment shows the greatest narrowing in osteoarthritis (Fig. 1.11).

In rheumatoid arthritis of the hip, uniform narrowing results in superomedial or medial migration of the femoral head (Fig. 1.12), whereas in osteoarthritis the superior weight-bearing aspect is most narrowed (Fig. 1.13). Arthritis in Paget's disease shows uniform joint space narrowing.

Erosions characterize some of the arthritides, whereas others are typically nonerosive. The absence of erosions in the hands is typical of Jaccoud arthritis, Reiter's syndrome, and systemic lupus erythematosus.

Rheumatoid erosions tend to be fuzzily marginated without a sclerotic margin. Erosions are initially located at joint margins in the bare areas (Figs. 1.14 and 1.15). There may be compression erosions with a "ball-in-socket" configuration (Fig. 1.16). Surface erosions may also occur (Fig. 1.17). Erosions of bone may also occur at tendinous insertions (Fig. 1.18).

Later in chronic disease, the articular cartilage is destroyed and the subchondral bone is eroded (Fig. 1.19) and may be destroyed (Fig. 1.20). Sarcoidosis can also result in bony erosions in the vicinity of a joint. The margins are

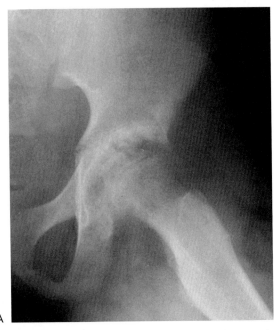
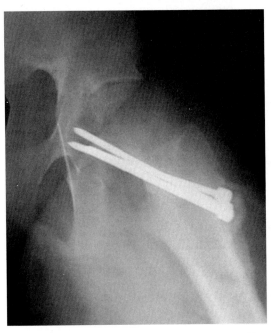

FIGURE 1.9. Slipped femoral capital epiphysis. **A:** Preoperative view of the hip shows rotation downward of the femoral head. Hip pinning was subsequently performed. **B:** Film 8 months after **(A)**. The patient complained of a painful hip and limitation of motion. The pins are seen to project outside of the femoral head. There has been narrowing of the hip joint space and local osteoporosis of the femoral head and neck. This represents acute chondrolysis.

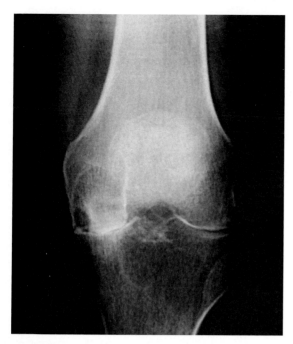

FIGURE 1.10. Rheumatoid arthritis. Knee. Uniform narrowing of the medial and lateral compartments is noted.

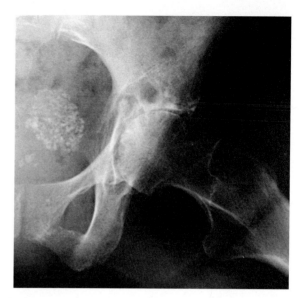

FIGURE 1.12. Rheumatoid arthritis. Hip. There is uniform narrowing of the joint space with medial drift of the femoral head. Subchondral sclerosis is also seen. A calcified fibroid is incidentally noted.

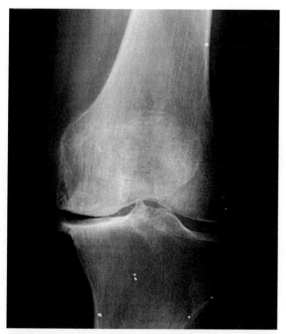

FIGURE 1.11. Osteoarthritis. Knee. Narrowing of the medial compartment of the joint space is seen. There is also medial spur formation, a vacuum sign in the medial compartment, and chondrocalcinosis.

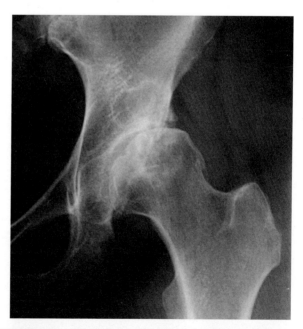

FIGURE 1.13. Osteoarthritis. Hip. There is narrowing of the superior aspect of the hip joint space with slight lateral migration of the femoral head. Subchondral sclerosis is also seen.

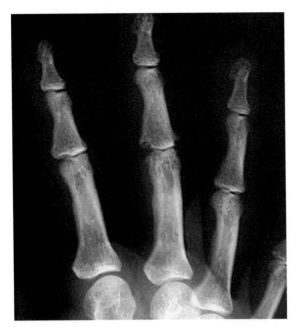

FIGURE 1.14. Rheumatoid arthritis. Hand. An early erosion is seen at the proximal interphalangeal joint of the middle finger. The erosion is poorly marginated.

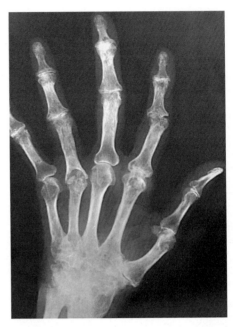

FIGURE 1.16. Rheumatoid arthritis. Hand. There is a compression erosion at the fourth metacarpophalangeal joint with a "ball-in-socket" configuration. Fusion at the wrist has also occurred.

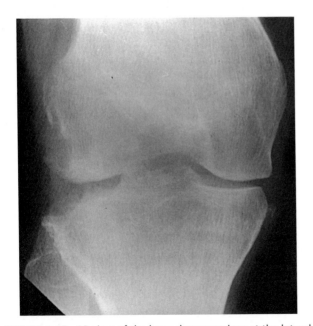

FIGURE 1.15. AP view of the knee shows erosions at the lateral margin of the knee joint. Joint space narrowing is also seen.

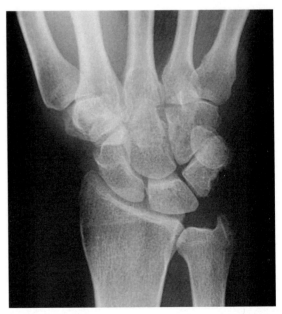

FIGURE 1.17. Rheumatoid arthritis. Wrist. Erosion along the outer surface of the triquetrum and the ulnar styloid process is noted.

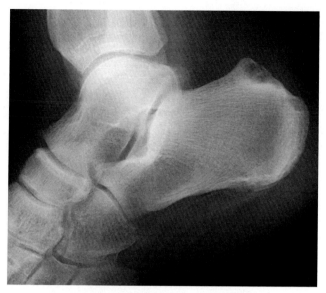

FIGURE 1.18. Rheumatoid arthritis. Calcaneus. There is a large erosion at the insertion of the Achilles tendon.

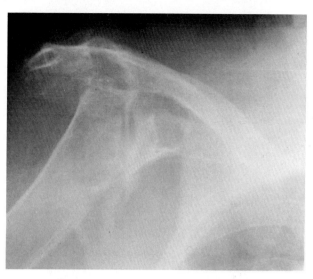

FIGURE 1.20. Rheumatoid arthritis. Shoulder. There has been extensive resorption and destruction of the humeral head.

poorly defined and there is an increased trabecular pattern of bone (Fig. 1.21).

In infectious arthritis, where cartilage is destroyed by proteolytic enzymes, erosions in contact areas occur (Fig. 1.22). Hemophilia in the knee is characterized by a large erosion in the intercondylar notch of the femur, as well as along the articular surface (Fig. 1.23), owing to hemorrhage.

Gouty erosions, in contrast to rheumatoid arthritis, tend to have a well-defined sclerotic margin with a characteristic overhanging edge (Fig. 1.24).[2] They can be expansile (Fig.

1.25). The first metatarsophalangeal is a typical location (Fig. 1.26). Erosions of bone remote from the articular surface also occur in gout.

Erosions in osteoarthritis also have well-defined margins (Fig. 1.27). Erosions visualized *en face* appear as cystic. Synovial fluid is forced by pressure of motion of the joint through a defect in the articular cartilage to form a cyst (Fig. 1.28). A cystlike appearance may also be caused by growth of granulation tissue into bone. These structures may become quite large and rarely may result in expansion of the

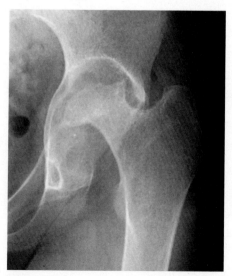
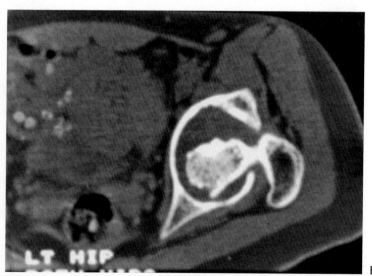

A   B

FIGURE 1.19. Juvenile rheumatoid arthritis. Hip. **A:** AP view of the left hip shows marked erosion of the acetabulum with acetabular protrusion. Erosion of the femoral head, to a large degree, is also noted. **B:** CT. Left hip. The erosion and expansion of the acetabulum are well demonstrated along with erosion of the femoral head.

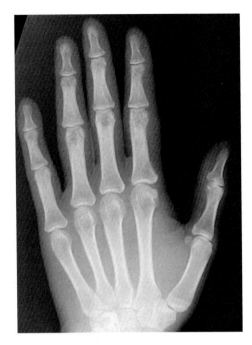

FIGURE 1.21. Sarcoidosis. Hand. Erosions are noted at the distal aspects of the proximal phalanges of the index, middle, and ring fingers. There is a coarsened trabecular pattern of the middle phalanx of the index finger. The erosions are poorly marginated.

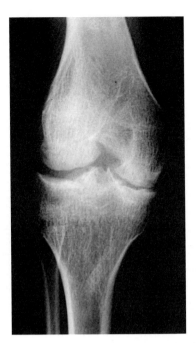

FIGURE 1.23. Hemophilia. Knee. A large erosion in the inter-condylar notch is seen as well as erosions of the articular surface.

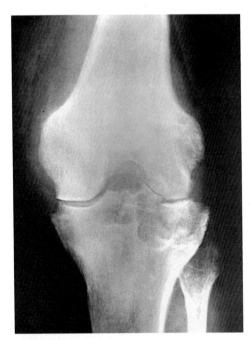

FIGURE 1.22. Tuberculosis. Knee. Extensive erosions and se-questrations of the articular surfaces are seen.

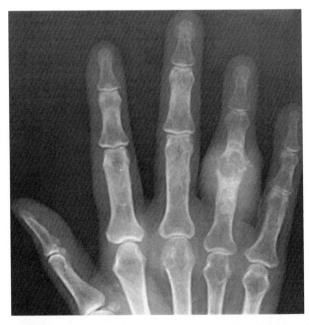

FIGURE 1.24. Gout. Hand. A well-defined erosion at the proximal interphalangeal joint of the ring finger is noted with sharp margination and an overhanging edge. A large amount of soft-tissue swelling is present.

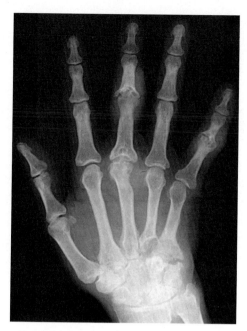

FIGURE 1.25. Gout. Hand. Erosions are seen in the carpus, at the base of the fourth and fifth metacarpals with expansile appearance and well-defined margins. They are also seen at the metacarpophalangeal joint and proximal interphalangeal joint of the middle finger, and at the proximal interphalangeal joint of the little finger.

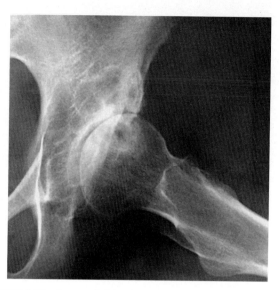

FIGURE 1.27. Osteoarthritis. An erosion at the upper aspect of the humeral head is seen with well-defined sclerotic margins. There is also narrowing of the superior surface of the hip joint and subchondral sclerosis as well as erosions and cysts in the acetabular roof.

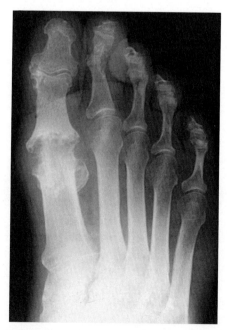

FIGURE 1.26. Gout. This is the typical location at the first metatarsophalangeal joint. The bone density is maintained.

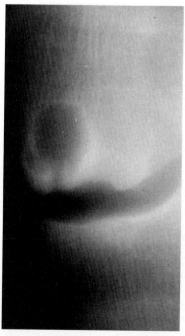

FIGURE 1.28. Osteoarthritis. Knee. Conventional tomogram. A cyst is seen with a narrow channel to the articular surface. A sclerotic margin is noted.

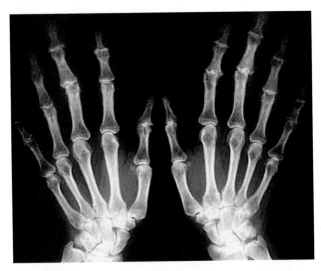

FIGURE 1.29. Erosive osteoarthritis. Hands. In addition to osteoarthritic changes in the distal interphalangeal joints, central erosions at the distal aspects of the middle phalanges are noted.

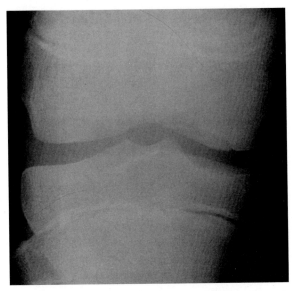

FIGURE 1.31. Osteochondritis dissecans. A defect is seen of the articular surface at the medial condyle of the distal femur.

cortex.[3] Large cysts are called *geodes*. Osteoarthritis in the hands may have an inflammatory component in the hands, in which case central erosions at the distal interphalangeal joints may be seen (Fig. 1.29). A small pit in the femoral neck may also be seen as a normal variant. Fungal infections may also cause erosions in joints without any other obvious changes on conventional radiographs (Fig. 1.30). Irregularities of the articular surface may also be caused by osteochondritis dissecans (Figs. 1.31 and 1.32). Pigmented

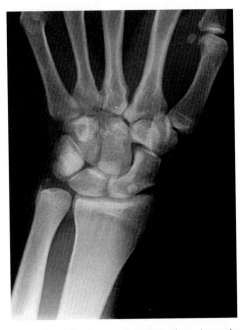

FIGURE 1.30. Coccidioidomycosis. Wrist. There is erosion of the ulnar styloid process without any other obvious changes.

villonodular synovitis results in well-marginated erosions on both sides of the joint, with preservation of joint cartilage and bone density (Fig. 1.33).

A cystlike expansile appearance may be seen in fibrous dysplasia.

Resorption of bone occurs in various conditions, including the collagen diseases. It is characteristic of the atrophic type of neuropathic arthropathy, or of a neurotrophic component of arthritis. Resorption of part (Fig. 1.34) or the entire humeral head may occur. Tapering of one side of the joint is seen in the hands and feet, along with exaggerated concavity of the opposite side, giving a "pencil-in-cup" appearance. Both sides of the joint may be tapered, particularly at the metatarsophalangeal joints, resulting in marked deformity. Resorption and dislocation at multiple joints of the hand cause shortening and deformity of the fingers, resulting in the "main-en-lorgnette" or "opera glass" hand of end-stage rheumatoid arthritis (Fig. 1.35).

Resorption of the distal clavicle may occur following trauma (Fig. 1.36) or in hyperparathyroidism (Fig. 1.37). Resorption and erosion of the distal clavicle occur in rheumatoid arthritis. These are not to be confused with hypoplasia, as can be seen in cleidocranial dysostosis (Fig. 1.38). Terminal phalangeal tuft resorption (Fig. 1.39) occurs in many conditions, including scleroderma and hyperparathyroidism (Fig. 1.40).

The *ossification centers and small bones* show changes in juvenile rheumatoid arthritis (JRA) (Fig. 1.41), juvenile articular infections (Fig. 1.42), and hemophilia, with changes in the time of appearance and fusion of the epiphyseal ossification centers. A characteristic appearance includes enlargement, irregularity of contour, squaring, osteoporosis, and coarsening of the trabecular pattern of the epiphyses. In

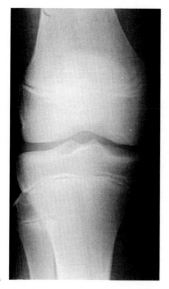 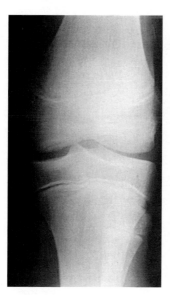 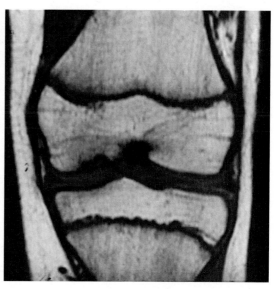

A
B

FIGURE 1.32. Osteochondritis dissecans. **A:** AP view of both knees reveals defects at the articular surface of the medial femoral condyle. This is a typical location. **B:** MRI. T1-weighted image. A low signal intensity defect is seen at the articular surface of the medial femoral condyle.

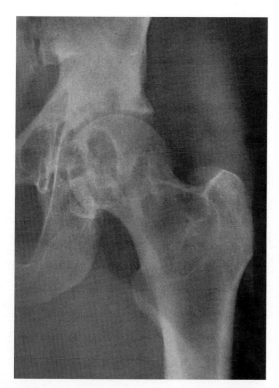

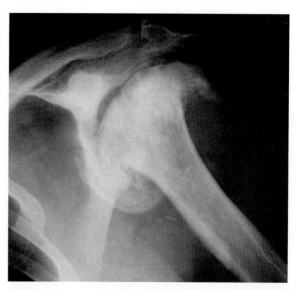

FIGURE 1.33. Pigmented villonodular synovitis. Hip. Multiple well-demarcated erosions are seen on both sides of the joint. The hip joint space is only slightly narrowed and the bone density is maintained.

FIGURE 1.34. Neurotrophic arthropathy. Shoulder. Resorption of the major portion of the humeral head and enlargement of the glenoid fossa is noted along with osteosclerosis and spur formation.

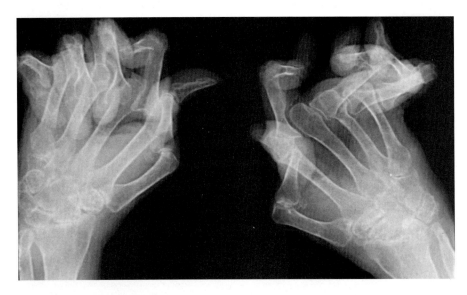

FIGURE 1.35. End-stage rheumatoid arthritis. Hands. Resorption of bone in the wrist and hands with multiple sub-luxations and malalignment is noted, as well as dislocations at the metacarpopha-langeal joints. This is the so-called "opera glass" hand.

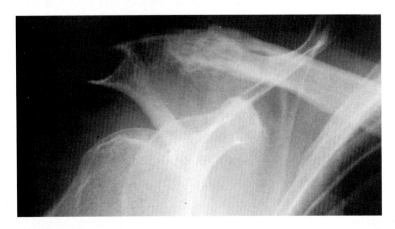

FIGURE 1.36. Shoulder. There has been resorption of the distal clavicle following trauma.

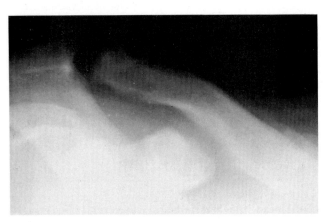

FIGURE 1.37. Hyperparathyroidism. Resorption of the distal clavicle with widening of the acromioclavicular joint is seen. There is also erosion at the undersurface of the clavicle. This patient is on dialysis.

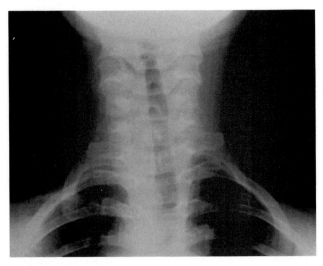

FIGURE 1.38. Cleidocranial dysostosis showing hypoplasia of the clavicles.

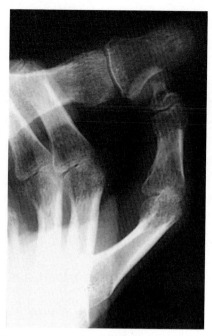

FIGURE 1.39. CRST syndrome. Resorption of the terminal tuft of the index finger is seen.

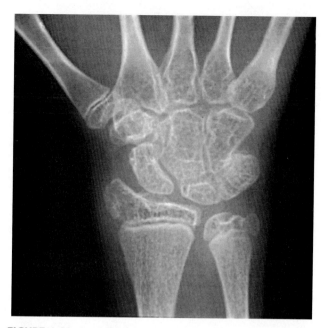

FIGURE 1.41. Juvenile rheumatoid arthritis. Wrist. There is enlargement of the epiphyseal ossification centers of the distal radius and ulna. Increased trabeculation in these centers as well as in the carpal bones is noted.

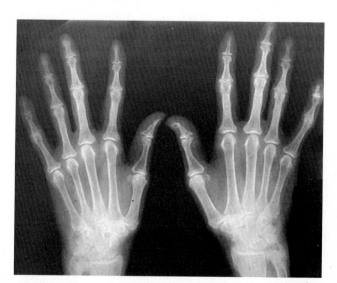

FIGURE 1.40. Hyperparathyroidism. Hand. Resorption of the terminal tufts is noted as well as subperiosteal bone resorption.

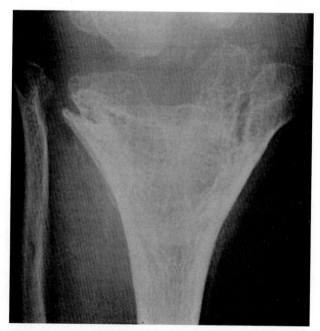

FIGURE 1.42. Postinfectious arthritis in the knee. There is shortening of the tibia and a cone-shaped epiphysis with irregularity of the articular surface.

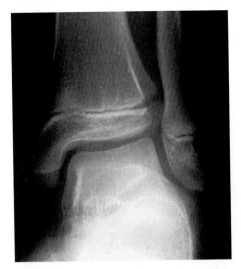

FIGURE 1.43. Hemophilia. Ankle. Tibiotalar slant is seen.

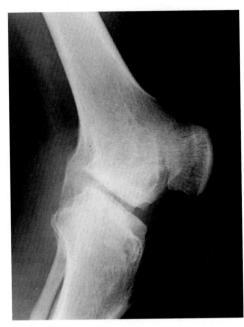

FIGURE 1.44. Hemophilia. Knee. Lateral view. A square inferior margin of the patella is seen. Flattening and erosions at the articular surface of the knee joint are also seen.

addition, alteration of the length of the extremity may occur.

Tibiotalar slant is a characteristic finding in the ankle in JRA, hemophilia, and multiple dysplasia (Fig. 1.43). Hemophilia also shows squaring of the inferior margin of the patella (Fig. 1.44). Bony proliferation of the epiphyseal ossification centers is seen in dysplasia epiphysealis hemimelica, or Trevor's disease.

Avascular necrosis (AVN) of the epiphyses may begin as a subchondral radiolucent fracture line (Fig. 1.45). It then proceeds to sclerosis and deformity (e.g., of the femoral head). MRI can demonstrate better detail of this process (Fig. 1.46). Later, collapse and cyst formation occur (Fig. 1.47). Legg Perthes' disease is a specific type of AVN that occurs in childhood (Fig. 1.48). AVN of the

small bones occurs frequently, and various eponyms have been applied. An example is Koehler's disease of the tarsal navicular (Fig. 1.49). Various congenital conditions may have features that overlap the arthritides. Examples are spondyloepiphyseal dysplasia (Fig. 1.50), spondylometaphyseal dysplasia (Fig. 1.51), and Madelung's deformity (Fig. 1.52).

Subchondral sclerosis is characteristic of osteoarthritis (OA) (Fig. 1.53). Rheumatoid arthritis in the weight-bearing joints may develop secondary osteoarthritis with sub-

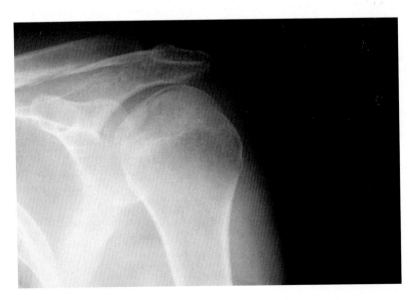

FIGURE 1.45. Avascular necrosis of the humeral head. The patient has lupus and is on steroids. A subchondral radiolucent line representing a fracture line and slight deformity of the humeral head are seen.

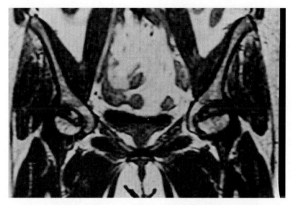
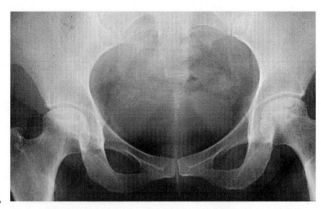

A   B

FIGURE 1.46. A: Avascular necrosis (AVN) of the hips in a patient on steroids. Bilateral sclerosis of the humeral heads is noted and there is a subchondral fracture line on the left side. The joint space is preserved and the acetabulum appears normal. **B:** MRI. T1-weighted image. The avascular segments of both femoral heads are demarcated from the normal marrow by a dark line of signal void.

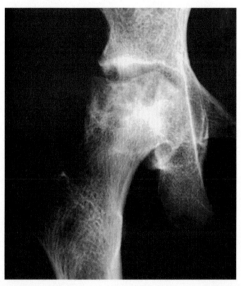

FIGURE 1.47. Sickle cell anemia. Hip. AVN. Cyst formation and collapse have occurred.

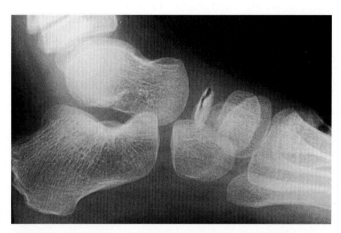

FIGURE 1.49. AVN of the tarsal navicular bone, or Koehler's disease. There is flattening and sclerosis of the navicular bone with a fracture line centrally.

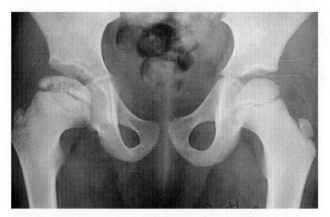

FIGURE 1.48. Legg Perthes' disease. There is sclerosis and flattening of the right femoral head and widening of the femoral neck. The joint space is also widened.

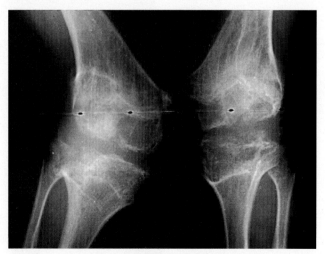

FIGURE 1.50. Spondyloepiphyseal dysplasia. Knees. Irregularities of the epiphyses are noted as well as genu valgus.

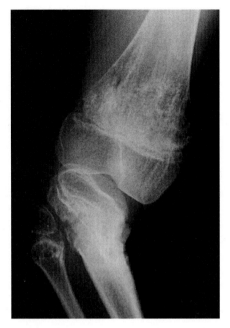

FIGURE 1.51. Spondylometaphyseal dysplasia. Metaphyseal irregularities at the distal femur and proximal tibia and fibula as well as deformity of the proximal tibial epiphysis is present. Genu varus is noted.

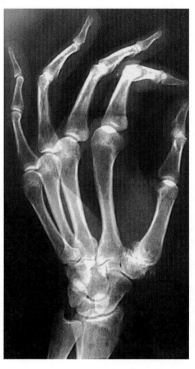

FIGURE 1.53. Osteoarthritis. Subchondral sclerosis and spur formation as well as joint space narrowing at the first carpometacarpal joint is noted. This is a typical location for osteoarthritis.

chondral sclerosis after cartilage destruction. Friction of opposing bone ends leads to osteosclerosis. Reactive osteitis of a sesamoid bone may be a cause of pain (Fig. 1.54). Rarely, osteoblastic metastases may involve a peripheral small bone (Fig. 1.55).

Sclerosis around a joint may also be seen in melorheostosis (Fig. 1.56).

Osteophytes at joint margins are a characteristic feature of OA. They extend horizontally from the articular margins. The cortex of the osteophyte or spur is continuous with

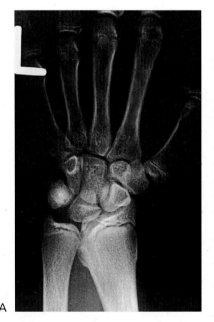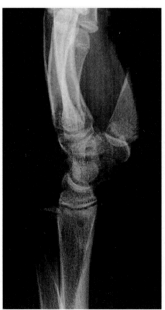

FIGURE 1.52. Madelung's deformity. **A:** AP view of the wrist shows a V shape of the radiocarpal articular surface. There is deformity of the ossification centers of the distal radius and distal ulna. **B:** Lateral view showing dorsal dislocation of the distal ulna.

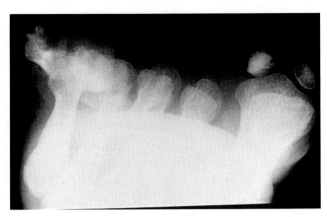

FIGURE 1.54. Patient with pain at the metatarsophalangeal joint of the great toe. Sesamoid-axial view. There is sclerosis of the lateral sesamoid bone indicating reactive osteitis.

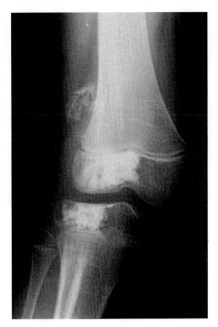

FIGURE 1.56. Melorheostosis. Knee. Osteosclerosis is noted in the distal femoral and proximal tibial epiphyses. Osteosclerotic strands in the proximal tibial metaphysis are also seen.

that of the adjacent bone (Fig. 1.57). The interior of the spur consists of trabeculae and fatty marrow, often covered by cartilage or periosteum. They represent reactive bone formation. In OA of the hand, osteophytes at the distal interphalangeal joints are known as Heberden's nodes (Fig. 1.58), whereas those at the proximal interphalangeal joints are known as Bouchard's nodes (Fig. 1.59). Hooklike osteophytes at the metacarpal heads are characteristic of hemochromatosis (Fig. 1.60) and calcium pyrophosphate deposition disease (CPPD) (Fig. 1.61).

Periosteal new bone may be seen in the reactive inflammatory arthritides. It is rare in adult onset rheumatoid arthritis, with less than 5% of patients showing this finding. Juvenile rheumatoid arthritis typically shows periosteal new bone. Reiter's syndrome also characteristically exhibits thick, fluffy periosteal new bone. The infectious arthritides also show new bone formation. Ankylosing spondylitis (AS) may be associated with irregular new bone formation at entheses, or sites of muscle attachments. Fluffy periosteal new

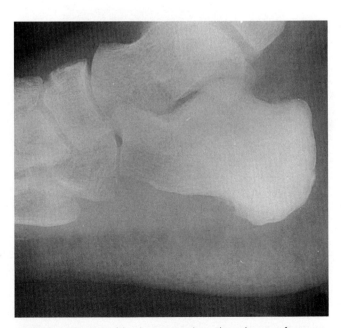

FIGURE 1.55. Osteoblastic metastasis to the calcaneus from carcinoma of the prostate.

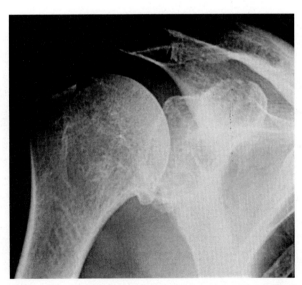

FIGURE 1.57. Osteoarthritis. Shoulder. Spur formation at the inferior margin of the humeral head and the glenoid fossa are noted. The cortex of the osteophyte at the inferior margin of the humeral head is seen to be continuous with that of the parent bone.

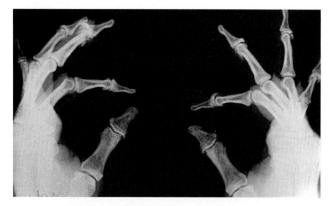

FIGURE 1.58. Osteoarthritis. Hands. Spur formation at the distal interphalangeal joints is noted. These are the Heberden's nodes.

bone formation at the base of the distal phalanx of the great toe can be seen in Reiter's syndrome and psoriatic arthritis. Septic arthritis and osteomyelitis also show new bone formation. Periosteal new bone is a characteristic feature of pulmonary hypertrophic osteoarthropathy (Fig. 1.62). This has a characteristic appearance on radioscintigraphy with increased activity of the periosteum on both sides of the bone, the "double rail" sign (Fig. 1.63). Various tumors in the vicinity of joints may also cause periosteal reaction (e.g., osteoid osteoma) (Fig. 1.64).

Malalignment may be seen as deviation, flexion, or hyperextension. Deviation is caused by muscular imbalance. Ulnar deviation of the fingers at the metacarpophalangeal joints is typically seen in rheumatoid arthritis (Fig. 1.65), systemic lupus erythematosus (Fig. 1.66), and Jaccoud's arthritis. In rheumatoid arthritis, ulnar deviation is not eas-

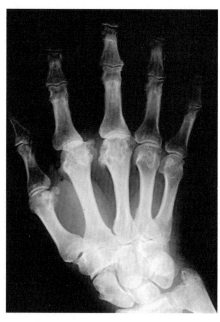

FIGURE 1.60. Hemochromatosis. "Hooklike" osteophytes are seen at the metacarpal heads. Cyst formation is also noted.

ily reversible and is usually associated with erosions. In the last two conditions the opposite is true.

Deformities of flexion and hyperextension include the boutonniere (Fig. 1.67) and the swan neck (Fig. 1.68) deformities of the fingers. The former consists of flexion of the proximal interphalangeal joint and hyperextension of the distal joint. It may be seen in RA, systemic lupus erythematosus, and Jaccoud's arthritis. The latter deformity is hy-

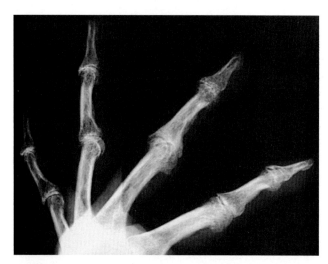

FIGURE 1.59. Osteoarthritis. Hands. Spur formation at the proximal interphalangeal joints of the index and middle fingers is noted. These are the Bouchard's nodes. Heberden's nodes are also seen.

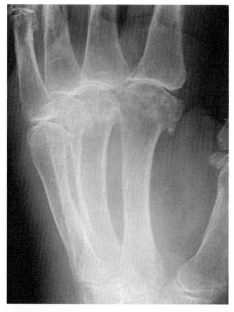

FIGURE 1.61. CPPD. "Hooklike" osteophytes are seen at the metacarpal heads.

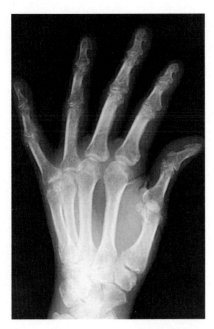

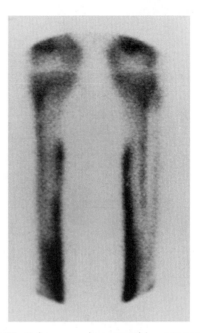

FIGURE 1.62. Pulmonary hypertrophic osteoarthropathy. Periarticular osteoporosis is noted as well as thin periosteal new bone formation at the radial side of all of the proximal phalanges.

FIGURE 1.63. Pulmonary hypertrophic osteoarthropathy. Radionuclide bone scan. There is increased activity of the periosteum on both medial and lateral aspects of the bone. This is the "double rail" sign.

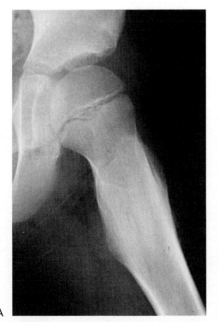

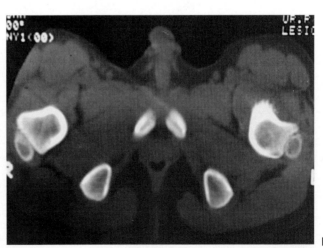

A

B

FIGURE 1.64. Osteoid osteoma. The patient had pain in the left hip. **A:** AP view of the hip shows an area of sclerosis in the trochanteric region, and there is a small radiolucency containing a more sclerotic center. This is the nidus. **B:** Computed tomogram showing a spiculated type of periosteal new bone formation at the left trochanter.

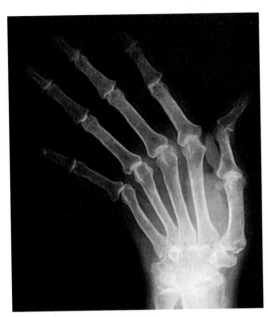

FIGURE 1.65. Rheumatoid arthritis. Hand. Ulnar deviation is noted at the metacarpophalangeal joints. Erosions at several metacarpal heads and proximal interphalangeal joints are seen as well as multiple erosions in the wrist. Osteoporosis is also noted.

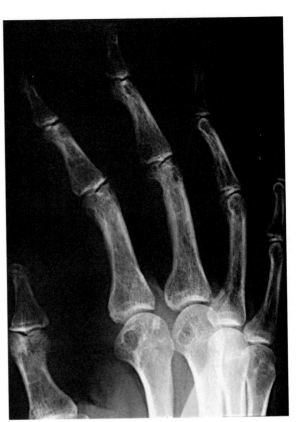

FIGURE 1.67. Rheumatoid arthritis. Hand. Boutonniere deformity of the ring finger is noted with flexion at the proximal interphalangeal joint and extension at the distal interphalangeal joint. Erosions at the metacarpal heads are also seen.

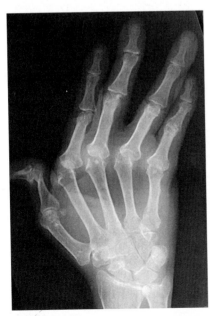

FIGURE 1.66. Systemic lupus erythematosus. Hand. Ulnar deviation of the fingers at the metacarpophalangeal joints is noted without erosions.

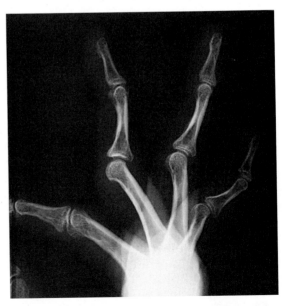

FIGURE 1.68. Rheumatoid arthritis. Hand. Swan neck deformity of the middle finger. There is hyperextension at the proximal interphalangeal joint and flexion at the distal interphalangeal joint.

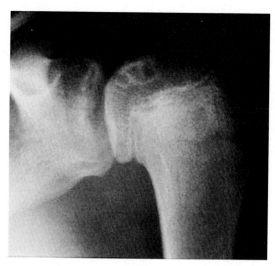

FIGURE 1.69. Hemophilia. Shoulder. There has been injury due to hemorrhage at the growth plate resulting in humerus varus and deformity of the epiphysis. A small cyst is also seen in the subchondral region.

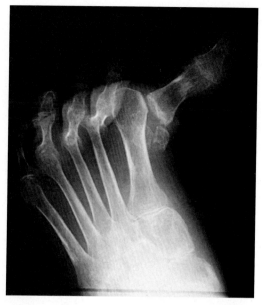

FIGURE 1.71. Rheumatoid arthritis. Foot. There has been dislocation at the metatarsophalangeal joint of the great toe.

perextension of the proximal interphalangeal joint and flexion of the distal joint.

Interference with the growth plate from injury or a disease process results in deformities (Fig. 1.69).

Subluxation and *dislocation* result from progression of malalignment, from large effusions (Figs. 1.70 and 1.71), pyogenic arthritis (Fig. 1.72), or erosion and destruction of the bone ends. Large effusions of the shoulder or hip in infants result in dislocations. Carpal malpositions may occur in RA and JRA (Fig. 1.73). Elevation of the humeral head

owing to erosion of the rotator cuff tendon occurs in RA (Fig. 1.74). Displacement can also occur at the epiphyseal cartilage plate, as in slipped capital femoral epiphysis (Fig. 1.75).

Disorganization of a large joint is typically seen in neurotrophic arthropathy. Fragmentation of bone, dislocation,

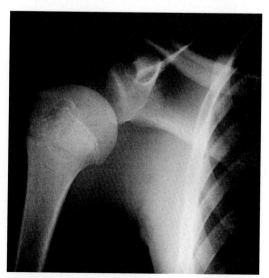

FIGURE 1.70. Hemophilia. Shoulder. There is a large effusion or hemorrhage within the shoulder joint resulting in subluxation. A cyst in the epiphysis and metaphysis is also seen.

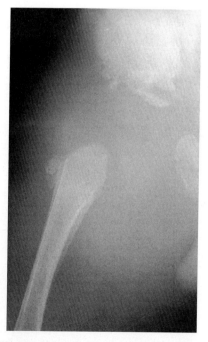

FIGURE 1.72. Pyogenic arthritis in an infant. Destruction of the acetabulum and the femoral head have occurred. Pus in the joint has distended it and there is now dislocation. Periosteal new bone formation at the proximal femur is also seen.

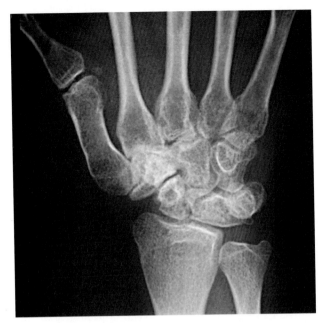

FIGURE 1.73. Juvenile rheumatoid arthritis. Wrist. Malposition of the carpal bones in the proximal carpal row is noted as well as erosion at the radial articular surface.

and soft-tissue debris occur (Figs. 1.76 and 1.77). Marked erosion may occur (Fig. 1.78). The fragments may later fuse into a bony mass (Fig. 1.79). Arthritis mutilans refers to a destructive end-stage arthritis of the hands or feet. It may result from RA (Fig. 1.80), JRA, psoriatic arthritis, leprosy, or diabetes mellitus.

Ankylosis has a different distribution and frequency pattern in the various arthritides. Interphalangeal bony ankylosis is more common in JRA and in psoriatic arthritis. It is

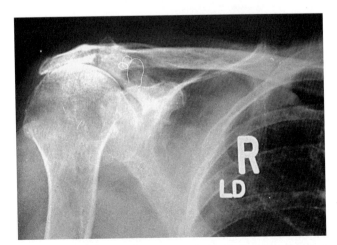

FIGURE 1.74. Rheumatoid arthritis. Shoulder. There is elevation of the humeral head owing to unopposed pull of the deltoid muscle because of erosion of the rotator cuff tendon. Erosion of the acromion process is also seen.

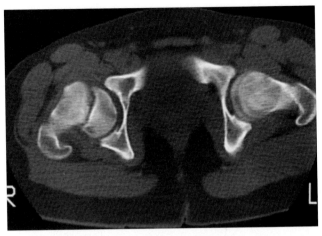

FIGURE 1.75. CT. Slipped capital femoral epiphysis. The right humeral head is seen to be rotated at the epiphyseal cartilage plate.

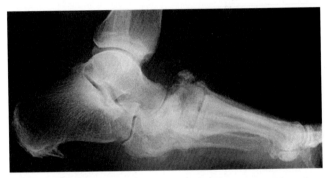

FIGURE 1.76. Neurotrophic joint in a diabetic patient. There has been fragmentation of the tarsal bones with bony debris at the dorsum.

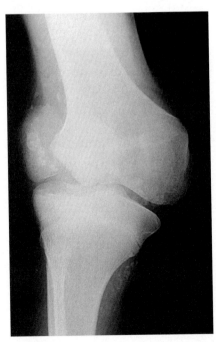

FIGURE 1.77. Neurotrophic joint. Knee. There are destructive changes at the lateral femoral condyle with soft-tissue debris and dislocation of the patella.

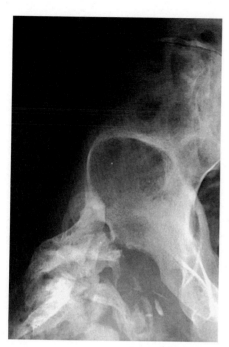

FIGURE 1.78. Neurotrophic joint. Congenital insensitivity to pain. Hip. There is marked erosion and enlargement of the acetabulum and destruction and fragmentation of the proximal femur.

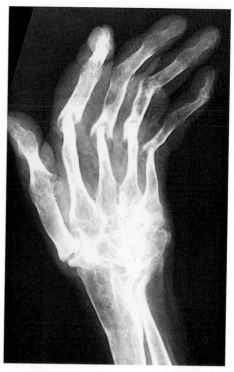

FIGURE 1.80. Rheumatoid arthritis. Hand. End-stage with compression erosions at the metacarpophalangeal joints and fusion of the interphalangeal joints with ulnar deviation and fusion of the wrist.

rare in adult onset rheumatoid arthritis. Carpal and tarsal bony ankylosis can be seen in adult and JRA (Fig. 1.81). Bony ankylosis of the hip and knee is most frequently seen in JRA. Bony ankylosis in osteoarthritis is very rare. In the sacroiliac joints, the inflammatory arthritides can ankylose the synovial-lined lower two-thirds (Fig. 1.82), whereas in DISH, ligamentous ossification can fuse the upper third (Fig. 1.83).

The *distribution* of joint involvement is important in diagnosis because sites of predilection of the various arthritides differ. In the hands the distal interphalangeal joints are often initially involved with primary osteoarthritis (Fig. 1.84) and psoriatic arthritis. The proximal interphalangeal

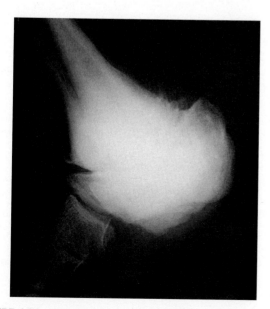

FIGURE 1.79. Congenital insensitivity to pain. Ankle. The bony debris has fused into a solid mass.

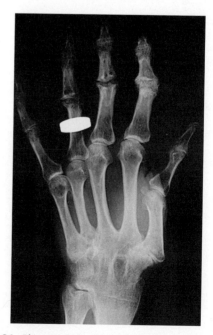

FIGURE 1.81. Rheumatoid arthritis. There has been fusion at the wrist.

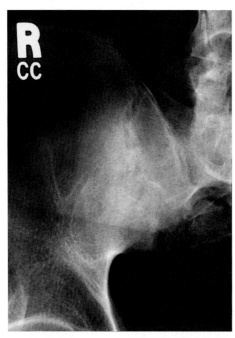

FIGURE 1.82. Ankylosing spondylitis. Sacroiliac joint. There is obliteration of the lower two-thirds of the sacroiliac joint.

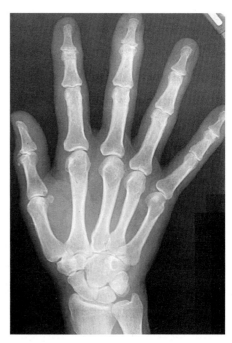

FIGURE 1.84. Osteoarthritis. Hand. Joint space narrowing and spur formation at the distal interphalangeal joints are noted.

joints are typically initially involved with rheumatoid arthritis. CPPD has a tendency to involve the radiocarpal compartment of the wrist, whereas gout tends to involve the carpometacarpal compartment. Primary osteoarthritis often involves the first carpometacarpal joint. Bilateral symmetrical distribution is typical of rheumatoid arthritis, whereas

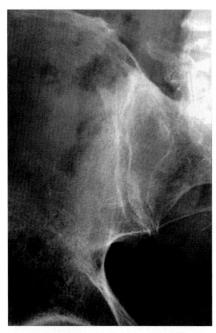

FIGURE 1.83. DISH. Sacroiliac joint. There is fusion of the superior aspect of the sacroiliac joint by ligamentous ossification.

gout is sporadically distributed. Bilateral symmetrical involvement of the sacroiliac joints is typical of AS. The typical distribution, however, does not occur in every case.

The *time* and *sequence of changes* are important for diagnosis and management. For example, the demonstration of early erosions is used by many rheumatologists as an indication to change therapy. The evolution of changes is important. For example, in pyogenic arthritis with rapid progress, destruction precedes osteoporosis, whereas in tuberculous arthritis the reverse is true (Fig. 1.85).

The *soft-tissues* may show edema, atrophy, or calcifications. Soft-tissue bony debris is characteristic of a neurotrophic joint. Clubbing of the terminal phalanges is seen in hypertrophic osteoarthropathy of various etiologies (Fig. 1.86), acromegaly, and hyperparathyroidism. Subungual hyperkeratosis occurs in psoriatic arthritis and Reiter's syndrome. Soft-tissue swelling representing tophi are seen in gout. Soft-tissue nodules may be seen in rheumatoid arthritis, amyloidosis, thyroid acropachy, and xanthoma. Diffuse soft-tissue swelling of an entire finger (sausage digit) can be seen in psoriatic and infectious arthritis (Fig. 1.87). This may also be seen in macrodactyly (Fig. 1.88). Diffuse soft-tissue enlargement of an entire limb may be seen in plexiform neurofibromatosis (Fig. 1.89). Soft-tissue prominence containing calcifications may be seen in vascular malformations and hemangioma.

Rheumatoid arthritis has a typical early distribution of soft-tissue swelling about the ulnar styloid process and the proximal interphalangeal joints, and later, the metacarpophalangeal joints (Fig. 1.90).

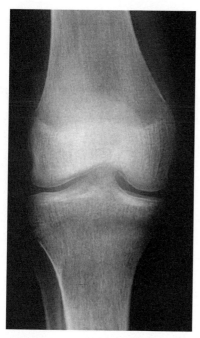

FIGURE 1.85. Tuberculosis. Knee. Marked local osteoporosis is present with a subchondral radiolucent band. Destruction has not yet occurred.

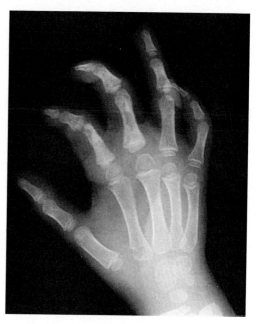

FIGURE 1.87. Septic arthritis and osteomyelitis. Hand. Diffuse swelling of the entire index and middle fingers is noted along with bony changes.

Soft-tissue masses in the popliteal fossa may represent Baker's cysts; however, tumors and aneurysms of the popliteal artery may also be present.

Soft-tissue atrophy is present in the terminal phalanges in scleroderma. Atrophy of the thenar and hypothenar muscles, giving a concave rather than convex hypothe-

nar border, is seen in systemic lupus erythematosus (Fig. 1.91).

Soft-tissue calcifications may be metabolic (called metastatic), calcifications, calcinosis (subcutaneous calcification), or dystrophic calcifications. They may be paraarticular

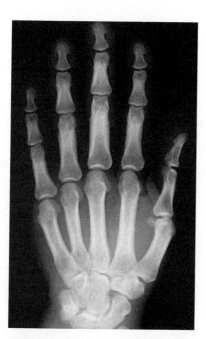

FIGURE 1.86. Idiopathic osteoarthropathy. Soft-tissue clubbing of the fingers is noted as well as periosteal new bone formation.

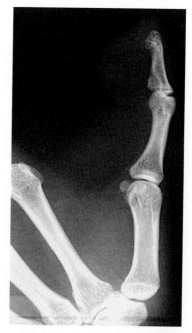

FIGURE 1.88. Macrodactyly. Thumb. Marked soft-tissue prominence of the thumb is noted. The bone is relatively uninvolved. Biopsy showed excess fatty tissue. A similar picture can be seen in plexiform neurofibroma.

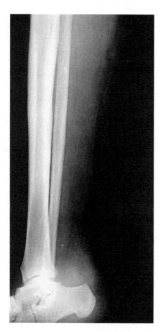

FIGURE 1.89. Plexiform neurofibromatosis. Lateral view of the leg shows diffuse soft-tissue enlargement. There is also an appearance simulating the subperiosteal resorption of hyperparathyroidism. This, however, is not generalized as is seen in that disease.

or in vessels, tendons, bursae, the joint capsule, articular cartilage, or fibrocartilage. Metastatic calcifications may be seen in chronic renal disease, hypoparathyroidism, and hyperparathyroidism. Calcinosis is often seen in scleroderma and in the Calcinosis, Reynolds, Sclerodactyly, and Telangiectasia

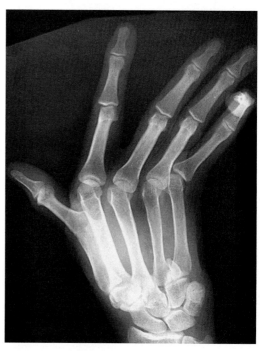

FIGURE 1.91. Systemic lupus erythematosus. Hand. Atrophy of the thenar and hypothenar musculature is noted, as well as nonerosive ulnar deviation of the fingers.

(CRST) syndrome (Fig. 1.92). Dystrophic calcification may be present in gouty tophi and tumoral calcinosis.

Hydroxyapatite deposition disease (HADD) is a cause of calcific tendinitis, bursitis (Fig. 1.93), and periarticular calcification. Vascular calcification occurs most frequently in atherosclerosis, diabetes mellitus, and renal osteodystrophy.

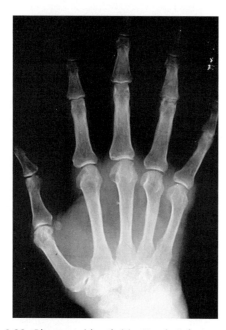

FIGURE 1.90. Rheumatoid arthritis. Hand. Soft-tissue swelling about the proximal interphalangeal joints, the metacarpophalangeal joints, and the ulnar styloid region is noted. Marginal erosions are also seen.

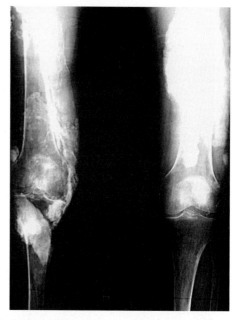

FIGURE 1.92. CRST syndrome. Extensive calcinosis is seen subcutaneously.

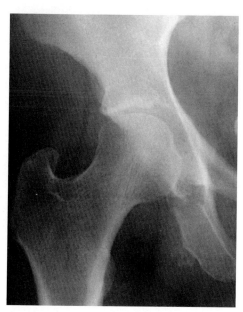

FIGURE 1.93. Calcific ischial bursitis. Calcification is seen at the ischial bursa.

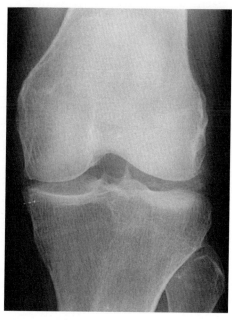

FIGURE 1.95. Chondrocalcinosis. Knee. Calcification of the lateral meniscus is seen.

Hyalin articular cartilage calcifications (Fig. 1.94) and meniscal calcifications (Fig. 1.95) are characteristic of chondrocalcinosis (CPPD). Synovial osteochondromatosis is a condition of intraarticular calcific bodies resulting from synovial chondrometaplasia (Fig. 1.96).

Each segment of the vertebral column consists of three joints: the amphiarthrodial intervertebral disk and the two diarthrodial facet joints. Only the facet joints are synovial-lined and subject to inflammatory arthritis.

The *vertebral body* shows various changes.

The vertebral *margin* can characterize several processes. Marginal osteophytes, or spondylosis, are mechanical reactive proliferations of cortical bone, with a medulla and a cartilaginous cap. They have a horizontal takeoff (Fig. 1.97), in contrast to syndesmophytes, which have a vertical orientation. CT shows osteophytes as linear osseous structures adjacent to the vertebral body (Fig. 1.98). Posterior osteophytes encroach on the intervertebral foramina, and may

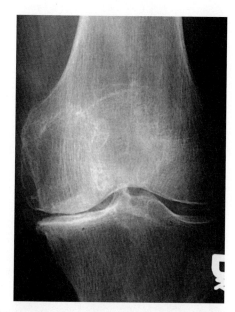

FIGURE 1.94. Chondrocalcinosis. Knee. Hyalin articular cartilage calcification is seen in the lateral compartment, whereas there is narrowing as well as calcification in the medial compartment.

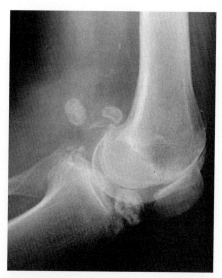

FIGURE 1.96. Synovial osteochondromatosis. Knee. Lateral view. Ossified loose bodies are seen within the knee joint. Osteoarthritis at the patellofemoral joint is also noted.

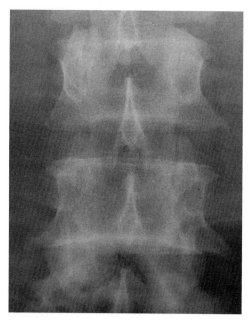

FIGURE 1.97. AP view of the lumbar spine showing osteophytes with a horizontal takeoff.

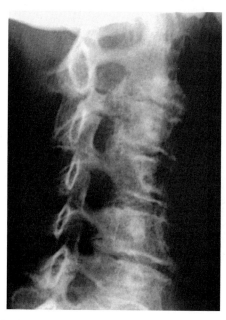

FIGURE 1.99. Cervical spine. Oblique view. Osteophytes projecting posteriorly seen to encroach into intervertebral foramina.

cause radiculopathy (Fig. 1.99). They may encroach on the neural canal (Fig. 1.100). Some osteophytes are 1 mm removed from the actual vertebral corner. These are called traction spurs and indicate segmental instability.

Thin marginal syndesmophytes are calcifications of the annulus fibrosus and the inner layers of the longitudinal ligament. They are characteristic of AS (Fig. 1.101) and reactive spondylitis. They can be seen on CT as a thin line adjacent to the vertebral body (Fig. 1.102). Thicker marginal syndesmophytes may also occur in the last two conditions (Figs. 1.103 and 1.104).

Thick nonmarginal syndesmophytes are seen in psoriatic arthritis (Fig. 1.105) and Reiter's syndrome. They extend from the midvertebral bodies.

Diffuse idiopathic skeletal hyperostosis (DISH) has a characteristic appearance of calcification or ossification of the anterior longitudinal ligament with a thin radiolucent line of separation from the vertebral body margin (Figs.

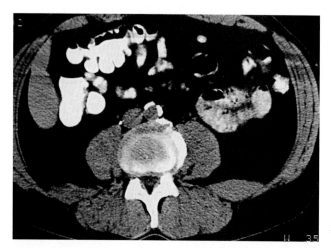

FIGURE 1.98. Lumbar spine. An osteophyte is seen at the left side of the lumbar vertebra.

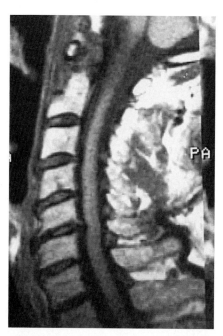

FIGURE 1.100. Cervical spine. MRI. T1-weighted image. A posterior osteophyte at C-5 is seen compressing the spinal cord.

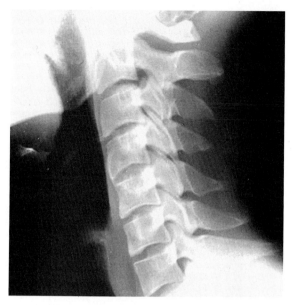

FIGURE 1.101. Ankylosing spondylitis. Cervical spine. Lateral view. A thin syndesmophyte is seen anteriorly between C-4 and C-5.

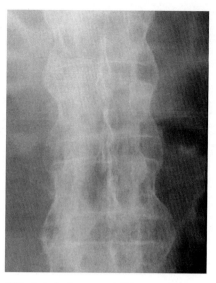

FIGURE 1.103. Ankylosing spondylitis. Lumbar spine. Marginal syndesmophytes are noted throughout, which are somewhat thicker.

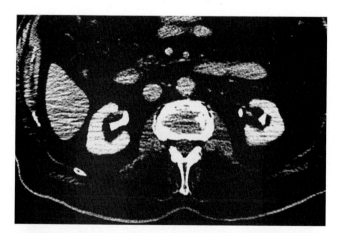

FIGURE 1.102. Ankylosing spondylitis. CT. A syndesmophyte is seen as a thin line on each side of the vertebral body.

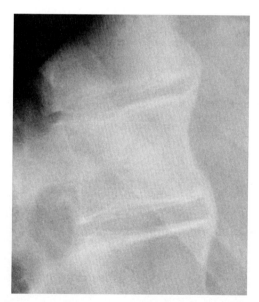

FIGURE 1.104. Ankylosing spondylitis. Lumbar spine. Lateral view. Thicker marginal syndesmophytes are seen.

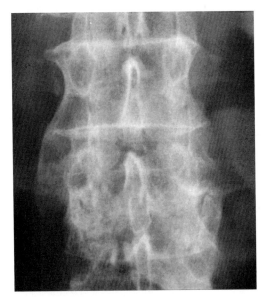

FIGURE 1.105. Psoriatic arthritis. Lumbar spine. Thick non-marginal syndesmophytes are seen.

1.106 and 1.107). Rarely, the posterior longitudinal ligament may become calcified (Fig. 1.108).

Changes in the shape and density of the vertebral bodies occur in various conditions. A specific appearance of AS is "squaring" of the vertebral bodies owing to bone resorption of the anterior margins, prior to visible syndesmophytes (Fig. 1.109). In late AS, squaring of all of the vertebral bodies and syndesmophyte formation cause a "bamboo spine" (Fig. 1.110).

Biconcavity of the vertebral bodies is seen in sickle cell disease (Fig. 1.111) as well as in homocystinuria (Fig.

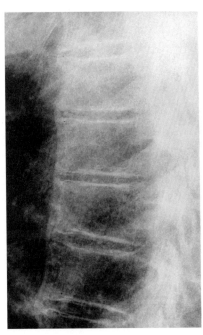

FIGURE 1.107. DISH. Thoracic spine. Ossification of the anterior longitudinal ligament is noted with a radiolucent line between the ossified ligament and the anterior vertebral body.

1.112). Collapse of vertebral bodies can occur, usually resulting from osteoporosis, but also from tumor metastases. Wedgelike collapse can be caused by trauma or metastases, and waferlike collapse can be caused by metastases or eosinophilic granuloma (Fig. 1.113).

Osteopenia can occur in metabolic bone disease (Fig. 1.114), along with flattening of the vertebral bodies

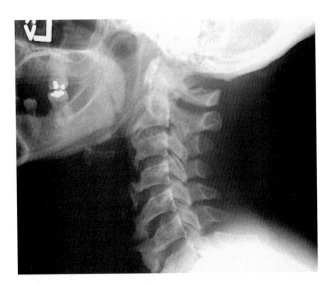

FIGURE 1.106. Diffuse idiopathic skeletal hyperostosis (DISH). Cervical spine. Exuberant anterior ossifications in the anterior longitudinal ligament are seen. There is no loss of bone density, and there is no narrowing of the intervertebral spaces.

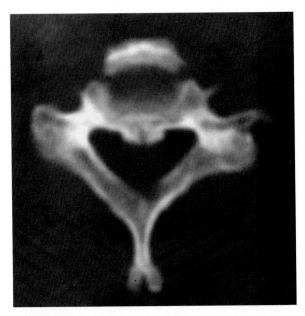

FIGURE 1.108. CT of the cervical spine. Ossification of the posterior longitudinal ligament is seen.

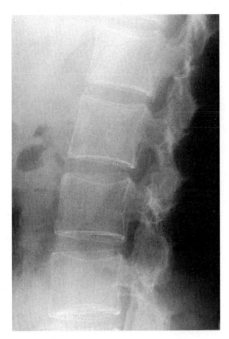

FIGURE 1.109. Ankylosing spondylitis. Lumbar spine. "Squaring" of the vertebral bodies. The anterior margins of the vertebral bodies have lost their concave appearance. Osteopenia is also noted.

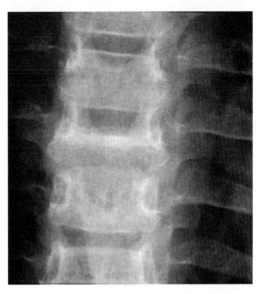

FIGURE 1.113. Eosinophilic granuloma of the eighth thoracic vertebral body, which has caused a "waferlike" collapse.

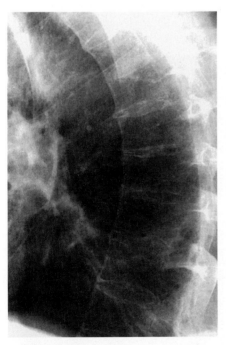

FIGURE 1.110. Ankylosing spondylitis. "Bamboo spine." Syndesmophyte formation, squaring of the anterior vertebral bodies, and kyphosis are noted.

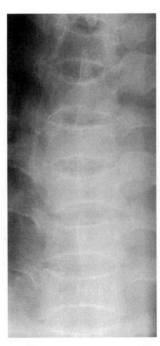

FIGURE 1.111. Sickle cell anemia. Thoracic spine. AP view. Biconcavity of the vertebral bodies is noted.

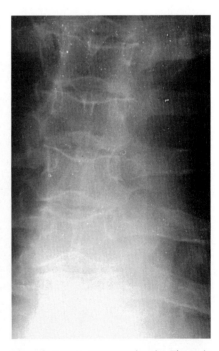

FIGURE 1.112. Homocystinuria. Thoracic spine. Biconcavity of the vertebral bodies is noted.

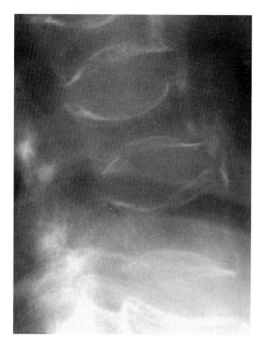

FIGURE 1.114. Advanced osteoporosis. Loss of bone density and deformities of the vertebral bodies with superior and inferior end plate compressions are seen.

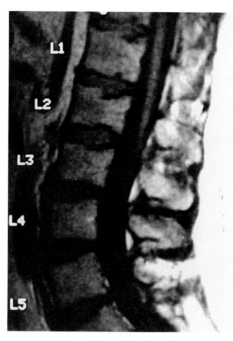

FIGURE 1.116. Lumbar spine. MRI. Schmorl's nodes are seen as end plate depressions of several vertebral bodies.

(Fig. 1.115). Focal end plate depressions are owing to Schmorl's nodes (Fig. 1.116). Osteosclerosis can occur in various patterns, including the "rugger jersey" spine of renal osteodystrophy (Fig. 1.117), the "picture frame" appearance of Paget's disease (Fig. 1.118), and the "bone within a bone"

appearance of osteopetrosis tarda (Fig. 1.119). Uniform sclerosis is seen in osteoblastic metastases, Hodgkin's disease (Fig. 1.120), and third-stage Paget's disease.

The *intervertebral disc* may show narrowing (Fig. 1.121), or contain gas (Fig. 1.122) or calcification

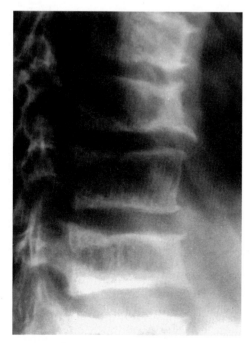

FIGURE 1.115. Renal osteodystrophy. Flattening of the vertebral bodies is noted as well as relative sclerosis of the end plates.

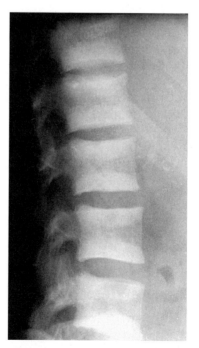

FIGURE 1.117. Renal osteodystrophy. "Rugger jersey" spine. Osteosclerosis at the end plates extending into the vertebral bodies is noted with a normal density centrally.

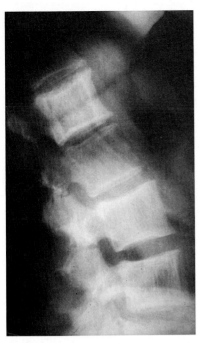

FIGURE 1.118. Paget's disease. Lumbar spine. L-1 shows the "picture frame" appearance of second-stage Paget's disease and L-4 shows the vertical striated appearance of second-stage Paget's disease. L-3 shows uniform sclerosis of third-stage Paget's disease.

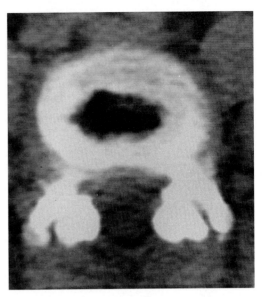

FIGURE 1.122. Degenerative disk disease. CT. Gas in the intervertebral disk is noted with a low density centrally.

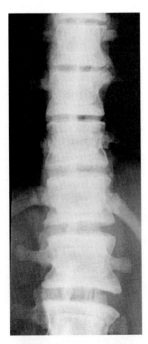

FIGURE 1.119. Osteopetrosis tarda. A "bone within a bone" appearance is seen in the vertebral bodies.

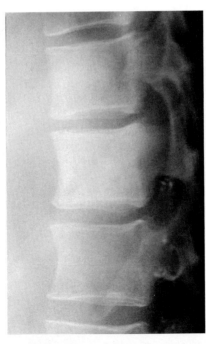

FIGURE 1.120. Hodgkin's disease. Lateral view of the spine shows dense sclerosis of a single vertebral body. The contour is not altered.

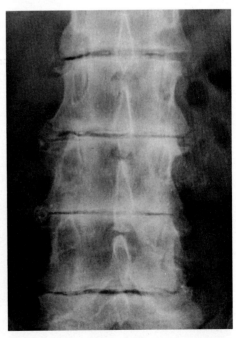

FIGURE 1.121. Ochronosis. Lumbar spine. There is narrowing of all of the intervertebral spaces with increased radiolucency indicating gas within the intervertebral disc. This is the "vacuum" sign.

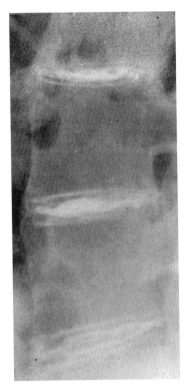

FIGURE 1.123. Ochronosis. Lumbar spine. Dense calcification of the intervertebral discs is seen.

(Fig. 1.123). Localized narrowing at one or more intervertebral spaces may be caused by herniation of the nucleus pulposus, disc degeneration, infection (Fig. 1.124), congenital anomaly, or atrophy accompanying fusion of the segmental apophyseal joints. Chronic diskitis and TB may result in reactive sclerosis (Figs. 1.124 and 1.125). General disc space narrowing is suggestive of ochronosis, which also typically causes generalized calcification of the intervertebral discs. Localized calcification of a disc may be idiopathic, posttraumatic, or infectious. The "vacuum sign," or gas seen within the intervertebral disk, indicates disc degeneration.

The *apophyseal joints* can be involved in synovial inflammatory disease. They may show narrowing and erosions in both RA and AS, which can progress to fusion. Ankylosing spondylitis typically involves the lower spine, whereas RA predilects the cervical spine. Apophyseal joint fusion is often accompanied by atrophic narrowing of the corresponding intervertebral disc. Osteoarthritis of the facet joints can cause spur formation and hypertrophy, which can be seen to encroach on the intervertebral foramina on oblique views (Fig. 1.126), and may be seen on CT (Fig. 1.127) or MRI as lateral recess stenosis.

A vacuum sign in the facet joint space may be demonstrated on CT (Fig. 1.128).

The *atlantoaxial articulation* is a critical area because of the subluxations that frequently occur in several conditions. The most common causal arthritis is rheumatoid, and it is common in Down's syndrome. In RA and JRA, erosions, destruction, and fractures (Fig. 1.129) of the odontoid pro-

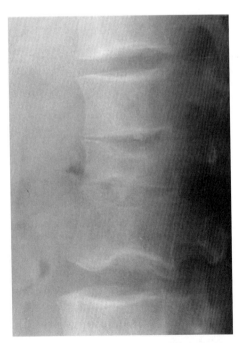

FIGURE 1.124. Sickle cell anemia with diskitis. Narrowing of the intervertebral spaces and end plate irregularity are seen. Biconcavity of the vertebral bodies is also noted.

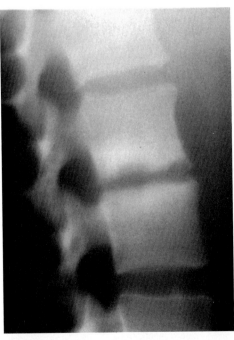

FIGURE 1.125. Tuberculosis of the spine. Intervertebral space narrowing, end plate irregularity, and reactive sclerosis are seen.

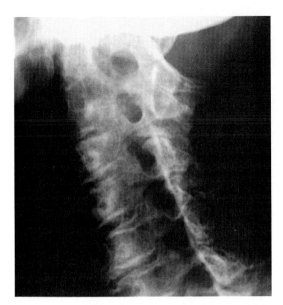

FIGURE 1.126. Facet joint osteoarthritis. Oblique view demonstrates posterior spurs encroaching into the intervertebral foramina, particularly at C3-4.

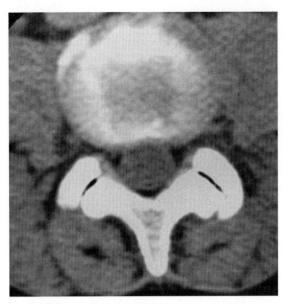

FIGURE 1.128. Facet joint osteoarthritis. CT. Lumbar spine. A vacuum sign is seen bilaterally at the facet joints.

cess may occur, as well as a large mass of pannus that encroaches on the neural canal. This region is best demonstrated with MRI.

Radiography of the neck *carefully* in flexion and extension lateral views is often required to demonstrate atlantoaxial instability.

The *paravertebral area* can be involved with coarse syndesmophytes in psoriatic arthritis or Reiter's syndrome. A soft-tissue mass can occur in association with various processes, including inflammatory masses and extramedullary hematopoiesis (Fig. 1.130). A calcified paravertebral mass is typical of tuberculous spondylitis, or Pott's disease.

The *differential diagnosis* of several features related to the arthritides is found in the following:[4]

Arthritis with Relative Lack of Osteoporosis
    Gout
    Jaccoud's arthritis
    Neurotrophic arthritis
    Pigmented villonodular synovitis
    Psoriatic arthritis
    Reiter's disease
    Sarcoidosis
    Septic arthritis (early)

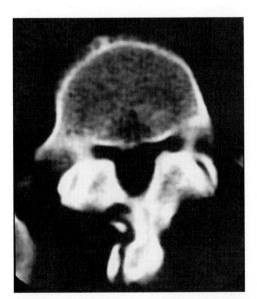

FIGURE 1.127. Facet joint osteoarthritis. CT. Lumbar spine. Hypertrophy of the facet joints has resulted in lateral recess stenosis.

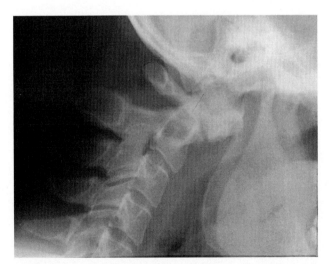

FIGURE 1.129. Fracture of the odontoid process. Flexion lateral view. There is forward displacement of C-1. Note the anterior displacement of the spinous process at C-2. The odontoid process is also displaced forward.

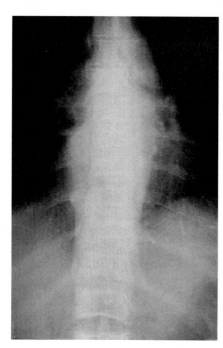

FIGURE 1.130. Sickle cell anemia. Thoracic spine. A paraspinal mass on both sides of the spine is noted representing extramedullary hematopoiesis. Biconcavity of the vertebral bodies is also noted.

Boutonniere and Swan Neck Deformities
Camptodactyly
Jaccoud's arthritis
Juvenile rheumatoid arthritis
Psoriatic arthritis
Rheumatoid arthritis
Systemic lupus erythematosus

Easily Correctable Ulnar Deviation
Jaccoud's arthritis
Systemic lupus erythematosus

Thicker Periosteal New Bone Formation
Juvenile rheumatoid arthritis
Psoriatic arthritis
Reiter's disease
Septic arthritis

Uniform Swelling of a Digit: Sausage Digit
Neurotrophic arthritis
Psoriatic arthritis
Reiter's disease
Septic arthritis

Arthritis Mutilans
Chronic infection
Diabetes mellitus
Juvenile rheumatoid arthritis
Leprosy

Lipoid dermatoarthritis
Psoriatic arthritis
Rheumatoid arthritis

Nonerosive Arthritis in the Hands
Jaccoud's arthritis
Reiter's disease
Systemic lupus erythematosus

Enlarged or Irregular Epiphyseal Ossification Centers
Hemophilia
Juvenile rheumatoid arthritis
Juvenile tuberculous arthritis

Cystic Erosions in Humeral Head
Ankylosing spondylitis
Gout
Hemophilia
Lipoid dermatoarthritis
Osteoarthritis (rare)
Pigmented villonodular synovitis
Rheumatoid arthritis
Tuberculous arthritis

Atlantoaxial Subluxation
Ankylosing spondylitis (rare)
Congenital hypoplasia or absence of the dens
Juvenile rheumatoid arthritis
Mongoloidism
Morquio's syndrome
Psoriatic arthritis
Rheumatoid arthritis
Systemic lupus erythematosus

Sacroiliac Joint Fusion
Ankylosing spondylitis
Enteropathic arthritis
Gaucher's disease
Juvenile rheumatoid arthritis
Paraplegia
Polyvinyl chloride intoxication
Psoriatic arthritis
Reiter's disease
Relapsing polychondritis

Unilateral Sacroiliac Involvement
Ankylosing spondylitis (early)
Gout
Septic arthritis
Tuberculous arthritis

Migration of Femoral Head (Usual)
Osteoarthritis—outward
Paget's arthritis—inward
Rheumatoid arthritis—inward

Erosion of Intercondylar Notch of Knee
   Hemophilia
   Juvenile rheumatoid arthritis
   Tuberculous arthritis

Tibiotalar Slant
   Hemophilia
   Juvenile rheumatoid arthritis
   Multiple epiphyseal dysplasia

Calcaneal Erosions
   Ankylosing spondylitis
   Hyperparathyroidism
   Lipoid dermatoarthritis
   Psoriatic arthritis
   Reiter's disease
   Rheumatoid arthritis

Premature Degenerative Joint Disease
   Acromegaly
   Amyloidosis
   Chondromalacia patellae
   Gout
   Hemochromatosis
   Hemophilia
   Ischemic necrosis
   Kashin—Bek's disease
   Neuropathic arthropathy
   Ochronosis
   Scheuermann's disease
   Septic arthritis
   Trauma
   Wilson's disease

Arthritis Often Associated with Periosteal Reaction
   Hemophilia
   Juvenile rheumatoid arthritis
   Psoriatic arthritis
   Reiter's disease
   Septic arthritis

"Apple Core" Femoral Neck Erosions[5]
   Amyloidosis
   Pigmented villonodular synovitis
   Rheumatoid arthritis
   Synovial osteochondromatosis

"Hooklike" Osteophytes at Metacarpal Heads
   Pseudogout
   Hemochromatosis
   Neurotrophic arthropathy
   Osteoarthritis (rare)

REFERENCES

1. Hall FM. Radiographic diagnosis and accuracy in knee joint effusions. *Radiology* 1975;115:49–54.
2. Martel W. The overhanging margin of bone: a roentgenologic manifestation of gout. *Radiology* 1968;91:755–756.
3. Glass TA, Dyer R, Fisher L, et al. Expansile subchondral bone cyst. *AJR* 1982;139:1210–1211.
4. Greenfield GB. *Radiology of bone diseases,* 5th ed. Philadelphia: JB Lippincott, 1990, pp. 968–969.
5. Goldberg RP, Weissman BN, Naimark A, et al. Femoral neck erosions: sign of hip joint synovial disease. *AJR* 1983;141:107–111.

INFLAMMATORY ARTHRITIDES

The synovial inflammatory arthritides include several distinct entities. The principal diseases are rheumatoid arthritis (RA), juvenile rheumatoid arthritis (JRA), ankylosing spondylitis (AS), and reactive arthritis. The last includes psoriatic arthritis, Reiter's disease, enteropathic arthritis, and miscellaneous conditions. They are discussed separately in the following.

RHEUMATOID ARTHRITIS

Clinical Considerations

Keith Kanik

Rheumatoid arthritis (RA) is an inflammatory arthropathy of unknown etiology.[1,3] The criteria for the classification of RA include morning stiffness, arthritis of three or more joint areas, arthritis of hand joints, symmetric arthritis, rheumatoid nodules, serum rheumatoid factor, and radiographic changes.[1] If a patient meets four or more of these seven criteria then the patient may be given the diagnosis of RA with the caveat that these criteria are only 90% sensitive and specific.

RA affects approximately 1% of the population, and is more common in women than men. Prevalence increases with age in both men and women.[2] A higher concordance rate in monozygous twins is present when compared with dizygous twins.[3] This suggests multiple factors responsible for the disease.

Typically, patients present with fatigue, weakness, and nonspecific musculoskeletal complaints. Most present gradually with symmetric involvement of hands, wrists, feet, and knees. Some present rapidly and acutely. Affected joints are swollen, tender, and stiff and are worse after prolonged inactivity. The joints usually feel better while using them. Patients may also complain of fatigue, weight loss, depression, and low-grade fevers. Signs of chronic disease include ulnar deviation, swan neck deformities, boutonniere defor-

mities, C-spine subluxation, and metatarsal subluxation. Extraarticular features may include rheumatoid nodules, rheumatoid vasculitis, keratoconjunctivitis sicca, pleuropulmonary disease, neuropathy, Felty's syndrome, and *Pyoderma gangrenosum*.

Laboratory testing will usually show some sign of acute phase reaction. This can take the form of thrombocytosis, elevated erythrocyte sedimentation rate (ESR), or elevated C-reactive protein (CRP). Although these can be useful to confirm systemic inflammation, they do not necessarily correlate with disease activity. Patients with fulminant RA may have no signs of acute phase reactant, whereas patients without rheumatic disease may have these tests elevated for other reasons.

Rheumatoid factor is positive in most cases of RA but is not independently specific for the disease. It may also be positive in other rheumatic diseases (systemic lupus erythematosus, sarcoid, cryoglobulins), as well as nonrheumatic diseases (cirrhosis, endocarditis, etc.).

Radiographic features correspond with the stage of the arthritis. Early RA may show only juxtaarticular osteopenia, particularly of metacarpophalangeal (MCP) and proximal interphalangeal (PIP) joints with some slight soft-tissue swelling. This can increase in intensity as the RA becomes more advanced. More advanced or aggressive disease demonstrates subarticular or articular erosions, symmetric joint space narrowing, osteoporosis with or without subchondral bone resorption, bone cysts, and ultimately fusion of some joints. Such changes are usually symmetric. Unlike psoriatic arthritis and osteoarthritis, RA is rarely associated with reactive bone formation.

The treatment of RA has shifted in the last 10 years. The use of disease modifying antirheumatic agents (DMARDS) early in the disease to prevent deformities is currently recommended. For this reason, documentation of radiographic findings early or progression of radiographic findings on therapy may prompt the clinician to use more aggressive therapy.

Radiologic Aspects

George B. Greenfield

Radiologically, osteoporosis is seen to be most severe in post-menopausal women, patients on steroid treatment, and those with advanced disease.[4] In the extremities there is a predilection for the proximal interphalangeal joints, the metacarpophalangeal joints, the intercarpal joints, and the distal radioulnar and radiocarpal joints to be involved. The acromioclavicular and sternoclavicular joints may also be involved, as well as the temporomandibular joints, knees, calcanei, ankles, hips, elbows, and shoulders.

In the spine, the cervical area is usually involved, and only minimal changes are seen in the thoracolumbar spine. Sacroiliac joint involvement is uncommon, but may occur late in the disease.

The distribution in adult onset disease is usually symmetrical.

Peripheral Joints. The *hands* show the earliest changes, including periarticular soft-tissue swelling, joint effusion, and synovitis. The swelling is most commonly seen in the proximal interphalangeal joints (Fig. 2.1) and the metacarpophalangeal joints.

Soft-tissue swelling at the ulnar styloid, loss of the lateral fat planes of the wrist, and radiocarpal joint narrowing usually occur prior to any bony changes.

Periarticular osteoporosis results from local hyperemia and disuse (Fig. 2.2). Joint effusion may result in widening of the joint space, seen only in early stages. Early cortical erosive changes are best seen at the metacarpal heads. Initially, cortical thinning is seen, progressing to a dot-dash pattern in the bare areas. Then there is loss of the cortical white line on the radial aspects of the metacarpal heads.[5] The "ball-catchers," or AP oblique view, can best demonstrate this. The most frequent erosion pattern is the distal first three metacarpals and the corresponding proximal phalangeal bases, the base of the distal phalanx of the thumb, and the proximal interphalangeal joint of the middle finger.[6]

The synovium is attached to the margins of the articular cartilage. On the metacarpals, it is reflected proximally along the neck of bone, forming synovial pouches that are largest on the dorsal surface, smallest on the volar surface. Thus, a pouch with a double layer of synovium lies directly on cortical bone (bare area) with no intervening articular cartilage. The thin cortical bone at these sites is perforated by vessels.

Pannus in the synovial pouches is in direct contact with the bare area. The invasion of pannus along the nutrient vessels follows, causing marginal erosions. It is very important to determine whether or not early erosions are present, because this finding changes the treatment plan (Figs. 2.3 through 2.7). The "ball-catcher's" view is helpful in this respect. MRI can show erosions earlier than conventional radiographs. The erosions then progress (Fig. 2.8). Some patients may show a coalescent collar of erosion around the metacarpal neck (Fig. 2.9).

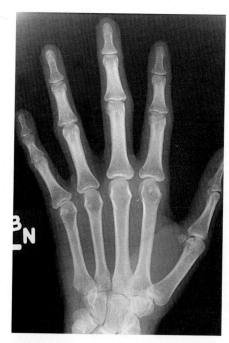

FIGURE 2.1. Early rheumatoid arthritis. Hand. Soft-tissue swelling about the proximal interphalangeal joints of the index, middle, and ring fingers is noted. There is also mild periarticular osteoporosis at these sites.

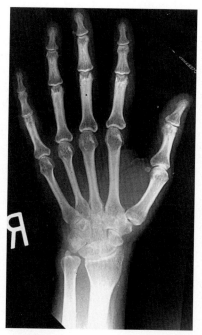

FIGURE 2.2. Rheumatoid arthritis. Hand. Periarticular osteoporosis is noted. No erosions are evident.

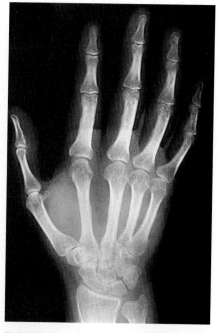

FIGURE 2.3. Rheumatoid arthritis. An early erosion at the second metacarpal head is noted. Periarticular osteoporosis is also seen.

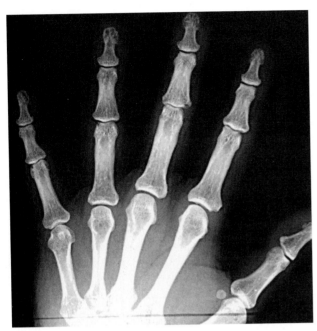

FIGURE 2.4. Rheumatoid arthritis. Hand. Early erosions. Erosions at the margins of the proximal interphalangeal joint of the middle finger noted on the radial side. The proximal phalanx of the index finger also shows a marginal erosion. The bone density is preserved.

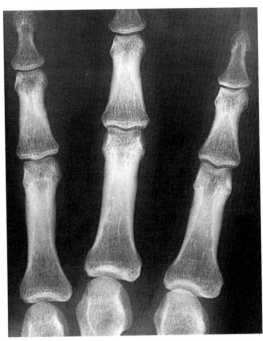

FIGURE 2.6. Rheumatoid arthritis. Hand. Small marginal erosions about the proximal interphalangeal joint of the middle finger are seen.

The patterns of erosions of the hand and wrist have been classified as marginal erosions, compressive erosions, superficial surface resorption, and pseudocyst formation.[6]

Marginal erosions are most evident at the radiovolar aspect of the metacarpal heads. Compressive erosions are

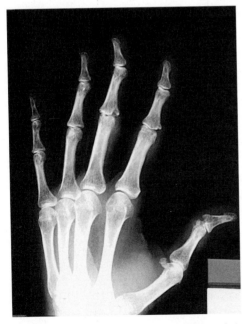

FIGURE 2.5. Rheumatoid arthritis. Oblique view of the hand. Erosions are noted at the proximal interphalangeal joints of the index and middle fingers, as well as at the interphalangeal joints of the thumb. Periarticular osteoporosis is also present.

owing to muscular forces acting on osteoporotic bone. As the proximal phalanges undergo volar subluxation and ulnar deviation, more articular cartilage on the dorsal and dorsoradial aspects lie in contact with diseased synovium, which destroys and replaces cartilage. Erosions of the metacarpal heads are greatest. Muscular forces may compress the bone ends into one another, causing bony invaginations, splaying, or irregular surfaces (Figs. 2.10, 2.11, and 2.12).

Superficial surface resorption occurs along the shaft and may be caused by tenosynovitis. It is seen as thinning and irregularity of the cortex somewhat resembling hyperparathyroidism. It may be accompanied by minimal periosteal new bone formation. The dorsal aspect of the first metacarpal and the proximal phalanx of the thumb are the most frequent sites.[6]

Pseudocysts are marginal erosions seen *en face.* They may attain large size and result from pressure erosion.

The joint space becomes narrowed because of cartilage atrophy and destruction. Joint space narrowing without erosions may be present in rheumatoid arthritis.

The typical malalignment at the metacarpophalangeal joints is ulnar deviation of the phalanges (Fig. 2.13) leading to subluxation (Figs. 2.14, 2.15, and 2.16). Ulnar deviation and subluxation in rheumatoid arthritis are usually erosive and are irreversible. Reversible, nonerosive ulnar deviation of the fingers suggests systemic lupus erthematosus (SLE) or Jaccoud's arthritis.

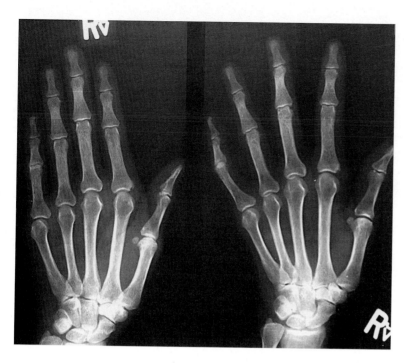

FIGURE 2.7. Rheumatoid arthritis. Hand. Marginal erosions at the metacarpophalangeal joint and distal interphalangeal joint of the index finger are seen.

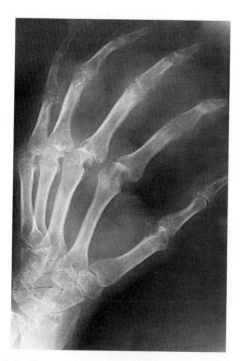

FIGURE 2.8. Rheumatoid arthritis. Hand. Large erosions at the metacarpal heads and bases of the proximal phalanges are seen. There is also soft-tissue swelling and osteopenia at the proximal interphalangeal joints and involvement of the distal interphalangeal joints as well.

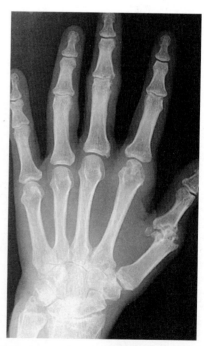

FIGURE 2.9. Rheumatoid arthritis. Erosions at the heads of the first and second metacarpals have formed a collar about the bones. Erosion at the proximal interphalangeal joint of the middle finger is seen with soft-tissue swelling, as well as erosions in the wrist.

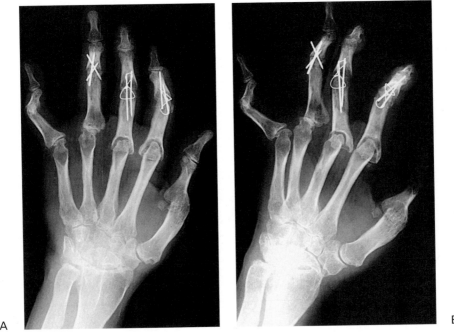

FIGURE 2.10. Rheumatoid arthritis. **A,B:** AP and oblique views of the hand. Compression erosions at the bases of the proximal phalanges of the index and middle fingers are seen as well as erosions of the metacarpal heads. There has been surgical fusion of three fingers, and a boutonniere deformity of the little finger. Marked erosions at the wrist are also seen.

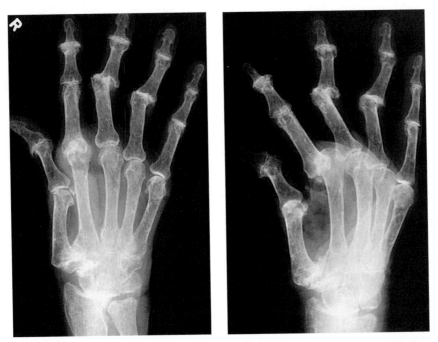

FIGURE 2.11. Rheumatoid arthritis. Hand. **A,B:** AP and oblique views of the hand. Compression erosions and subluxation at the proximal interphalangeal joints of the middle and ring fingers are seen as well as subluxation at the metacarpophalangeal joint of the index finger. There are also erosive changes at the distal interphalangeal joints. Marked osteoporosis is seen as well as erosions at the wrist and the distal radioulnar joint.

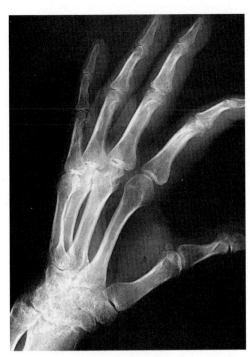

FIGURE 2.12. Rheumatoid arthritis. Hand. Oblique view. A collarlike erosion at the third metacarpal head is noted, as well as multiple erosions at the wrist.

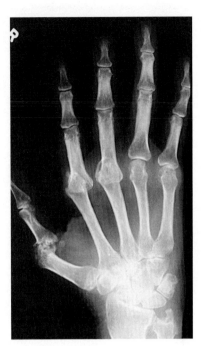

FIGURE 2.14. Rheumatoid arthritis. Hand. Compression erosions and subluxation of the metacarpophalangeal joints of the thumb, index finger, and middle finger are seen.

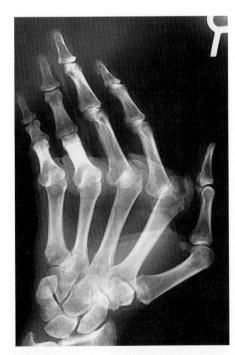

FIGURE 2.13. Advanced rheumatoid arthritis. Hand. There is ulnar deviation of all of the fingers, and subluxations at the second and third metacarpophalangeal joints.

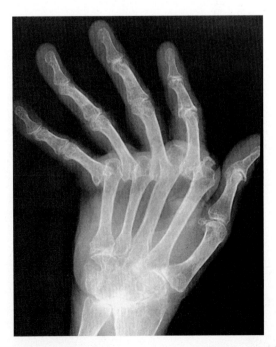

FIGURE 2.15. Advanced rheumatoid arthritis. There are subluxations and dislocations at the metacarpophalangeal joints of the index through to the little finger.

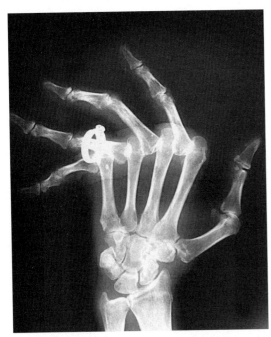

FIGURE 2.16. Advanced rheumatoid arthritis. There are subluxations and dislocations at the metacarpophalangeal joints of the index through to the little finger. Erosions at the first metacarpal head are also seen.

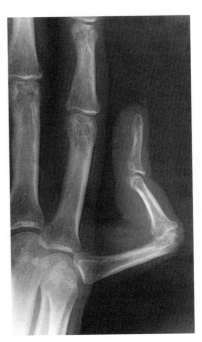

FIGURE 2.17. Rheumatoid arthritis. Boutonniere deformity of the little finger.

Metacarpophalangeal bony ankylosis does not occur. Soft-tissue atrophy is common later in the disease.

The earliest signs in the proximal interphalangeal joints are fusiform soft-tissue swelling and joint space narrowing. Marginal erosions of the proximal phalanx and the base of the middle phalanx occur, most commonly in the middle finger. Compressive erosions, with "ball-in-socket" configurations may occur in all proximal interphalangeal joints.

Characteristic deformities of the fingers, the boutonniere deformity and the swan neck deformity, occur in RA. They may also be associated with SLE and Jaccoud's arthritis.[7]

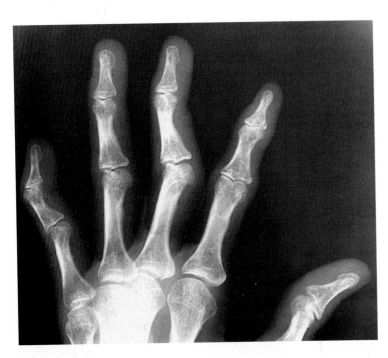

FIGURE 2.18. Rheumatoid arthritis. Hand. There is a "swan neck" deformity of the middle and ring fingers with hyperextension at the proximal interphalangeal joints and flexion at the distal interphalangeal joints.

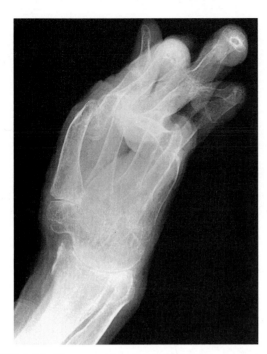

FIGURE 2.19. Rheumatoid arthritis. Hand. Advanced changes with osteoporosis, and subluxations at the metacarpophalangeal joints result in shortening of the fingers. This is the "opera glass" hand. Involvement of the wrist with carpal bone fusion is also seen.

There is flexion of the proximal interphalangeal joint and extension of the distal interphalangeal joint, giving the appearance of securing a carnation in a lapel, or boutonniere (Fig. 2.17). This is owing to detachment of the extensor tendon from the middle phalanx with volar displacement, and paradoxical action as a flexor.

The opposite is the swan neck deformity (Fig. 2.18); it occurs when the extensor tendon is shortened, resulting in hyperextension of the proximal interphalangeal joint and compensatory flexion of the distal interphalangeal joint. In the thumb, the distal phalanx is often subluxed dorsally, with flexion of the metacarpophalangeal joint.

Bony ankylosis of the interphalangeal joints may occur very rarely. The disease may progress to extensive destruction of the bone ends, with a clinical appearance of telescoping of the fingers, called a "main-en-lorgnette" or "opera glass" hand (Fig. 2.19) and severe dislocations and destruction at the end stage, called arthritis mutilans.

MRI can show erosions several months earlier than conventional radiographs. Erosions are well demonstrated as low signal intensity foci on T1W images. Pannus enhances with gadolinium (Fig. 2.20).

Periosteal new bone formation, rarely present, is sparse and thin. Secondary osteoarthritis may develop with subchondral sclerosis and marginal osteophyte formation, but it usually does not overshadow the features of rheumatoid arthritis.[6]

In the *wrist,* soft-tissue swelling is the earliest change, most pronounced around the ulnar styloid process, with obliteration of the adjacent fat planes (Fig. 2.21). The soft tissue swelling can progress to involve the entire wrist, and small erosions may be seen (Fig. 2.22). Periarticular osteoporosis follows. There is general involvement of the carpus, in contrast to gout, which sometimes involves the carpometacarpal area, and calcium pyrophosphate deposition disease (DPDD), which has a predilection for the radiocarpal region. Narrowing of the radiocarpal joint may occur (Fig. 2.23). Cyst formation in the distal radius may follow (Figs. 2.24 and 2.25).

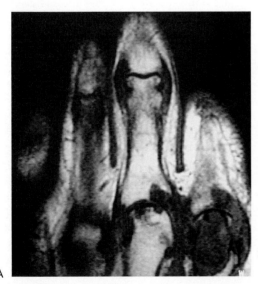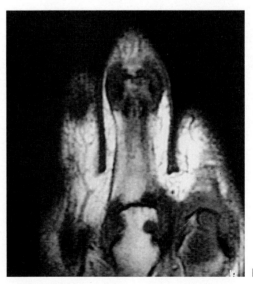

A

B

FIGURE 2.20. Middle-aged woman with active, aggressive rheumatoid arthritis. Left hand. MRI. **A,B:** T1-weighted images. Erosions about the metacarpophalangeal joints are seen as low signal intensity involving, principally, the margins.

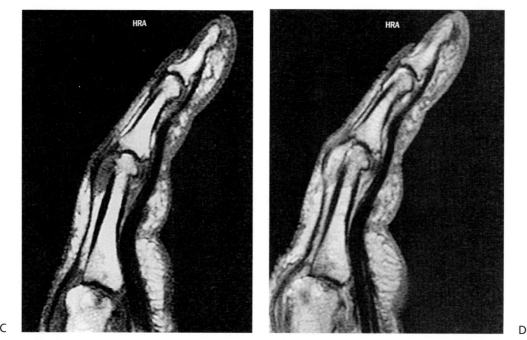

C

D

FIGURE 2.20. *(continued)* C,D: Pregadolinium and postgadolinium images show pannus eroding bone at the dorsal margin of the proximal interphalangeal joint. Gadolinium infusion shows increase in signal intensity of the pannus. (Photo, courtesy of Dr. Iain Watt, Bristol, UK.)

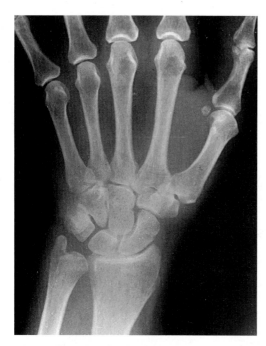

FIGURE 2.21. Rheumatoid arthritis. Wrist. Early change. There is soft-tissue swelling about the ulnar styloid process, with obliteration of the fat planes. No osteoporosis or erosions are as yet evident.

Frequent sites of erosion in RA are the distal trapezium (Fig. 2.26), triquetrum and pisiform, the ulnar styloid and the groove or notch of the distal ulna (Fig. 2.27), the midscaphoid at its radial aspect, any proximal carpal bone, capitate, radial styloid (Fig. 2.28), the distal ulna itself (Fig. 2.29), and the distal radioulnar joint with "notching" of the distal radius (Figs. 2.30, 2.31, and 2.32).

A pattern of bone fragmentation involving the scaphoid, distal radius, and ulna (Figs. 2.33 and 2.34), and an elongated bony spicule overlying the radiocarpal joint, associated with carpal fusion, has been described.[8] The carpal bones progress to malposition.[9] Widening of the spaces of the distal radioulnar joint, the scaphoid-capitate joint, and the scaphoid-lunate joint is characteristic (Figs. 2.35 and 2.36). Posterior subluxation of the lunate may occur.

The wrist may progress to volar dislocation at the radiocarpal joint. Diastasis of the radioulnar joint with dorsal displacement of the distal ulna may follow. Deviation of the wrist, causing the scaphoid to lie in the hollow of the distal radius, may also occur.

The changes progress to bony ankylosis in the intracarpal, carpometacarpal, and intermetacarpal joints (Fig. 2.37). Radioulnar ankylosis may rarely be seen. Erosion of the distal ulna may occur. Patients with severe wrist changes and minimal hand changes may show progress of disease in the hand to overtake that in the wrist.[10]

The *shoulder* is not usually involved at first. Narrowing of the glenohumeral joint occurs (Fig. 2.38). Erosions occur in

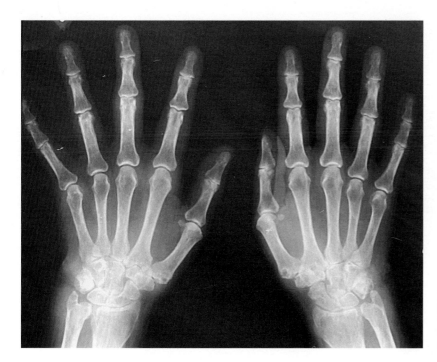

FIGURE 2.22. Rheumatoid arthritis. Wrist. Bilateral soft-tissue swelling is noted involving the entire wrists, more so on the right side. Small erosions are seen at the bases of the first metacarpals bilaterally.

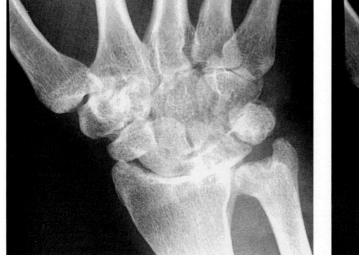
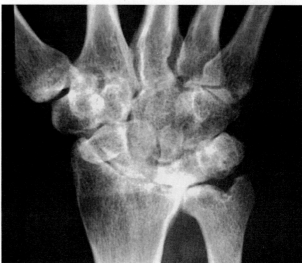

A   B

FIGURE 2.23. Rheumatoid arthritis. Wrist. **A:** There is narrowing of the radiocarpal joint. **B:** Same patient 1 year later. There has been progression of narrowing at the radiocarpal joint with rotation of the scaphoid and lunate. Erosions at the ulnar notch are also seen.

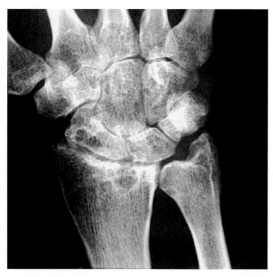

FIGURE 2.24. Rheumatoid arthritis. Wrist. A cyst in the distal radius is seen as well as narrowing of the radiocarpal joint and erosions in the carpal bones.

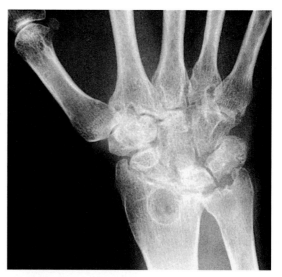

FIGURE 2.25. Rheumatoid arthritis. A large cyst is seen in the distal radius and there is destruction involving the scaphoid and lunate bones. Erosions in the ulnar styloid and ulnar notch are also seen, as well as small erosions in the metacarpal bases.

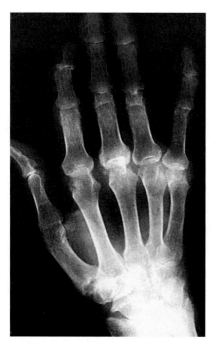

FIGURE 2.26. Rheumatoid arthritis. Wrist and hand. There is general involvement of the carpus with a large erosion at the trapeziometacarpal joint. Erosions at the metacarpal heads and interphalangeal joints are also seen as well as osteoporosis.

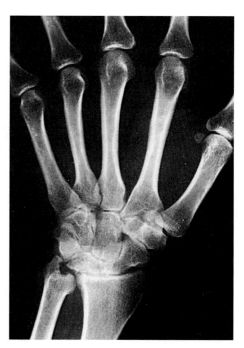

FIGURE 2.27. Rheumatoid arthritis. Wrist. There is erosion of the ulnar styloid and notch of the distal ulna. There is also loss of the radiocarpal joint space and erosions of the scaphoid and lunate.

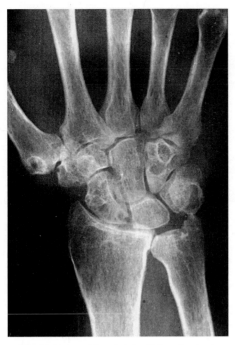

FIGURE 2.28. Rheumatoid arthritis. Wrist. Cystic changes in the carpal bones are noted as well as an erosion at the base of the first metacarpal. There is erosion in the notch of the distal ulna.

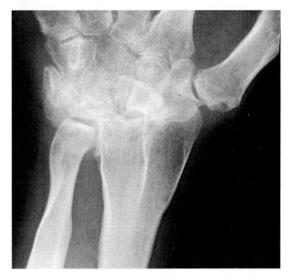

FIGURE 2.29. Rheumatoid arthritis. Wrist. Destructive changes in the carpal bones are noted as well as an erosion at the base of the first metacarpal. There is smooth erosion with narrowing of the distal ulna.

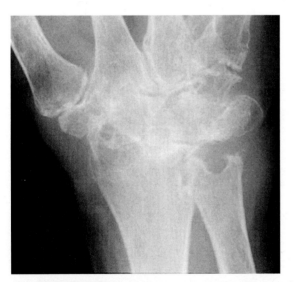

FIGURE 2.30. Rheumatoid arthritis. Wrist. There is marked destruction of the carpal bones and erosion at the radial styloid. A small amount of erosion at the distal radioulnar joint is seen.

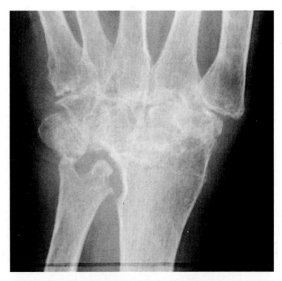

FIGURE 2.31. Rheumatoid arthritis. Wrist. There is marked destruction of the carpal bones. A larger erosion at the distal radioulnar joint is seen than on previous figure. Erosions at the distal ulna are also seen.

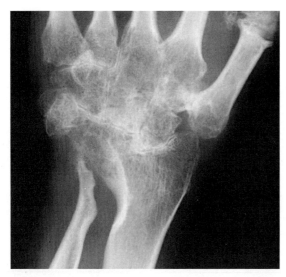

FIGURE 2.32. Rheumatoid arthritis. Wrist. There is destruction of the carpal bones and erosion of the radial articular surface. A larger erosion at the distal radioulnar joint is seen with a pencil-like deformity of the distal ulna.

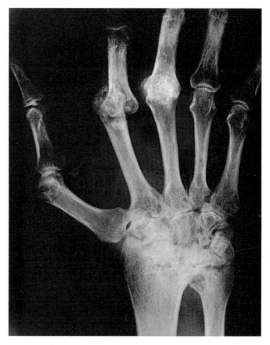

FIGURE 2.33. Rheumatoid arthritis. Wrist and hand. There is destruction involving the scaphoid, lunate, distal radius, and ulna. Subluxations at the metacarpophalangeal joints are also seen.

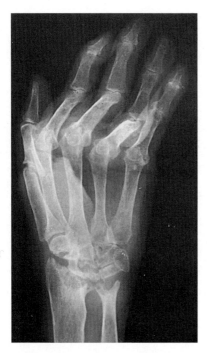

FIGURE 2.34. Rheumatoid arthritis. Wrist. Multiple erosions in the carpal bones including the scaphoid, pisiform, trapezium, hamate, and base of the first metacarpal are seen. There is erosion at the notch of the ulna as well.

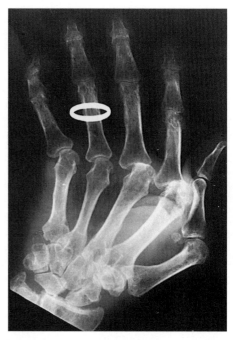

FIGURE 2.35. Rheumatoid arthritis. Wrist. Scaphoid-lunate separation is noted as well as cyst formation. The second and third metacarpophalangeal joints are subluxed.

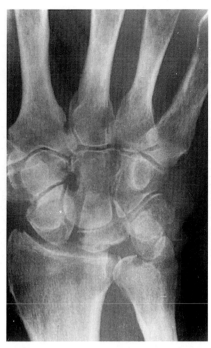

FIGURE 2.36. Rheumatoid arthritis. Wrist. Scaphoid-lunate separation and multiple erosions are present.

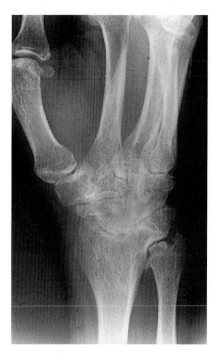

FIGURE 2.37. Rheumatoid arthritis. Wrist. Block fusion of the carpus has occurred.

the humeral head, initially marginal and often seen above the greater tuberosity at the inferior margin of articular cartilage (Fig. 2.39). Large erosions and pseudocysts may develop (Fig. 2.40), some with sclerotic margins.

Erosion of the glenoid fossa (Fig. 2.41) and humeral articular surface occasionally may be seen.

Destruction and tear of the rotator cuff tendon allows upward displacement of the humeral head by the unopposed pull of the deltoid muscle. This results in erosion of the inferior aspect of the distal clavicle and the acromioclavicular joint. Severe erosion and resorption occur in advanced disease. Pressure erosion of the humeral neck results in a "hatchet-shaped" appearance (Fig. 2.42). Resorption of a part or all of the entire humeral head may occur, with subsequent dislocation (Fig. 2.43).

Erosion on the undersurface of the distal clavicle may be seen at the site of attachment of the coracoclavicular ligament.[11]

In the *elbow,* three fat pads are present between the synovial membrane and the capsule: two anterior and one posterior. These fill the olecranon fossa of the distal humerus. The posterior fat pad is the largest and is pressed deeply into the olecranon groove by the triceps tendon. The anterior fat pads on lateral view may be normally visible. In any condition leading to joint hemorrhage, effusion, or synovitis, the anterior fat pad may be displaced anteriorly and the posterior fat pad displaced posteriorly so that it becomes visible. This is called the positive "fat pad sign," which frequently occurs in rheumatoid arthritis (Figs. 2.44 and 2.45). It may precede bony changes. A positive fat pad sign in the absence

of trauma most probably indicates rheumatoid arthritis.[12] This may also be present in hemophilia and gout.[13]

A large noncommunicating bursa is located posterior to the olecranon, with bursitis frequently present. It can be seen as a soft-tissue mass, and may cause erosion of the posterior aspect of the olecranon process.

Rheumatoid nodules are common about the elbow. These are well-circumscribed, painless masses in the subcutaneous tissue, of up to several centimeters.

There is uniform narrowing of the entire joint. Symmetrical bilateral involvement is typical. Marginal erosions (Fig. 2.46) develop, with loss of the articular cortex. Erosion of the olecranon fossa may occur (Fig. 2.47). Subchondral cysts, large in number and size, may be prominent. Spontaneous fracture of the olecranon process may occur, usually through the midpoint of the trochlear notch. Extensive destruction and erosion may follow, with subluxation and a destructive end stage. Bony ankylosis rarely may occur, although this is more common in juvenile onset rheumatoid arthritis.

In the *hips,* rheumatoid arthritis is characterized by uniform narrowing of the joint space, followed by erosions and secondary osteoarthritis (Figs. 2.48 and 2.49). This is in contrast to osteoarthritis, where narrowing occurs at the superior portion. Because of narrowing also of the medial portion of the joint space, there is superomedial or medial drift of the femoral head.[14,15] This leads to erosion and remodeling of the acetabulum to cause acetabular protrusion (Fig. 2.50). A pathological fracture may occur (Fig. 2.51). Osteoporosis occurs along with the bone and joint changes.

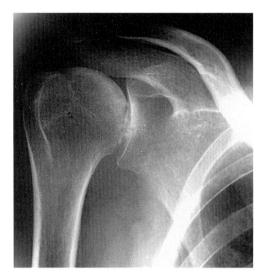

FIGURE 2.38. Rheumatoid arthritis. Shoulder. Narrowing of the glenohumeral joint space is seen.

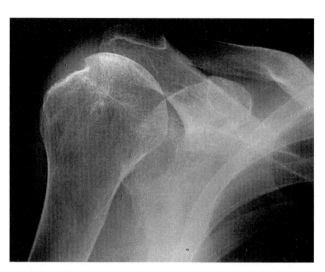

FIGURE 2.39. Rheumatoid arthritis. Shoulder. Erosion at the outer margin of the humeral head is seen.

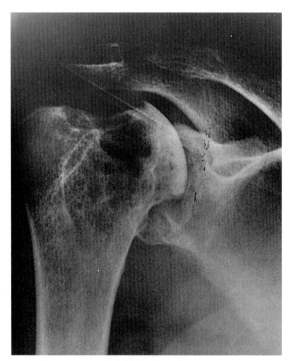

FIGURE 2.40. Rheumatoid arthritis. Shoulder. Erosions are seen as a collar about the humeral neck.

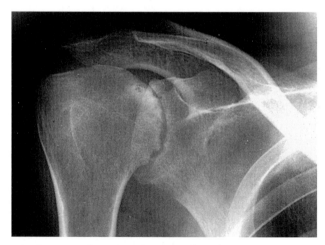

FIGURE 2.41. Rheumatoid arthritis. Shoulder. Erosions of the glenoid fossa and of the articular surface of the humeral head are seen.

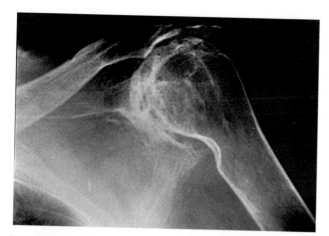

FIGURE 2.42. Rheumatoid arthritis. Shoulder. There is elevation of the humerus. Erosions are seen at the acromioclavicular joint and at the humeral neck. This leads to a "hatchet-shaped" appearance.

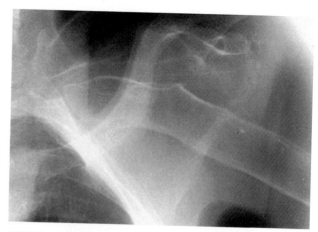

FIGURE 2.43. Advanced rheumatoid arthritis. Shoulder. Resorption of the humeral head has occurred and there is medial dislocation of the humerus. New bone formation about the glenoid is also seen.

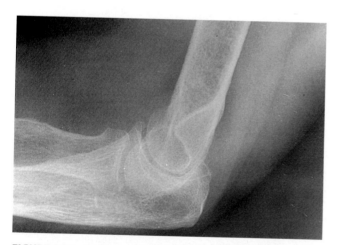

FIGURE 2.44. Rheumatoid arthritis. Elbow. A positive "fat pad" sign is seen with fat planes anterior and posterior to the distal humerus.

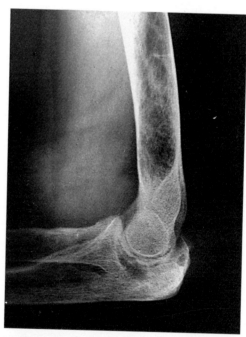

FIGURE 2.45. Rheumatoid arthritis. Elbow. A positive "fat pad" sign is seen with displacement of fat planes anteriorly.

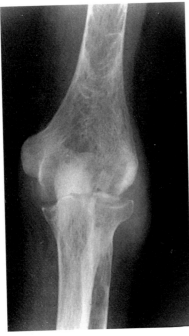

FIGURE 2.46. Rheumatoid arthritis. Elbow. Erosion at the radial aspect with soft-tissue swelling is seen.

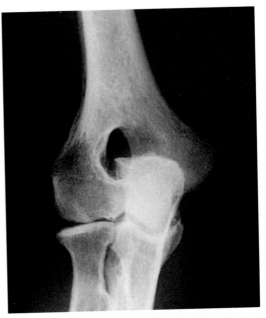

FIGURE 2.47. Rheumatoid arthritis. Elbow. There is erosion of the olecranon fossa. Periosteal new bone formation along the medial aspect of the distal humerus is noted. Erosion at the proximal radioulnar joint is also seen, as well as joint space narrowing and irregularity at the capitulum.

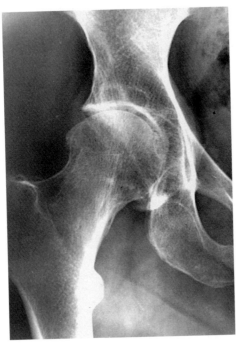

FIGURE 2.48. Rheumatoid arthritis. Hip. There is uniform narrowing of the joint space with subchondral sclerosis and small cyst formation.

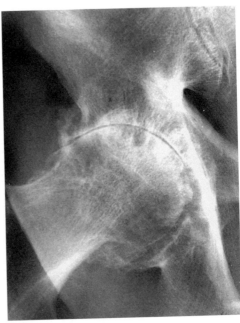

FIGURE 2.49. Rheumatoid arthritis. Hip. Uniform joint space narrowing is noted. Subchondral cysts at the acetabulum are seen as well as secondary spurring at the margin of the femoral head. Osteoporosis is also present.

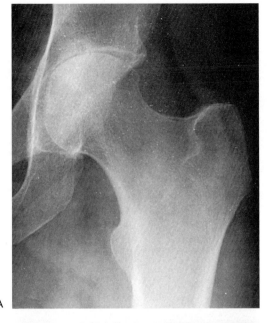

A

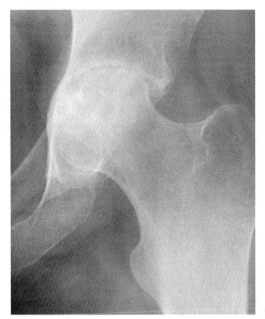

C

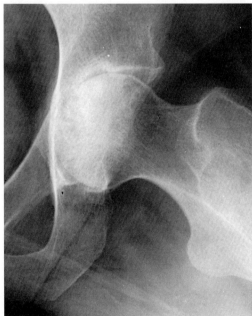

B

FIGURE 2.50. Rheumatoid arthritis of the hip. **A:** Uniform narrowing of the hip joint space with medial migration of the femoral head are seen. **B:** Same patient eight months later. There has been further narrowing of the hip joint space. Cyst formation and sclerosis in the femoral head is noted. **C:** Same patient 2 years later. Acetabular protrusion is seen as well as increase in the size and number of cysts in the femoral head. The joint space is further narrowed.

Erosions and subchondral cysts in both the femoral head and acetabulum occur. Destructive changes and avascular necrosis of the femoral head may result. Large pelvic retroperitoneal or inguinal soft-tissue masses owing to massive enlargement of the iliopsoas bursa, which communicates with the hip joint, may occur.[16,17] Piriformis bursitis, communicating with the hip joint, causing pressure on the sciatic nerve and with pain referred to the knee has been reported.[18] A stress fracture of the ischium may mimic the symptoms of arthritis of the hip (Fig. 2.52).

In the *knees,* early changes include periarticular osteoporosis and joint effusion (Fig. 2.53). This is seen as supra-

patellar fullness, with displacement of fat planes.[19] There may also be massive distension of the popliteal bursae, if communication with the capsule exists.[20] A huge distended bursa may extend down the calf. Synovial fluid may leak, causing severe pain, and simulate deep vein thrombosis.

RA in the knee uniformly narrows all three compartments: the medial, lateral, and patellofemoral (Fig. 2.54). In osteoarthritis, the joint space is usually narrowed only in one, the medial compartment.

Marginal erosions may develop, although they are not usually prominent (Fig. 2.55). Erosions of the central portion of the medial femoral condyle may progress to destruc-

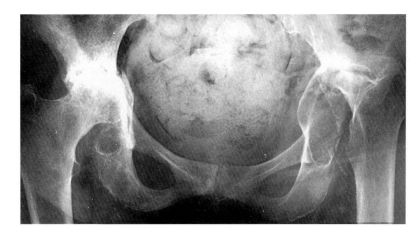

FIGURE 2.51. Rheumatoid arthritis. AP view of both hips shows erosion of both acetabula, with acetabular protrusion and a pathological fracture of the acetabulum on the right side. There is also marked erosion with almost complete disappearance of the left femoral head and a large amount of acetabular erosion and protrusion.

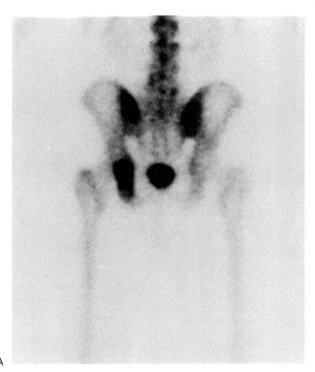

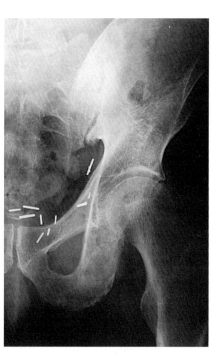

A   B

FIGURE 2.52. Arthritic patient who has left hip pain. **A:** Radionuclide bone scan shows increased activity in the left ischium and inferior aspect of the acetabulum. There is greater activity in the right sacroiliac joint than in the left on this posterior scan. **B:** Conventional radiograph shows a stress fracture of the left ischium. Sacroiliitis is also seen.

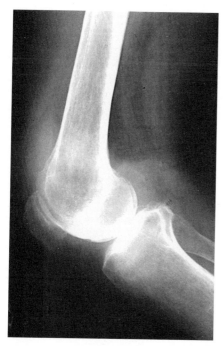

FIGURE 2.53. Rheumatoid arthritis. Knee. Effusion in the suprapatellar region is noted as well as posteriorly. A Baker's cyst is present.

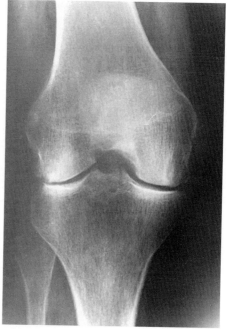

FIGURE 2.55. Rheumatoid arthritis. Knee. Narrowing of both medial and lateral compartments of the knee joint space is noted as well as marginal erosions at the lateral margins. A cyst is seen at the medial tibial condyle. Osteoporosis is noted.

tion of major portions of the articular cortex (Fig. 2.56). Geodes may form later (Fig. 2.57).[21] Sclerosis of the subarticular cortex may result. Delicate periosteal new bone may be seen at the distal femoral metaphyses. The intercondylar notch may appear enlarged.

The proximal tibiofibular joint communicates with the knee joint in 10% of adults.[22] It may be involved, with narrowing and erosions.

In the *ankles,* there is uniform narrowing of the ankle joint, with possible eburnation and subchondral cyst formation, usually bilateral. Erosion at the medial aspect of the distal fibula within the tibiofibular syndesmosis may be seen. Erosions and sclerosis at the talonavicular joint may be seen, as well as tarsal bone erosions (Fig. 2.58). Subluxation

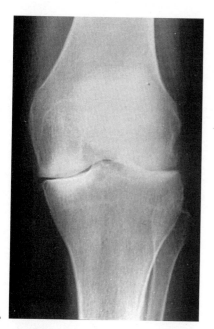

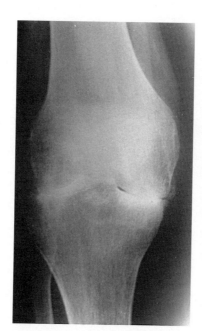

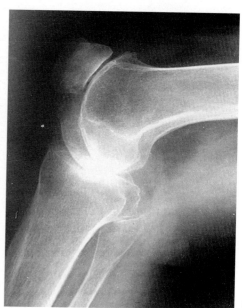

A

B

FIGURE 2.54. Knees. **A:** AP view showing narrowing of both compartments of the knee joint with subchondral sclerosis. **B:** Lateral view showing narrowing of the patellofemoral joint and secondary spur formation.

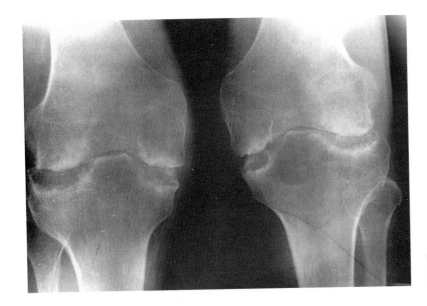

FIGURE 2.56. Rheumatoid arthritis. Knees. There is destruction of major portions of the articular cortex as well as osteosclerosis of the subarticular cortex.

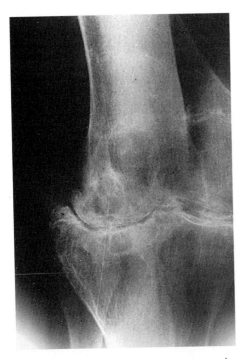

FIGURE 2.57. Rheumatoid arthritis. Knee. Large geodes are seen at the distal femur and proximal tibia. Marked joint space narrowing is noted.

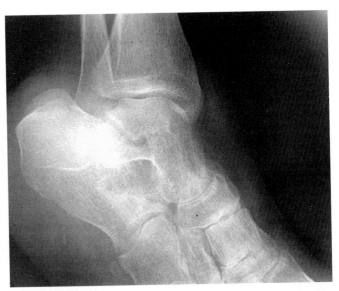

FIGURE 2.58. Rheumatoid arthritis. Erosion in the subtalar joint and subchondral sclerosis are seen.

is occasionally seen.[23] Late changes may include bony anky-losis of the tarsals, as well as large cysts (Fig. 2.59).

The posterior aspect of the calcaneus at the site of the Achilles tendon bursa frequently shows changes with edema (Fig. 2.60) and obliteration of the triangular radiolucency that is normally present.[24] The tendon becomes thickened and erosion at this site follows (Fig. 2.61). Erosion also may be seen at the calcaneal plantar surface and is often associated with a bony spur.

The *feet* are commonly involved, and show changes similar to those in the hands.[25,26] Hallux valgus (Figs. 2.62 and 2.63) and valgus deviation of the toes at the meta-tarsophalangeal joints occur with crossing. Metatarsopha-langeal joint erosions are frequent, and are most marked in the metatarsal heads (Fig. 2.64). Subluxations (Fig. 2.65) and dislocations of the toes (Fig. 2.66) may also occur.

Flexion deformities of the proximal and distal interpha-langeal joints may occur, associated with hyperextension at the metatarsophalangeal joints, resulting in "cocked-up" toes. There may be pes planus. There may be spreading of the metatarsal heads. Superimposed infection may result in draining sinuses (Fig. 2.67).

Central Skeleton. *Spinal* involvement in RA predilects the cervical region. The changes include the following:

1. Cysts[27]
2. Erosions
3. Facet joint arthritis and fusion
4. Granulomatous vertebral lesions (rare)[28]
5. Intervertebral disc narrowing
6. Osteoporosis
7. Subluxation[29,31]

The most important point of subluxation is at the atlantoaxial joint. The normal upper limit of separation between the odontoid process and the ring of C-1 in adults is 2.5 mm. In children it is up to 4 mm, because of unossified cartilage that is not visible on conventional radiographs. The odontoid process is secured firmly by

the strong transverse ligament that attaches to each side of the ring of C-1, preventing separation during flexion and extension.

Two separate synovial joints are present, anterior and posterior to the odontoid process. Synovial inflammation and pannus lead to loosening of the ligamentous attach-ments and laxity of the transverse ligament, allowing at-lantoaxial subluxation. This is most often associated with RA, but may also occur in AS and psoriatic arthritis. Severe neurological symptoms and death may follow because of cord compression. Subluxation is best demonstrated in flexion lateral views, where a C1-2 space of greater than 2.5 mm in adults is seen (Fig. 2.68). The dentate line is inter-rupted with anterior displacement of C-1 on C-2. There may be odontoid erosions (Fig. 2.69), circumferential ero-sion of the odontoid, pathological fracture (Fig. 2.70), or rarely the entire odontoid process may be amputated by erosions.[32]

Upward displacement of the odontoid process in RA has been recorded as a cause of severe neurological syndromes and death.[33–36] MRI can demonstrate the bone and soft-tis-sue abnormalities in the cervical spine and also can show the effects on the spinal cord and brainstem.

Subluxations may be present at other levels in the cervi-cal spine, most often at C4-5. Occasionally multiple sub-luxations occur, often accompanied by intervertebral disc narrowing, showing a "stepladder" pattern. Typically no os-teophytes are seen. Frequent sites of erosion other than the odontoid process include the vertebral end plates, where the lesions may resemble Schmorl's nodes, the apophyseal joints, and the spinous processes, which may taper.

Ankylosis, when present, usually involves the apophyseal joints at one or a few levels, but general ankylosis is rare in adult onset disease.

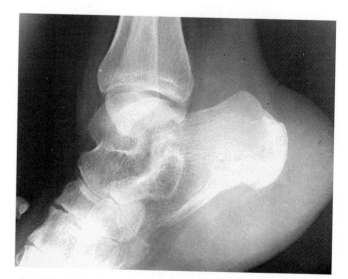

FIGURE 2.60. Rheumatoid arthritis. Soft-tissue swelling about the calcaneus is see along with slight erosion posteriorly.

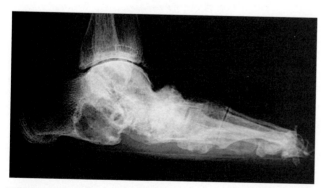

FIGURE 2.59. Rheumatoid arthritis. Ankle. Destruction and fu-sion in the tarsus has resulted in pes planus. There is a large cyst in the anterior calcaneus.

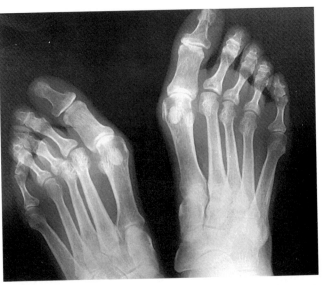

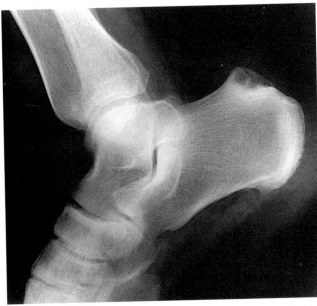

FIGURE 2.61. Rheumatoid arthritis. Calcaneus. Erosion at the insertion of the Achilles tendon is noted.

FIGURE 2.62. Rheumatoid arthritis. Feet. Hallux valgus is noted bilaterally, as well as erosions at multiple metatarsal heads. Joint space narrowing at the right third metatarsophalangeal joint with slight subluxation is evident.

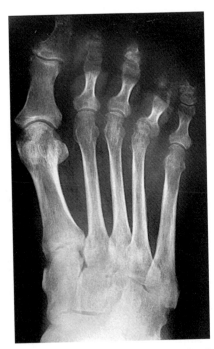

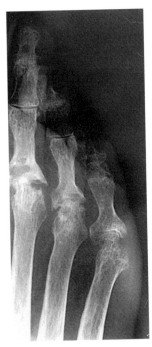

FIGURE 2.63. Rheumatoid arthritis. Foot. Erosions at the metatarsophalangeal joints are seen, as well as hallux valgus.

FIGURE 2.64. Rheumatoid arthritis. Foot. Erosions at the metatarsophalangeal joints are seen, as well as hallux valgus.

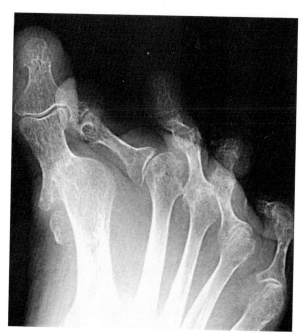

FIGURE 2.65. Rheumatoid arthritis. Foot. There are subluxations at the metatarsophalangeal joints of the second and fourth toes. Fusion across this joint in the great toe has also occurred.

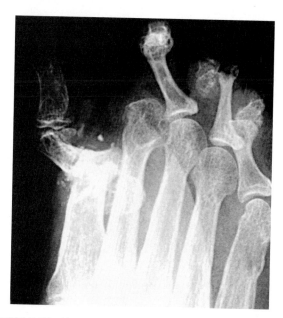

FIGURE 2.66. Rheumatoid arthritis. Foot. There is dislocation and bony resorption along the first metatarsophalangeal joint. The second toe has been amputated.

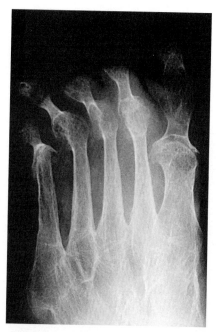

FIGURE 2.67. Rheumatoid arthritis. Foot. Dislocations at metatarsal heads 2-4 are seen. Soft-tissue swelling about the second metarsophalangeal joint is seen, which is the site of a draining sinus.

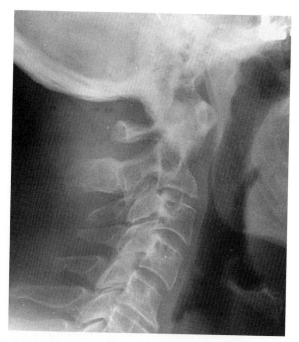

FIGURE 2.68. Rheumatoid arthritis. Upper cervical spine. Erosion of the anterior aspect of the odontoid process and forward displacement of C-1 is noted.

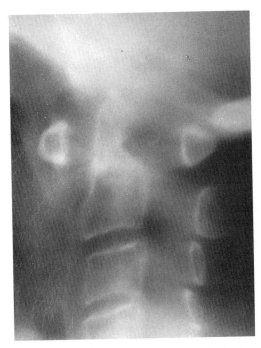

FIGURE 2.69. Rheumatoid arthritis. Upper cervical spine. Linear tomogram. There is widening of the joint space between the dens and the anterior arch of C-1. Posterior erosion at the base of the dens is seen. The dentate line is interrupted with anterior displacement of C-1 on C-2.

A large intracranial mass of rheumatoid granulation tissue, causing brainstem compression, and a pseudomeningocele prolapsing into the atlantoaxial space on flexion, has been reported.[37] Cervical cord compression owing to extradural granulation tissue may occur, and may be directly demonstrated by MRI.[36]

The thoracic and the lumbar spine show osteoporosis, which may have been made worse by steroid therapy. Rarely, rheumatoid nodules occur in the vertebral bodies. In the thoracic and lumbar spine, rheumatoid lesions consist of facet joint and end plate erosions, instability, lumbar nerve root compression, and vertebral body collapse.[38]

The *sacroiliac joints,* late in the course of this disease, rarely exhibit minimal erosions, with a unilateral or a bilateral asymmetrical distribution. Joint space narrowing without reactive sclerosis or, very rarely, fusion of an SI joint has been reported.[39]

Smooth erosion of the superior margins of the upper *ribs* occurs in rheumatoid arthritis (Fig. 2.71) , as well as in scleroderma and hyperparathyroidism.

A reported complication of rheumatoid arthritis is necrotizing vasculitis with occlusion and resulting gangrene.[40]

The *temporomandibular joint* is involved in a large percentage of patients with rheumatoid arthritis. Joint space narrowing or erosion of the condyle and fossa, along with limitation of range of motion, may be seen.

The *sternoclavicular joint* is frequently involved, with widening and erosions (Fig. 2.72).

The *manubriosternal joint* is sometimes involved in rheumatoid arthritis, as well as in AS, psoriatic arthritis, and Reiter's syndrome.

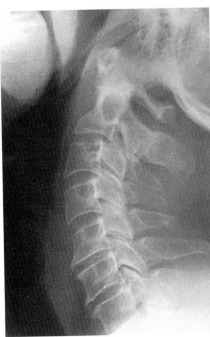
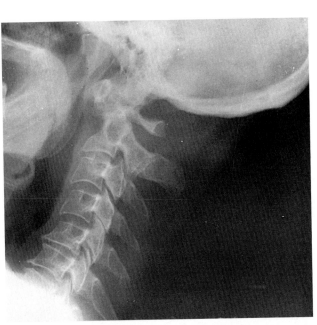

A   B

FIGURE 2.70. Rheumatoid arthritis. Cervical spine. Flexion and extension views. Fracture of the base of the odontoid process. **A:** Lateral view in extension showing normal position of the odontoid process. **B:** Flexion view showing anterior displacement of the odontoid process with the ring of C-1.

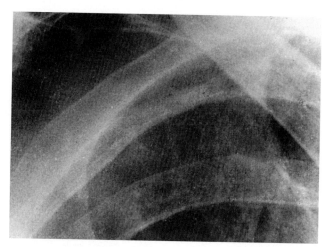

FIGURE 2.71. Rheumatoid arthritis. Erosion at the superior aspect of the third rib is noted.

Felty's syndrome is rheumatoid arthritis with associated splenomegaly and neutropenia.[41] Patients suffer from recurrent infections.

Septic arthritis and stress fractures are complications of rheumatoid arthritis.[42–44]

Unilateral rheumatoid arthritis may be seen in patients with hemiplegia, because the immobilization of paralysis seems to prevent arthritic changes from advancing.[45,46]

The radionuclide bone scan is a sensitive indicator of activity in rheumatoid arthritis. The pattern is symmetrical activity of peripheral joints (Fig. 2.73). Other inflammatory arthritides tend to have a more central involvement with asymmetrical peripheral joint uptake. Involvement of the sacroiliac joints can be detected by radioscintigraphy, although the normal increase in activity at this site can cause difficulties in interpretation.[47]

MRI has the ability to show early changes, particularly pannus formation in the preerosive stage. T1-weighted images with gadolinium infusion show high signal intensity of hypervascular pannus, whereas T2W-like images show high signal intensity in joint fluid, but not in pannus or areas of fibrosis.[48]

Haglund's syndrome is characterized by a prominent calcaneal bursa, retrocalcaneal bursitis, thickening of the Achilles tendon, and convexity of the superficial soft tissues at the Achilles tendon insertion.[49] Erosion at the posterior calcaneus is seen. It is a common cause of posterior heel pain, and is thought to result from irritation from wearing stiff-backed low-heeled shoes. Both bursae surrounding the Achilles tendon, the superficial and the retrocalcaneal, are involved (Fig. 2.74).

Case Reports

Keith Kanik

Case 1. A 33-year-old man who complained of joint pain and stiffness was seen. Two years prior to the visit he developed bilateral wrist pain and was treated with NSAIDs. The symptoms resolved after a few weeks. Two months prior to the visit the patient noticed increasing joint pain involving the bilateral shoulders, elbows, knees, hands, and wrists associated with more than 1 hour of morning stiffness. He also began to develop swelling of his proximal interphalangeal joints.

The physical examination revealed 2+ swelling of his right third MCP, second and third PIPs, and left third PIP, along with 1+ swelling of his wrists.

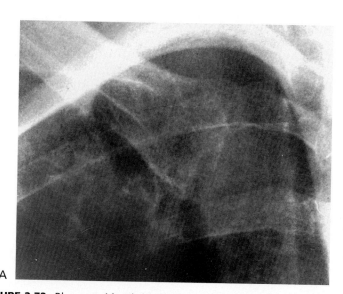

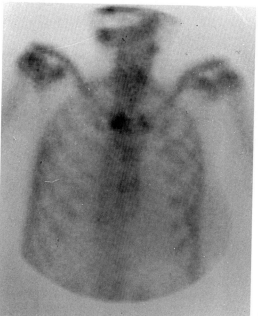

A

B

FIGURE 2.72. Rheumatoid arthritis. Sternoclavicular joint. **A:** Irregular erosions at the articular surface of the head of the clavicle are noted. **B:** Radionuclide bone scan showing increased activity at the right sternoclavicular joint.

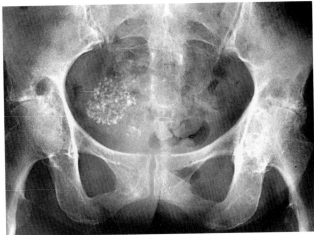

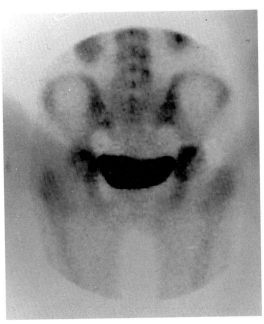

A

B

FIGURE 2.73. Rheumatoid arthritis. Hip joints. **A:** Uniform joint space narrowing and erosions are seen in both hips. A calcified fibroid is incidentally noted. **B:** Radionuclide bone scan showing increased activity in both hip joints.

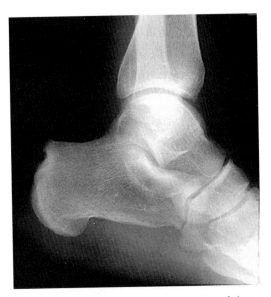

FIGURE 2.74. Haglund's syndrome. Lateral view of the os calcis shows an erosion at its superior aspect with surrounding reactive sclerosis. The superior aspect forms a spur.

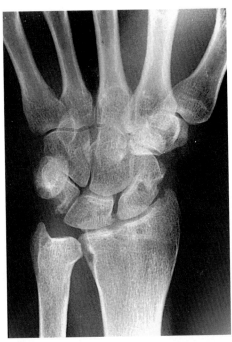

FIGURE 2.75. Rheumatoid arthritis. Wrist. Multiple erosions are seen at the proximal carpal row and distal radius and ulna.

Laboratory tests revealed an elevated ESR of 43 (normal <15), elevated CRP (normal <0.8), mild anemia, and an elevated rheumatoid factor of 120 (normal <39).

Radiographic examination of hands and wrists revealed multiple erosions bilaterally. There was narrowing of the radiocarpal joints bilaterally with multiple subchondral cysts formations at the left distal radius and ulna. A large erosion was noted at the triangular bone on the left side, with a smaller erosion on the right at the same site. Erosions were noted on the left as well as on the right distal fifth metacarpal and right distal proximal phalanx (Fig. 2.75).

The patient was treated with sulfasalazine (SSZ) (3 g/day) and methotrexate (MTX) (7.5 mg/week). The patient's anemia, ESR, and CRP all returned to normal within 2 months of therapy. The patient began to clinically improve after 2 months, with almost complete resolution of symptoms after 6 months of therapy. The patient continues on MTX (7.5 mg/week) and SSZ (2 g/day).

Case 2. A 49-year-old man with a 30-year history of rheumatoid arthritis was seen. He failed multiple treatment regiments and was currently maintained on ibuprofen and propoxyphene. The patient had only 15 minutes of morning stiffness, and described the majority of his arthritic complaints to be related to overactivity. Physical examination revealed marked deformities as well as Heberden's and Bouchard's nodes. Radiographic examination of his right hand and wrist revealed multiple abnormalities. These in-

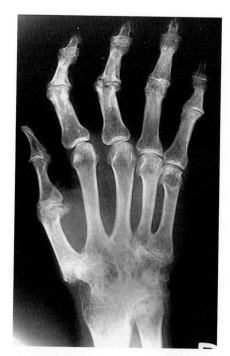

FIGURE 2.76. Rheumatoid arthritis. Hand and wrist. There is fusion of the carpus and ulnar deviation at the proximal interphalangeal joints of the index and middle fingers, as well as erosions at these sites.

cluded fusion and ankylosis of the carpal bones, radiocarpal and metacarpal joints, erosions at the head of the proximal phalanx of the second and third fingers, ulnar deviation at the PIP joints of the second and third fingers, PIP soft-tissue swelling, and severe joint space narrowing (Fig. 2.76). Similar changes were seen on the left. These marked destructive changes are typical for advanced rheumatoid arthritis.

JUVENILE ARTHRITIS

Clinical Aspects

Gail D. Cawkwell

The most common form of chronic childhood arthritis is juvenile rheumatoid arthritis (JRA).[50] JRA is considered by many to be a misnomer, because only about 8% of children with JRA are rheumatoid factor-positive; they make up a subset of JRA that is similar in many ways to adult rheumatoid arthritis.[51] The remaining children have an illness that differs very much from adult rheumatoid arthritis in presentation, complaints, complications, radiographic findings, and outcome. To make a diagnosis of JRA, a child must be less than 16, have arthritis in at least one joint for at least 6 weeks, and other causes of arthritis must be eliminated.[52] Laboratory and radiographic evaluation may be suggestive of JRA but are not part of the diagnostic criteria. Radiographs and laboratory tests are helpful at presentation for eliminating other causes of arthritis. In Europe, JRA is called juvenile chronic arthritis (JCA), and the term juvenile rheumatoid arthritis is reserved for the rheumatoid factor-positive subpopulation. In addition, the definition of JCA differs from JRA in that the duration of arthritis must be at least 3 months in Europe, compared to 6 weeks in North America.[52,53] Juvenile ankylosing spondylitis (AS) and juvenile psoriatic arthritis are included in JCA, but are excluded from the case definition of JRA. These differences in case definition in Europe and North America make the study of these diseases more complex. The prognosis in JRA overall is better than in rheumatoid arthritis. However, certain subtypes of JRA have a poor prognosis, and the remission rate is not as high as was previously thought, ranging from 8.7% for rheumatoid factor-positive polyarticular onset to 45% for systemic onset in a recent study.[54]

The incidence of JRA is about 14/100,000 per year, and the prevalence is 113/100,000.[50] JRA can be divided into three onset types by signs and symptoms present in the first 6 months of illness: pauciarticular, polyarticular, and systemic.[52] Further delineation of disease type is made by defining JRA in terms of disease course after the first 6 months, serologic markers (e.g., antinuclear antibodies and rheumatoid factors) and genetic markers.

Pauciarticular JRA mainly affects preschool-aged girls. By definition, pauciarticular JRA affects fewer than five joints at 6 months after onset. Articular symptoms are generally mild; however, approximately 20% of patients with pauciarticular JRA may develop iridocyclitis, a subacute, chronic anterior eye inflammatory disease that can have serious visual sequelae.[55–57] Although rheumatoid factor is rarely positive, the antinuclear antibody is often positive at a low or moderate titer and is indicative of increased risk of iridocyclitis. Typically a child with pauciarticular JRA presents insidiously with joint swelling and a morning limp. Joint pain and systemic signs such as poor growth, fatigue, and anorexia are often mild or absent. Systemic inflammatory markers such as C-reactive protein and erythrocyte sedimentation rate are often normal. Almost 40% of all children with pauciarticular JRA achieve prolonged or permanent remission.[54] About 30% of cases transition to polyarticular disease.[55] The most common bone and joint sequelae of pauciarticular JRA are growth abnormalities, including bony enlargement and leg length discrepancies. Erosive disease is not common.

Polyarticular JRA is most common in school-aged and teenaged girls and can be severe and lifelong. Polyarticular JRA affects more than five joints at 6 months after the onset and may be divided into rheumatoid factor-positive and rheumatoid factor-negative subgroups.[52] Children with polyarticular JRA may have more articular complaints, including pain and stiffness with inactivity, and commonly have mild systemic manifestations including fatigue, anorexia, poor growth, and mild pubertal delay. Anemia of chronic disease and markers of systemic inflammation may be present. Children with polyarticular JRA who are rheumatoid factor-positive are more likely to have symmetric disease affecting small joints of the hands with erosive changes, and are more likely to have rheumatoid nodules and other systemic manifestations such as pulmonary vasculitis.

Systemic JRA has no predilection for age or gender and is characterized by high spiking fevers once or twice daily and a salmon-colored evanescent rash.[58,59] The arthritis of systemic JRA can be similar to pauciarticular or polyarticular JRA. A subset of children with systemic onset JRA, typically those who start in the preschool age group, has very aggressive, erosive arthritis that is poorly responsive to most conventional therapy presently available. Additional manifestations of systemic-onset JRA include leukocytosis, often with a leukemoid-type reaction, thrombocytosis, significant anemia, serositis, interstitial lung disease, and hemophagocytic syndrome. Antinuclear antibodies and rheumatoid factor are rarely positive, and iridocyclitis rarely occurs.

The most common childhood arthritides are acute and short-lived. Postinfectious reactive arthritis is a self-limited form of arthritis that usually lasts less than 6 weeks. Reactive arthritis is typically painful and migratory, and is not accompanied by bony changes on radiographs. Bone and joint infections can present with arthritis, as can other infections such as Lyme disease and parvovirus B19. Malignancies, especially leukemia, lymphoma, disseminated neuroblastoma, and primary bone, synovial, and cartilage tumors can present with arthritis. In addition, systemic diseases such as cystic fibrosis can be accompanied by arthritis. Chronic rheumatic diseases of childhood can present with arthritis or be accompanied by arthritis, including systemic lupus erythematosus, juvenile dermatomyositis, scleroderma, vasculitis, and the spondyloarthropathies.

Growth Abnormalities. Children with JRA have local overgrowth of involved joints. This can be a significant problem in young children with pauciarticular JRA of one knee because they are in a period of rapid growth and their disease is often mild and may go undetected for a prolonged period of time. A significant leg length discrepancy may develop in children with unilateral knee arthritis because about 70% of leg growth comes from the growth plates around the knee.[60] In contrast, arm growth is more evenly divided among upper extremity growth plates; thus, less significant discrepancies are noted with pauciarticular involvement of an upper extremity joint. Rapid growth of an involved leg may also hinder contracture resolution as arthritis improves; thus, the child may maintain abnormal gait mechanics unless the leg length discrepancy is corrected. Ultimately, if arthritis is very aggressive, a growth plate may close early or be destroyed, resulting in a permanently shortened extremity.

In one of the earliest published descriptions of JRA, George Frederick Still noted that JRA patients are small and thin.[61] The mechanism underlying the poor growth is not understood. Pulsatile and stimulated growth hormone secretion are normal in most children with JRA, even those with short stature.[61,62] Insulinlike growth factor (IGF)-1 tends to be lower than expected in children with JRA; however, it is uncertain whether or not low IGF-1 correlates with short stature.[62,63] Nutritional status does not seem to account for poor growth in JRA, as it does in Crohn's disease (another inflammatory disease), and levels of IGF-1 do not correlate with nutritional status. Treatment with glucocorticosteroids clearly contributes to short stature; however, children who have not been treated with glucocorticosteroids may also have short stature.[63–65]

Radiographs. Radiographs are mainly helpful at the onset of arthritis in children to assess for causes other than chronic rheumatic diseases, such as tumor and infection. Except for effusions, few changes are seen early in JRA on plain radiographs. After several months of arthritis, however, periarticular osteopenia and accelerated bony maturation may be noted. These may be difficult to detect on a unilateral film. Thus, it is best to assess bilaterally so that a developmentally appropriate comparison can be made. In cases where the presence of effusions or synovitis is unclear by physical examination, such as an irritable hip, ultrasound can be very helpful. Three phase Technetium-99 bone scans can be useful for determining the presence of active arthritis, as well as assessing for other causes of arthritis, such as malignancy, infection, and trauma.

In patients where range of motion is lost, deformities are noted, or a significant change in a medical regimen is considered, follow-up radiographs may be helpful in assessing disease progression. As accelerated maturation increases, other osseous changes may be noted, including squaring off of carpals and tarsals, osseous crowding, and changes in bone morphology. Erosive changes are seen very late on plain radiographs because children have a much thicker cartilage layer than adults, and magnetic resonance imaging may be helpful in assessing for early erosive changes or other abnormalities. Late in aggressive disease, erosive changes can be seen on plain radiographs along with growth plate destruction. These late findings are seen in the minority of patients with JRA.

Local and generalized decreased bone mineralization is seen in all types of JRA.[66,70] Osteocalcin, a marker of bone turnover, has been found to be decreased in several studies of JRA patients.[68,71,73] This suggests that decreased bone turnover may be related to decreased bone mineralization in JRA patients. However, the cause of the decreased rate of bone turnover is not well understood. Medications, dietary deficiencies, abnormal calcium metabolism, poor growth, inflammatory mediators, and decreased exercise have all been implicated in the pathogenesis of decreased bone mineral density in JRA.

Radiologic Aspects

George B. Greenfield

Juvenile rheumatoid arthritis refers to rheumatoid disease with an onset before the age of 16 years. Girls are affected more often than boys. There are three types of presentations: pauciarticular arthritis with fewer than five joints involved 6 months after onset; polyarthritis with more than five joints involved; and systemic involvement. Most patients are seronegative for rheumatoid factor.

About 20% of patients have systemic symptoms of high-spiking fevers, polyarthralgia, hepatosplenomegaly, lymphadenopathy, rash, pleuropericarditis, and possibly myocarditis. This condition is known as *Systimic JRA*; it has also been reported as a rare occurrence in adults.[74,75]

JRA has findings that differ from those of adult onset disease.[76] The distribution of involvement differs, with a predilection for those joints undergoing rapid growth. Monarticular disease is more common in children than in adults. Periosteal new bone formation and soft-tissue swelling are frequently seen. The epiphyseal ossification centers are enlarged with an increased trabecular pattern.

About 8% of patients are positive for rheumatoid factor. These seropositive patients have early erosions at the metacarpal, interphalangeal, and metatarsal joints.[77] Progressive destruction occurs in untreated cases. Some consider these cases the only true JRA.

Peripheral Skeleton. Growth stimulation may result in an increase in bone length, and early epiphyseal fusion may cause a decrease of length. Brachydactyly is common (Fig. 2.77). Metaphyseal radiolucent bands may be present.

Overconstriction of the diaphyses occurs. The articular cartilage is destroyed relatively late. Carpal and tarsal ankyloses are frequent. Ankylosis or dislocations of large joints may occur. Erosions occur later in the disease process than in adult onset RA.

The knee, ankle, and wrist are most frequently involved, followed by the hand, elbow, hip, foot, shoulder, and cervical spine.[76]

In the *hand,* all of the joints are involved. The diaphyses are overconstricted and epiphyses are enlarged and osteoporotic with an increased trabecular pattern (Fig. 2.78). Periosteal new bone formation and epiphyseal compression fractures may occur. There is a lack of erosions. Brachydactyly may ensue. The *foot* shows similar changes.

In the *wrist,* soft-tissue swelling and osteoporosis are followed by premature appearance of enlarged, irregular, or squared carpal bones, secondary to erosions and repair. The end result is usually ankylosis, most often the carpometacarpal and midcarpal joints (Fig. 2.79).

The *shoulder* may rarely show erosions of the humeral head and glenoid fossa. There may be elevation of the

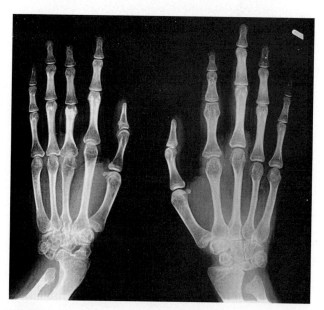

FIGURE 2.77. Juvenile rheumatoid arthritis (hands and wrists). Brachydactyly of several metacarpals and phalanges is seen, as well as shortening of both ulnas and deformities at the radiocarpal joints.

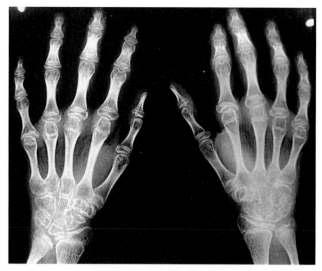

FIGURE 2.78. Juvenile rheumatoid arthritis (hands and wrists). Osteoporosis is noted in a periarticular pattern. The carpal bones and epiphyseal ossification centers are enlarged with an increased trabecular pattern. Narrowing and irregularity at the radiocarpal joints are noted. Overconstriction of several metacarpals bilaterally is seen.

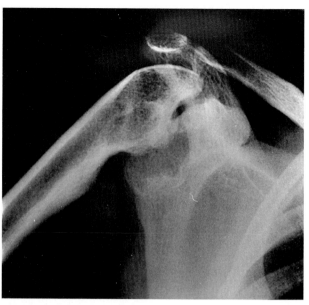

FIGURE 2.80. Juvenile rheumatoid arthritis. Shoulder. Destructive changes of the humeral head and neck, as well as of the glenoid fossa are noted. There is elevation of the humerus indicating destruction of the rotator cuff tendon.

humerus owing to rupture of the rotator cuff tendon and erosion of the undersurfaces of the distal clavicle and acromion (Figs. 2.80, 2.81, and 2.82).

The *elbow* may also be involved (Fig. 2.83), showing erosions.

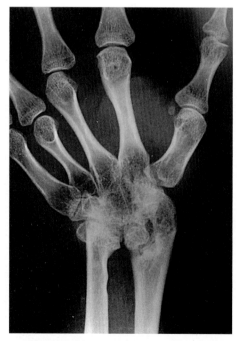

FIGURE 2.79. Juvenile rheumatoid arthritis. Wrist. Advanced changes are seen with destruction at the radiocarpal joint as well as ankylosis at the radius, carpals, and proximal metacarpals. Brachydactyly at the fourth metacarpal is also noted indicating juvenile onset.

The *hips* show early periarticular osteoporosis followed by enlargement of the femoral capital epiphysis and premature fusion of the physis. Coxa valga is present. Late changes include uniform joint space narrowing, acetabular protrusion, hip dislocation, and joint ankylosis. Erosions and irregularity of the femoral head and acetabulum (Fig. 2.84), acetabular dysplasia, and iliac hypoplasia may also occur (Fig. 2.85). Avascular necrosis of the femoral head, possibly related to steroid therapy, can sometimes be seen (Fig. 2.86). A ring of osteophytic proliferation at the junction of the femoral head and neck has been reported.[78]

The *knees* show soft-tissue swelling, periarticular osteoporosis (Fig. 2.87), enlarged epiphyses with an increased trabecular pattern, squaring of the inferior margin of the patella, diaphyseal overconstriction, erosions, and joint space narrowing.[79] The early appearance is similar to tubercular arthritis, whereas the late appearance is similar to hemophilia, with erosion of the femoral intercondylar notch (Fig. 2.88).

The *ankle* may show joint effusion (Fig. 2.89), tibiotalar slant, and narrowing of the joint space. Generalized osteoporosis is present in late stages. The tarsal bones may be deformed and irregular, and later fused.

Deformities caused by growth disturbances, subluxations, and contractures may result. Joint narrowing leads to secondary osteoarthritis. Periarticular, intraarticular, and capsular calcification have been reported following intraarticular steroid injection.[80]

Central Skeleton. The cervical region is predilected in the spine. Atlantoaxial subluxations are common (Fig. 2.90).

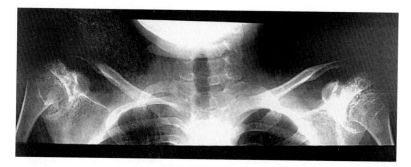

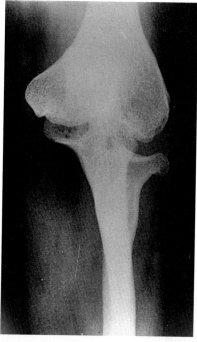

FIGURE 2.81. Juvenile rheumatoid arthritis. Shoulders. Osteoporosis is noted. There are erosions of the humeral head and glenoid fossa bilaterally, as well as erosion of the undersurface of both distal clavicles. An upward position of the humeri is noted. More marked on the right.

There is a tendency to develop apophyseal joint ankylosis (Fig. 2.91), which begins at a higher level and proceeds inferiorly. Undergrowth of vertebral bodies and intervertebral discs occur, which may be associated with block fusion. The spinous processes may be tapered. Compression fractures may occur, possibly secondary to osteoporosis aggravated by steroid therapy. Scoliosis may occur in advanced disease.[81] The changes somewhat overlap Klippel-Feil's syndrome, where block vertebrae and facet joint fusion are also seen (Fig. 2.92).

Sacroiliac joint fusion may occur.

Micrognathia is often present, with erosion of the mandibular condyle and condylar fossae.

Juvenile Spondylarthropathies

George B. Greenfield

When spondylarthropathies have an onset in patients under 16 years of age, they are prefaced with the term juvenile.[82] This group comprises juvenile AS, juvenile psoriatic arthri-

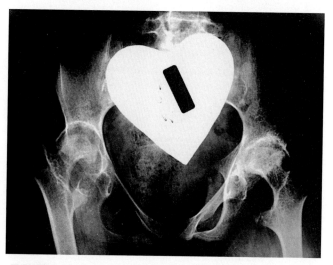

FIGURE 2.83. Juvenile rheumatoid arthritis Elbow. AP view shows resorption and irregularity at the articular surfaces.

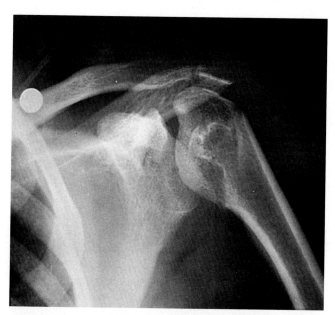

FIGURE 2.82. Juvenile rheumatoid arthritis. Shoulder. There is deformity of the humeral head resulting from erosions. There is an upward position of the humerus eroding the undersurface of the acromioclavicular joint.

FIGURE 2.84. Juvenile rheumatoid arthritis. Hips. Erosions at the acetabulum are seen causing enlargement. Erosions at the femoral necks bilaterally are also noted as well as irregularity of the femoral heads. There is joint space narrowing with secondary osteoarthritis on the left.

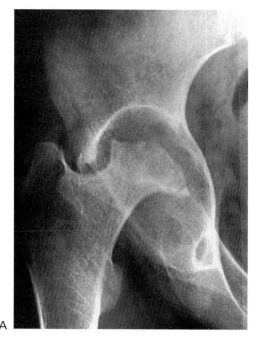

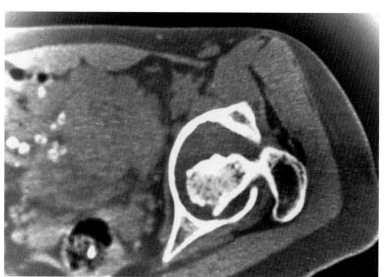

FIGURE 2.85. Juvenile rheumatoid arthritis. **A:** AP view of the left hip shows marked erosion of the acetabulum with acetabular protrusion and erosion of the femoral head. **B:** CT showing the marked erosions as seen in **(A)**.

tis, and juvenile reactive arthritis, including inflammatory bowel disease. These are seronegative with absence of rheumatoid factor and antinuclear antibodies.

Juvenile AS is predominantly seen in boys.[83] The mean age of onset is 10 to 12 years. Juvenile patients also have the presence of HLA-B27 antigen. The distribution of involvement is different than that in adults.[84] The appendicular joints are more frequently involved and may predominate

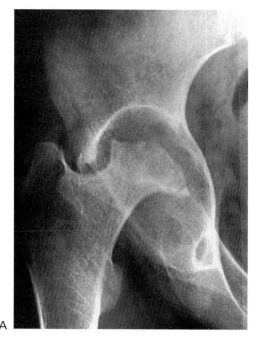

FIGURE 2.86. Juvenile rheumatoid arthritis. AP view of the pelvis reveals avascular necrosis of both femoral heads. There is narrowing of the joint spaces bilaterally. Cystic and sclerotic changes in the right acetabular roof are also seen. Fusion of the sacroiliac joints has occurred.

throughout the course of the disease. There is a tendency toward arthritis of the hip, shoulder, elbow, wrist, knee, ankle, and foot. The metatarsophalangeal joints are the most frequently involved of the small joints. Enthesitis commonly occurs.

At times it is not possible to define the exact diagnosis. The terms *juvenile chronic arthritis* and *juvenile spondyloarthropathy* are used, particularly in the European literature.

Case Reports

Gail D. Cawkwell

Case 1: Polyarticular-onset JRA. An 11-month-old white girl presented with right knee swelling that progressed over the subsequent 4 months to polyarthritis affecting both knees, the right wrist, several toes, the right ring finger, and the left thumb. Lyme serology and rheumatoid factor were negative and the antinuclear antibody was positive at a titer of 1:320 with a homogenous pattern. Lupus-related serologies were negative and the erythrocyte sedimentation rate was increased. By age 3 years she had been treated with a variety of NSAIDs, intraarticular corticosteroids, hydroxychloroquine, and low-dose oral corticosteroids with only modest success. Bilateral AP wrist radiographs were obtained at that time to assess for the presence of early aggressive disease. These radiographs showed early changes typical of JRA, including accelerated osseous maturation, local overgrowth, and periarticular osteopenia, but no erosions (Fig. 2.93). Methotrexate was initiated based on a poor clin-

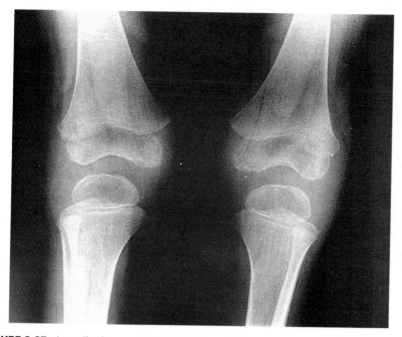

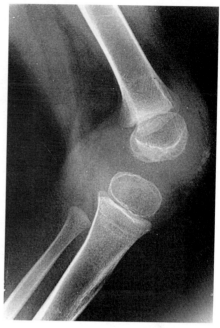

FIGURE 2.87. Juvenile rheumatoid arthritis (knees). **A:** AP view of both knees reveals soft-tissue swelling, osteoporosis, and irregularities at the articular surfaces. **B:** Lateral view shows soft-tissue swelling around the knee as well as irregularity at the distal femoral articular surface.

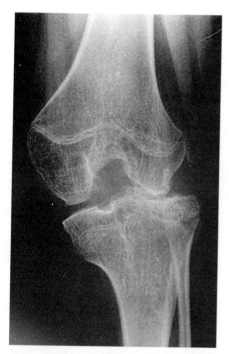

FIGURE 2.88. Juvenile rheumatoid arthritis. Knee. Enlargement of the distal femoral epiphyseal ossification center is seen with erosion of the intercondylar notch, as well as erosion along the articular surface of the tibia. Considerable osteoporosis is also noted.

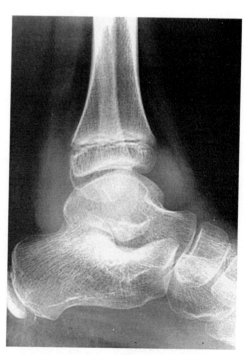

FIGURE 2.89. Juvenile rheumatoid arthritis. Ankle. A large effusion is seen both anterior and posterior to the tibiotalar joint.

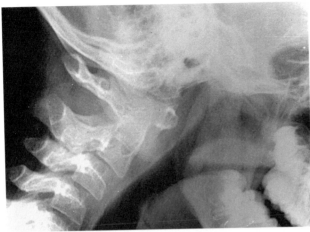
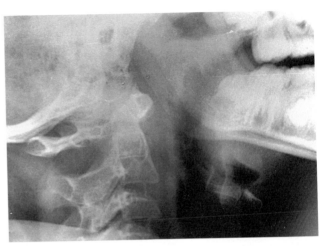

A   B

FIGURE 2.90. Juvenile rheumatoid arthritis. Cervical spine. **A:** Flexion. There is anterior displacement of C-1 on the odontoid process. **B:** Extension view showing return to normal C1-2 relationship, indicating instability.

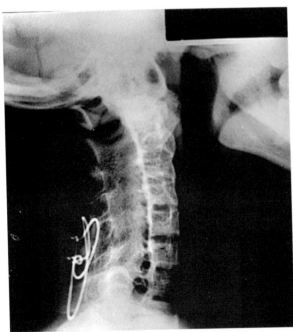

FIGURE 2.91. Juvenile rheumatoid arthritis. Cervical spine. There is fusion of the apophyseal facet joints between C-2 and C-7. There is enlargement of the anterior ring of C-1. Fusion across the intervertebral discs in the upper cervical spine is also seen as well as erosion at the anterior aspects of the vertebral bodies. A laminectomy has been performed.

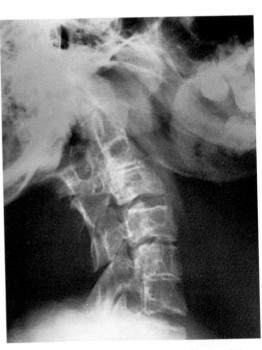

FIGURE 2.92. Klippel-Feil syndrome. Lateral view of the cervical spine shows block vertebra in both upper and lower cervical spine as well as upper facet joint fusions.

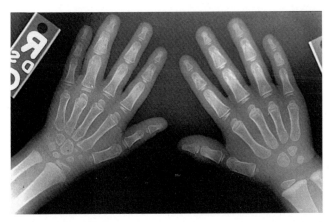

FIGURE 2.93. Bilateral AP wrist radiographs in a 3-year-old girl with a 2-year history of polyarticular JRA affecting the right wrist. Early radiographic changes typical of JRA are noted, including accelerated osseous maturation, local overgrowth, and local osteopenia, but no evidence of erosive disease.

ical course, despite lack of erosive disease. The patient had a minimal response to methotrexate and it was discontinued. Multiple intraarticular corticosteroid injections were performed under anesthesia with good symptomatic relief for several months. By age 4 years, she developed significant anterior uveitis, necessitating systemic therapy. Methotrexate was reinstituted at a higher dose in a subcutaneous fashion and systemic corticosteroids were used. Unfortunately, with steroid tapering, both the uveitis and arthritis worsened. A new experimental therapy was considered just prior to the patient starting kindergarten, and radiographs were obtained to assist in the decision to embark on this new, experimental therapy (Fig. 2.94). Again wrist radiographs showed accelerated bony maturation with squaring off of the carpals and crowding but without erosive disease. Despite the absence of erosive disease, the bony changes, along with the clinical arthritis and uveitis, were of sufficient concern to support initiation of experimental therapy.

Case 2: Severe Systemic-onset, Systemic-course JRA. A 21-month-old Middle Eastern boy presented with high spiking fevers, rash, arthritis, hemoglobin of 7 g/dL, white blood count (WBC) of 50,000/HPF, platelet count of 1.6 million, and a normal bone marrow aspirate and biopsy. A diagnosis of systemic onset JRA was made. Despite progressively more aggressive therapy, the patient failed to show more than a trivial clinical response to treatments, including a variety of NSAIDs, intravenous immunoglobulin, and methotrexate. Brief clinical responses to intravenous and oral corticosteroids were noted; however, toxicity of these therapies limited their utility. At age 7 years, a clinical deterioration with marked decrease in functional abilities prompted referral to a tertiary care center for evaluation for a more aggressive physical program or a more aggressive medical regimen. Radiographs were obtained at that time and compared with

previous radiographs. Based on the presence of marked erosive disease, a more aggressive medical regimen was initiated with higher-dose parenteral methotrexate, cyclosporin A, hydroxychloroquine, and intraarticular and oral corticosteroids. Despite some initial improvement, with corticosteroid tapering, the patient again deteriorated over the subsequent 3 years, and at age 10 hip MRI and plain radiographs were obtained in order to consider hip arthroplasty, other surgical therapies, or other aggressive medical regimens. Based on the radiographic findings and clinical deterioration, combined with familiar reluctance to perform arthroplasty at such a young age, intravenous cyclophosphamide therapy was initiated. Again, only a very modest clinical response ensued, and the patient was started on an experimental medical regimen at age 10. The new therapy resulted in improvement in constitutional symptoms and arthritis, and decreased gastrointestinal toxicity, but continued elevated acute phase reactants and a continued marked limitation of functional abilities because of hip pain. At age 11 hip radiographs were obtained and the hip was arthroscoped to differentiate secondary osteoarthritic changes from active inflammatory arthritis. Extensive proliferative synovitis was noted on arthroscopy as well as multiple bone fragments, a complete loss of femoral articular cartilage, and a marked degradation of pelvic articular cartilage. An arthroscopic synovectomy was performed with improvement in pain and functional abilities.

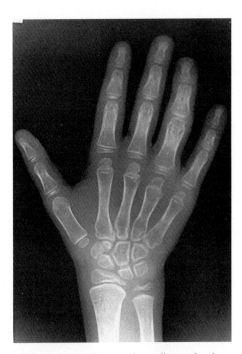

FIGURE 2.94. Two years later, wrist radiographs show progressive changes of JRA, including accelerated boney maturation, crowding, and squaring off of the carpals, but no erosive disease.

ANKYLOSING SPONDYLITIS

Clinical Aspects

Frank B. Vasey

AS is the most predictable of the spondyloarthropathies.[85] Persistent dull aching lumbar pain and stiffness begins typically in young men. Initially it may be difficult to separate lumbar strain from inflammatory backache. Hallmarks of ankylosing spondylitis include morning stiffness lasting 1 hour or longer and persisting for over 3 months. Typically, in peripheral previous radiographs, joints are not affected initially. Eventually hips, shoulders, and knees are involved in the majority of patients. Rarely patients may seem to have a combination of rheumatoid arthritis and ankylosing spondylitis. This condition occurs in women, but less often and with less tendency to spinal fusion. Involvement of the ribs (costovertebral joints) may be painful as well as lead to restriction of thoracic excursion and restrictive lung disease by pulmonary function testing.

Extraarticular manifestations most commonly include iritis, which affects about 20% of patients. Rarely aortitis can lead to aortic insufficiency with heart block. Upper lobe pulmonary fibrosis can simulate tuberculosis, and the cauda equina syndrome can lead to perirectal numbness and incontinence.

Laboratory testing is nonspecific with mild elevation of the erythrocyte sedimentation rate, the anemia of chronic disease in severe cases, and elevated serum IgA levels in some patients.[86] B27 testing is not usually clinically performed.[87]

Some investigators believe *Klebsiella* in the colon is the immune activating event in ankylosing spondylitis. Patchy inflammation in the colon has been seen by colonoscopy in AS patients even in the absence of bowel symptoms.[88] Elevated serum IgA levels further support the possibility of immune activation occurring in the bowel.

Radiographs of the pelvis and sacroiliac joints are central to making an early diagnosis. A Ferguson view (x-ray beam lowered to aim up along the sacroiliac joints) is a useful screening test in an individual with persistent back pain. Oblique x-ray views, CT scans, and MRIs can all contribute to making the diagnosis in equivocal cases.

X-ray findings in early disease may be limited to irregularity and sclerosis of the sacroiliac joints in typically symmetrical fashion.[89] Asymmetric involvement should raise the question of another form of spondyloarthritis, particularly psoriatic or Reiter's syndrome. Spinal involvement begins as inflammation in the annulus fibrosus. Rarely, this process may progress to such severity as to lead to erosions of the vertebral margins. This is known as spondylodiskitis and may mimic osteomyelitis. Spinal fusion occurs by calcification of the annulus fibrosus. This leads to the typical marginal syndesmophytes, and the end point is a "bamboo spine." Clinically it should be noted that the spine is brittle and subject to fracture. Onset of pain in a previously fused area of the spine should raise the question of a fracture. Careful plain radiographic evaluation will usually show the fracture. Onset of persistent headache in a patient with established cervical spine disease should suggest the possibility of atlantoaxial subluxation. A special order of a lateral flexion view (not usually included in routine cervical spine films) may reveal the C1-2 subluxation. Surgical fusion is recommended at times if paralysis is imminent.

Radiologic Aspects

George B. Greenfield

AS is a chronic, progressive spondylarthropathy characterized by involvement of the sacroiliac joints, the spinal apophyseal joints, the annulus fibrosus, and the deep layers of the anterior longitudinal ligament.[90–92] The hallmark is ankylosis of joints.

Approximately 90% of patients are men. The peak onset is between 25 and 35 years of age. Almost all patients have positive HLA-B27 antigen.

The sacroiliac joints are almost always affected early in the disease, typically bilaterally and symmetrically, but the earliest changes may be unilateral.

The histologic features of the proliferative chronic synovitis involving the diarthrodial joints are indistinguishable from those seen in rheumatoid arthritis. There is a tendency toward capsular fibrosis and relatively rapid bony ankylosis. Amyloidosis has been reported at autopsy in a small percentage of patients.

The lower two-thirds of the sacroiliac joints and the spine are the principal sites of involvement. Other areas include the hips, shoulders, knees, ankles, costovertebral joints, manubriosternal joint, symphysis pubis, rarely the temporomandibular joints,[93] and the os calcis. Involvement of the small joints of the hands and feet is unusual.

Peripheral Skeleton. *Radiologically,* the *hands and feet* are not often involved. In comparison with RA, there is less osteoporosis, fewer erosions, no subluxations, asymmetrical involvement, periostitis, and ankylosis. Bony ankylosis predominates rather than erosions; however, plain film findings similar to those of RA may be seen in a significant number of patients.[94] Arthritis mutilans does not occur.

When the large joints, particularly the hips, shoulders, and knees, are involved differences from rheumatoid arthritis are shown. There is less osteoporosis and erosions and more reactive sclerosis.

The *shoulder* is involved in about one-third of patients. Erosions may occur, starting out small (Fig. 2.95), rarely progressing to the "hatchet-shaped" humeral head seen in RA. There may be progression to ankylosis of the glenohumeral joint with or without erosions. Ossification of the coracoclavicular ligament also can be seen.[95]

Bony ankylosis at the *acromioclavicular joints* may also occur.

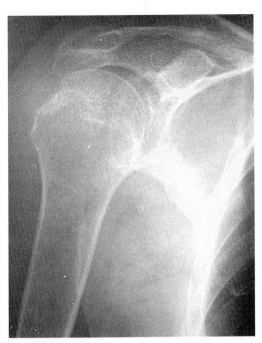

FIGURE 2.95. Ankylosing spondylitis. Shoulder. Erosion at the greater tuberosity is seen with reactive sclerosis.

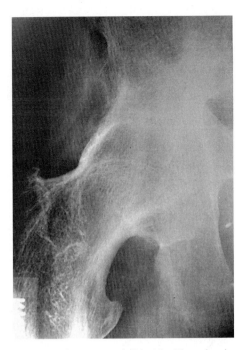

FIGURE 2.97. Ankylosing spondylitis. Hip. There has been ankylosis of the hip joint. No bony spurs are evident about the femoral head.

The *hip* is involved in about one-half of patients, usually bilaterally but sometimes unilaterally. There may be early loss of joint space as seen in RA. Shallow erosions are more common than large cysts and gross irregularity of the femoral head. A bony spur at the superior aspect of the junction between the femoral head and neck is sometimes seen. A ring of proliferative osteophytes at this junction is common (Fig. 2.96). Ankylosis then occurs, followed by osteoporosis and resorption of the osteophytes (Fig. 2.97).

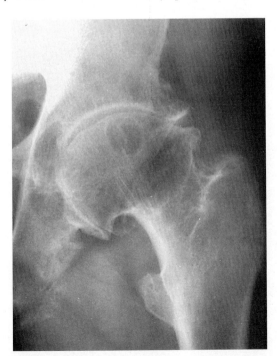

FIGURE 2.96. Ankylosing spondylitis. Hip. There is uniform narrowing of the hip joint space with flattening of the femoral head, as well as osteophytes at the junction of the femoral head and neck.

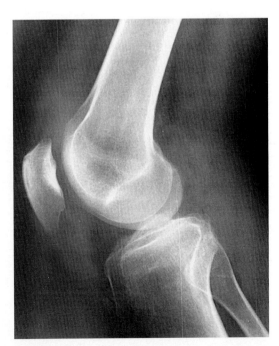

FIGURE 2.98. Ankylosing spondylitis. Lateral view of the knee shows knee joint effusion. There is fullness in the suprapatellar pouch, as well as widening of the patellofemoral joint.

The *knee,* which is involved in about one-third of cases, often shows only transient synovitis (Fig. 2.98). Erosions and sclerosis are not prominent. The end stage is bony ankylosis.

The *os calcis* may show erosions and reactive sclerosis above the site of attachments of the Achilles tendon, as in rheumatoid arthritis and Reiter's disease.

Progressive *ossification* of extraspinal joint capsules and ligaments is common. The sternomanubrial joint, costovertebral articulations leading to limited chest expansion, iliac crest, greater trochanter, knee, and coracoclavicular ligaments may be involved.[95]

Central Skeleton. In the *spine,* AS usually begins in the lumbar region and progresses superiorly. The thoracolumbar and lumbosacral regions are commonly involved. The cervical spine is involved last. The spine is prone to fracture, which may be caused by minor falls. The most common sites are C-5 to T-1, followed by T-10 to L-2.[96]

Osteitis of the vertebral bodies occurs with early sclerosis at their anterior corners (Fig. 2.99). Later resorption of the vertebral margins causes a loss of the normal anterior concavity, resulting in a square appearance of the bodies (Figs. 2.100 and 2.101), particularly in the lumbar spine. The corner sclerosis disappears. Both or only the superior margins may be affected.

The formation of thin vertical bony bridges between adjacent vertebral bodies, or *syndesmophytes,* is characteristic. They represent ossifications of the outer lamellae of the anulus fibrosus (Fig. 2.102) and the immediately adjacent anterior longitudinal ligament, which later blend with the pe-

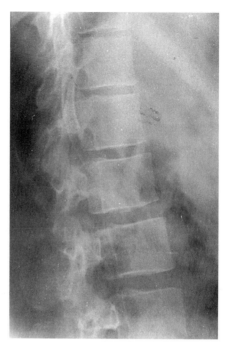

FIGURE 2.100. Ankylosing spondylitis. Lumbar spine. There is "squaring" of the anterior aspects of the vertebral bodies.

riosteum. They are seen anteriorly and laterally (Fig. 2.103), and can be seen on CT (Fig. 2.104). They can be differentiated from osteophytes by their vertical rather than horizontal origin. They can be differentiated from diffuse idiopathic skeletal hyperostosis (DISH) by their lack of a radiolucent line between the calcified ligament and the an-

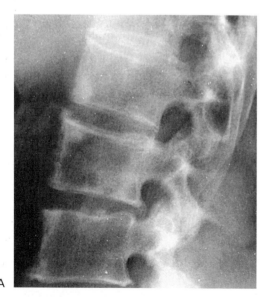
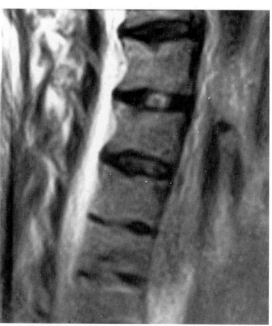

FIGURE 2.99. Ankylosing spondylitis. Spine. **A:** Lateral view of the spine shows sclerosis at the corners of the vertebral bodies. A syndesmophyte is seen at T11-12. "Squaring" of the anterior vertebral bodies is also noted. **B:** MRI T-2 weighted image. Squaring of the anterior vertebral bodies, low signal intensity at the corners in the lower aspects of L-1 and L-2 are seen as well as calcifications of the annulus fibrosus.

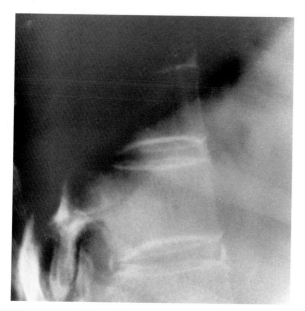

FIGURE 2.101. Ankylosing spondylitis. Lateral view of the spine shows calcification of the annulus fibrosus as well as "squaring" of the vertebral bodies.

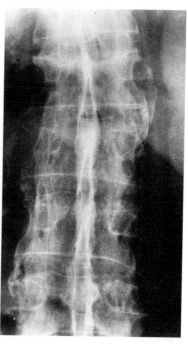

FIGURE 2.102. Ankylosing spondylitis. AP view of the lumbar spine. Syndesmophytes bridging the bony margins of several lumbar vertebral bodies are seen as well as ossification of the posterior spinal ligament. These are thin, marginal syndesmophytes.

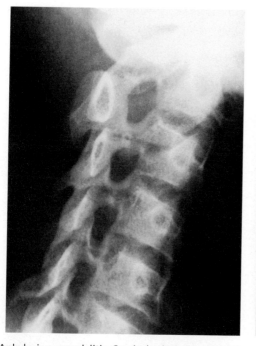

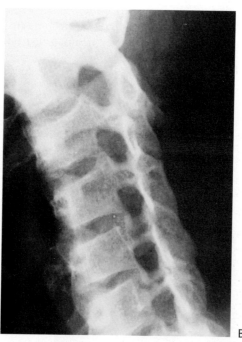

A

B

FIGURE 2.103. Ankylosing spondylitis. Cervical spine. **A:** Left oblique view shows syndesmophytes at the C4-5 level which are projected over the intervertebral foramen. **B:** Right oblique view showing projection of syndesmophytes anteriorly and posteriorly at C4-5 and C5-6.

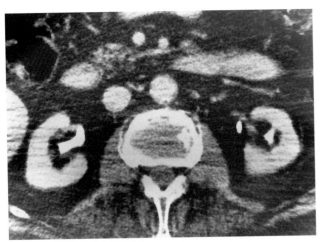

FIGURE 2.104. Ankylosing spondylitis. CT shows a thin line of a syndesmophyte at the lateral and anterior aspects of the vertebral body.

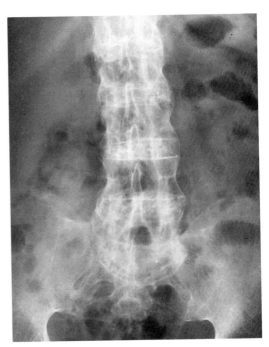

FIGURE 2.106. Ankylosing spondylitis. Lumbar spine. A "bamboo spine" is seen along with calcifications of the intervertebral discs.

terior margin of the vertebral body. Secondary degenerative spondylosis may result in osteophyte formation, particularly at levels between fused segments, where motion is possible. The end result is a "bamboo spine" with universal ligamentous ossification (Figs. 2.105, 2.106, and 2.107).

Other changes consist of arthritis of the apophyseal joints, generalized ligamentous ossification, disc degeneration, erosions, kyphosis (which may be marked), subluxations, ankylosis, pathological fractures, and vertebral destructive lesions.

The posterior facet joints of the thoracolumbar spine are involved with an inflammatory synovitis, resulting first in

haziness, then erosions, and subchondral sclerosis. This process proceeds to ankylosis, which may be general (Figs. 2.108 and 2.109). The cervical spine is involved later in the disease. Osteoporosis progresses after ankylosis has taken place.

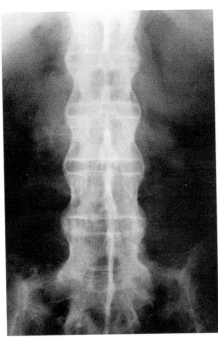

FIGURE 2.105. Ankylosing spondylitis. A "bamboo spine" is noted.

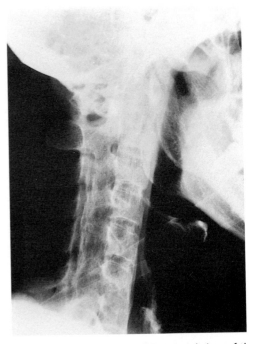

FIGURE 2.107. Ankylosing spondylitis. Lateral view of the cervical spine shows fusion of the posterior elements, "squaring" of the vertebral bodies, and general syndesmophyte formation.

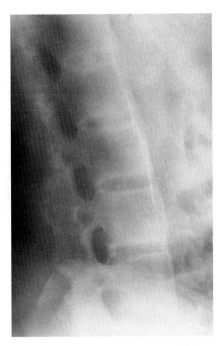

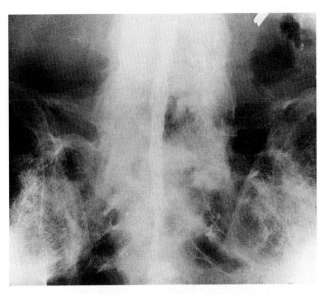

FIGURE 2.110. Ankylosing spondylitis. AP view of the lumbosacral region. A solid midline stripe is seen representing ossification of the posterior interspinous ligament. There is obliteration of both sacroiliac joints and calcification of ligaments in their superior portion.

FIGURE 2.108. Ankylosing spondylitis. Lateral view of lumbar spine. There is mass fusion of the posterior facet joints. General syndesmophytosis is seen as well as narrowing of the intervertebral space between T-12 and L-1. Calcification in the intervertebral spaces in the upper lumbar spine is also noted.

The posterior interspinous ligament ossification fuses the spinous processes and is seen on frontal projections as a solid midline linear vertical density (Fig. 2.110). Costovertebral ankylosis may also occur. The thoracic spine is involved (Fig. 2.111), often with marked kyphosis.

Superficial erosions of the vertebral end plates, and erosions of the spinous processes leading to tapering may occur. Bone resorption at the anterior surface of the cervical spine causing narrowing of the vertebral bodies may be seen in late stages (Fig. 2.112).

Intervertebral disc space narrowing accompanies posterior facet joint ankylosis. Rarely subluxation at the atlantoaxial joint may occur.

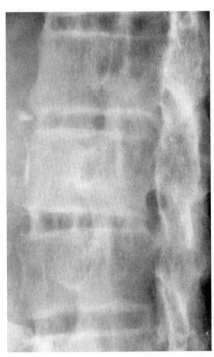

FIGURE 2.109. Ankylosing spondylitis. Lumbar spine. There is fusion of the posterior elements as well as calcifications in the annulus fibrosus.

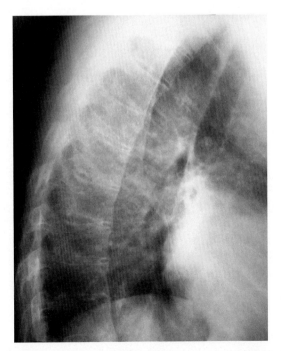

FIGURE 2.111. Ankylosing spondylitis. Thoracic spine. Kyphosis, "squaring" of the anterior vertebral bodies and syndesmophytes are seen. Calcifications in several intervertebral discs are also present.

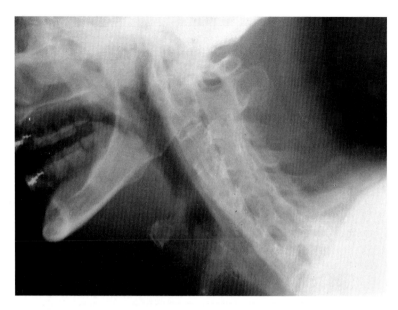

FIGURE 2.112. Ankylosing spondylitis. Cervical spine. There has been resorption of the anterior aspects of the vertebral bodies causing narrowing. Fusion of the posterior elements is also seen.

The rigid osteoporotic spine is prone to fractures (Figs. 2.113 and 2.114). The cervical spine readily fractures following minor trauma. These are predominantly at the lower cervical levels and are of the "chalk stick" type, with the fracture line passing horizontally through the spine, commonly through the intervertebral disc.[96,97]

Spinal cord compression may occur from disc herniation, encroachment of fracture fragments, or epidural hematoma. Fusion of the spine may occur in the displaced position. The thoracolumbar region is also a common site of fracture.

Destructive lesions in the vertebral bodies also may occur.[98,99] If there is an unfused segment between two larger ankylosed elements, destructive changes involving an intervertebral disc and contiguous portions of vertebral bodies result from spinal motion at this site.[101] Similar findings result from fracture of the fused posterior elements, which results in pseudarthrosis.[102] Multiple sites may be involved.[103] CT is more accurate than conventional tomograms in demonstrating this condition. It can define irregular discovertebral osteolysis, reactive sclerosis, vacuum sign,

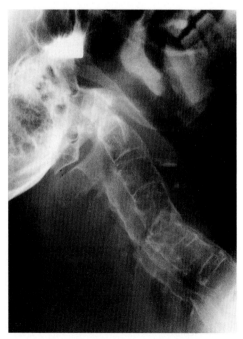

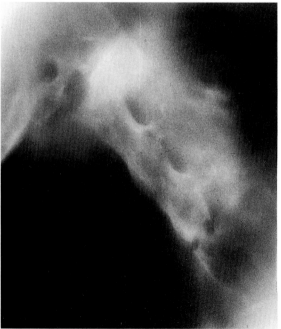

A

B

FIGURE 2.113. Ankylosing spondylitis. Cervical spine with fracture. **A:** Lateral view shows a fracture with acute angulation of the cervical spine at the C4-5 level. Marked osteoporosis and a "bamboo spine" are evident. **B:** Linear tomogram shows a fracture between the fused blocks of posterior elements.

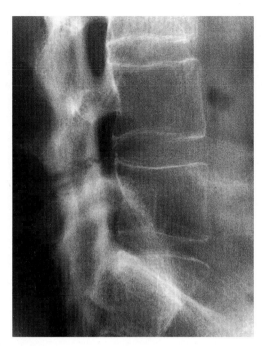

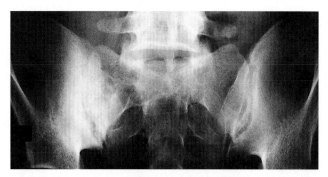

FIGURE 2.116. Ankylosing spondylitis. Sacroiliac joints. The right sacroiliac joint is involved with advanced changes. The left sacroiliac joint appears normal.

FIGURE 2.114. Ankylosing spondylitis. Lateral view of the lumbar spine. There has been fusion of all of the posterior facet joints. A fracture line is seen through the fused block at the L4-5 level. Osteopenia and "squaring" of the vertebral bodies is also noted.

paraspinal involvement, and a fracture or mobile facet joints.[104] Radioscintigraphy is useful in detecting spinal pseudarthrosis in chronic AS with late onset of back pain.[93]

In the *sacroiliac* (SI) joints, the process is bilateral, most often symmetrical, and changes often are present at the time the earliest lesions are seen in the spine. Earliest changes may be unilateral (Fig. 2.115). More advanced changes may remain unilateral (Fig. 2.116). The initial finding is loss of definition of the joint margins (Fig. 2.117). Erosions and marginal irregularity then occur (Figs. 2.118 and 2.119).

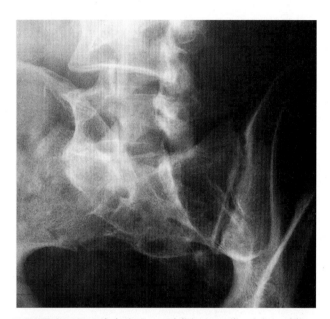

FIGURE 2.117. Ankylosing spondylitis. Sacroiliac joint. Oblique view. There is loss of the white cortical line on the iliac side of the sacroiliac joint with slight marginal irregularity.

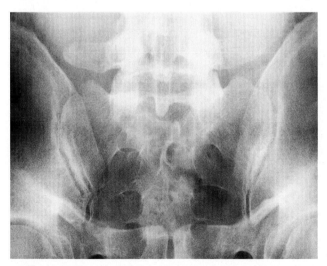

FIGURE 2.115. Ankylosing spondylitis. Sacroiliac joints. Early change. There is serration at the iliac side of the right sacroiliac joint.

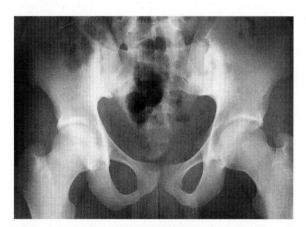

FIGURE 2.118. Ankylosing spondylitis. Sacroiliac joints. Bilateral sacroiliac sclerosis on both sides of the joint with resorption is noted.

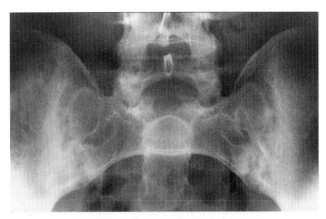

FIGURE 2.119. Ankylosing spondylitis. Sacroiliac joints. Bilateral sacroiliac joint involvement is seen with a picture of predominantly erosions bilaterally as well as sclerosis.

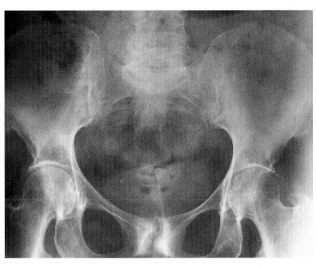

FIGURE 2.120. Ankylosing spondylitis. Pelvis. Involvement of the symphysis pubis is seen with irregularity and reactive sclerosis. Bilateral sacroiliitis is also noted.

The iliac side is affected before the sacral margins. Early involvement may be unilateral. CT and MRI can demonstrate findings earlier than conventional radiographs. Cartilage abnormalities, adjacent marrow edema, erosions, and effusion can be well demonstrated.[105] The joint spaces become narrowed and reactive sclerosis may be present on both sides of the SI joint. Some patients progress to fibrous and bony ankylosis, with regression of the reactive sclerosis if it was present. Ossification of the ligamentous upper one-third may follow. A thin sclerotic line may be the only residual of the SI joint, or complete disappearance may occur. Osteoporosis follows.

Ossification of the amphiarthrodial upper one-third of the sacroiliac joint without involvement of the synovial lower two-thirds is a manifestation of DISH.

The radionuclide bone scan may show increased uptake in early sacroiliitis, but this is difficult to appreciate because normally there is increased activity in this region. The sacroiliac joints may show normal or decreased activity at the time ankylosis is seen on radiographs. The last represents an inactive stage of the disease.

MRI can show early changes.

Osteitis pubis, which is common in women, may be seen. The symphysis pubis shows erosions, reactive sclerosis, and later ankylosis (Fig. 2.120).

Enthesitis is seen as irregular new bone proliferation, giving a "whiskering" effect at the sites of muscle and tendon attachments, sometimes associated with reactive sclerosis. This often occurs at the ischial tuberosities, iliac margins, and calcaneus.

Juxtaarticular masses of inflammatory tissue that are minimally painful have been reported as an uncommon occurrence.[106]

AS associated with primary hyperparathyroidism has been reported.[107,108]

Atrophy of the psoas and the posterior spinal muscles, demonstrated by CT, has been reported in AS, in which the normal muscle was replaced by fat.[109] Intersternal costoclavicular ossification has also been reported.[11]

Case Report

Frank B. Vasey

A 43-year-old white man had developed back pain and stiffness at age 28. Initially, the lumbar pain and stiffness was mild and ignored by the patient. The process gradually ascended his spine including his neck. The diagnosis was made 2 years after inception based on lumbar spine films, which showed sacroiliac fusion. A B27 test was positive. His illness rapidly progressed to cervical spine fusion a year later. His neck was so flexed that a resection extension osteotomy was performed in 1994 with a good result, allowing him to see straight ahead.

His medications included sulindac, oxycodone, methotrexate, and folic acid. In January 1998, he stooped forward to pick up a light box and had an immediate mild pain, but 4 hours later his back began to hurt. Several radiographs showed a fracture. The fracture took 1 year to heal but did not require surgery.

REACTIVE ARTHRITIS

Frank B. Vasey

Reactive arthritis includes several distinct entities that share some features with each other. They involve both the spine and other joints; hence, they are referred to as spondylarthropathies or spondylarthritis. They are considered to be a reaction to various agents. This category includes psoriatic arthritis, Reiter's disease, enteropathic arthritis, acne arthritis, and several miscellaneous conditions. These are discussed in this section.

The forms of inflammatory peripheral arthritis that have the potential to fuse the entire spine from the pelvis, including the sacroiliac joints to the cervical spine, are the focus of this section. Rheumatoid arthritis (RA) affects the cervical spine but not, oddly, the lumbar or thoracic spine. Osteoarthritis (OA) affects the lumbar and cervical spine. Neither of these common forms of arthritis actually leads to spinal fusion in the fashion of spondyloarthritis. DISH syndrome fuses the spine by calcifying the anterior spinal ligament but does not cause inflammatory peripheral arthritis.

The term spondyloarthropathy refers to conditions including ankylosing spondylitis (AS), psoriatic arthritis (PsA), Reiter's syndrome (reactive arthritis) (RS), and the arthritis of inflammatory bowel disease (AIBD).

Unusual arthropathies that share features in common with the spondyloarthropathies include Behçet's syndrome (oral and genital ulcers and arthritis), acne arthritis, the arthritis of hydradenitis suppurativa, and a syndrome encompassing synovitis, acne, pustulosis, hyperostosis, and osteitis (SAPHO). All of these forms of arthritis share common extraarticular features, such as eye inflammation (iritis in AS, conjunctivitis in Reiter's syndrome) and skin disease (psoriasis in psoriatic arthritis, and circinate balanitis and keratoderma blennorrhagicum in Reiter's syndrome). They also share a genetic predisposition. HLA-B27 remains the major histocompatibility antigen that is most closely linked to a disease. Ninety percent or more of patients with AS are also B27 positive. There is also an association between B27 and spinal disease in the other forms of spondyloarthritis; however, the association is not as strong as in AS.

Another apparent common thread is the importance of environmental factors, which include trauma and bacteria. Injured joints tend to evolve into chronically inflamed joints in a manner not seen in rheumatoid arthritis or osteoarthritis.

Suspect bacteria vary according to the syndrome and do not represent direct infection, as in septic arthritis. The bacteria seem to mysteriously activate the immune system into an attack on certain joints in an asymmetric distribution. It seems likely that macrotrauma or microtrauma overuse dictates which joints are affected.

HIV infection alters the clinical manifestation of traditional rheumatic diseases and represents a new rheumatic disease. It may mimic SLE even to the point of a positive antinuclear antibody test (ANA). The virus seems to suppress clinical RA, but interestingly exacerbates spondylarthritis. This author has observed rapid development of deforming psoriatic arthritis in patients with concurrent HIV and PsA. Similarly, Reiter's syndrome seems more severe and frequent; however, this is contested.

In younger patients, the differential diagnosis includes the muscle pain and tenderness of fibromyalgia. Observable joint swelling should not occur in fibromyalgia. Polymyalgia rheumatica (PMR) is a concern in patients older than 50 years. The sedimentation rate is usually elevated in PMR but may not be in spondylarthritis. Thyroid function (TSH hormone level) should be proven normal in all age groups.

Psoriatic Arthritis

Clinical Aspects

Frank B. Vasey

Psoriatic arthritis is a variable inflammatory arthropathy that may affect one or more joints.[111] The typical patient does not have a symmetrical polyarthritis as in rheumatoid arthritis. Psoriatic arthritis is most often an asymmetric oligoarthritis (four or fewer joints in value). Macrotrauma or microtrauma likely dictates which joints are affected. Five percent of patients may have a predominantly spinal disease similar to but not identical to ankylosing spondylitis. Most patients develop the psoriatic plaques before the arthritis. Men and women are affected approximately evenly.

The finding of the psoriatic skin disease is critical in making the appropriate diagnosis. The papulosquamous plaques may be hidden in the scalp, the gluteal cleft, or even the umbilicus. Typically they are obvious over the extension surfaces of elbows or knees. The esthesias or site of tendinous insertion into bone is an inflammatory target, as is the case in other forms of spondyloarthritis (Reiter's syndrome, reactive arthritis, and the arthritis of inflammatory bowel disease). The usual forms of tendinitis and bursitis are common in these patients.

Laboratory tests are nonspecific. The rheumatoid factor is absent. This author believes that this form of arthritis is a reactive process to group positive cocci, primarily Group A streptococci. Guttate psoriasis (droplike plaques of psoriasis) are well known to develop after streptococcal pharyngitis. We have also shown anti-DNAase B (a Group A streptococcal exotoxin) antibodies in the majority of psoriatic arthritis patients.[112] Most recently we found evidence of Group A streptococcal RNA in peripheral circulation in slightly less than one-half in a series of psoriatic arthritis patients.[113] These observations suggest that the course of the disease is as yet poorly understood chronic immune activation, which results in joint, tendon, and bursa tenderness and swelling. The process eventually causes radiographic changes.

Radiologically, a number of features are characteristic; others overlap with rheumatoid arthritis.[114] Erosions in the joints of the hands may mimic rheumatoid arthritis and occur in the bare areas (lacking cartilage) at the sides of the bone. Juxtaarticular osteoporosis, noted in RA, is typically not seen and radiologic involvement is asymmetric. Distal interphalangeal joint findings favor psoriatic arthritis or OA.[115] An uncommon but characteristic finding is terminal whittling of a phalanx, resulting in the "pencil-in-cup" deformity. Periosteal involvement, seen as fluffy periostitis, is also unusual but characteristic. The chronic inflammatory process eventuates in loss of joint space, but there is a greater propensity for the joints to ultimately fuse. Similarly, the synovium is more fibrotic than in RA, but in early stages it is more vascular.

The disease may cause unilateral or bilateral involvement of the sacroiliac joints, known as sacroiliitis.[116] Radiographically, it appears as an irregularity, widening or narrowing, with eventual bony thickening called sclerosis, evolving in some patients to fusion of the lower two-thirds of the spine. The fusion of the spine occurs in the form of bony bridges known as syndesmophytes. These typically do not arise from the margin of the vertebra as in ankylosing spondylitis, but closer to the midportion of the vertebral body. As with the peripheral joint and sacroiliac disease, the process is unpredictable and may affect one vertebra but not the next.

Radiologic Aspects

George B. Greenfield

Psoriatic arthritis represents a specific entity.[117–119] Up to 7% of patients with psoriasis may be affected, usually between the ages of 30 to 50 years.

There are three major forms of psoriatic arthritis.

First, and most common, is an asymmetrical peripheral polyarthritis with predominantly destructive changes of the distal interphalangeal joints, a relative lack of osteoporosis, and bone proliferation. Involvement of the spine and sacroiliac joints may also occur. A characteristic spondylitis also occurs in this condition.

Second, a single ray only may be involved, with soft-tissue swelling along the entire digit owing to tenosynovitis, called a "sausage digit."

Third, there is a form with a pattern similar to that of RA.

Psoriatic arthritis may precede skin lesions by a long interval. There is a relationship between nail and proximal interphalangeal joint involvement.

The hands and feet, and the spine and sacroiliac joints are principally involved.

Histologically, the synovitis is similar to that of rheumatoid arthritis. Rheumatoid factor and rheumatoid nodules are typically not present.

Peripheral Skeleton. *Radiologically,* in the *hands,* erosive and destructive arthritis is seen, which is bilaterally asymmetric, involving predominantly the distal interphalangeal joints with wide joint spaces and sharply demarcated adjacent bony surfaces (Figs. 2.121 and 2.122). Erosions begin at the margins (Fig. 2.123) and are preceded by soft-tissue swelling. Fluffy, irregular, or solid reactive marginal bone formation and periosteal reaction along the shaft may be seen.

Advanced cases may proceed to tapering and a "pencil-in-cup" appearance (Figs. 2.124 and 2.125).

There is said to be relatively little osteoporosis; however, established cases do show this finding. There is lack of ulnar deviation. Periosteal reaction of a linear or a fluffy type, near the joints and along the shafts, is seen occasionally. Soft-tissue swelling of an entire finger, or a "sausage digit," may be present in oligo or single ray involvement, as a result of tenosynovitis (Fig. 2.126).

Progression to bony ankylosis of the interphalangeal joints of the hands and feet occurs in up to 15% of patients.

Resorption of the terminal tufts may occur without arthritis as well as sclerosis of a distal phalanx.

A smaller group of patients develops subluxations and arthritis mutilans, with extreme resorption and erosion of the metacarpals and phalanges, shortening of the digits with "telescoping" of the fingers (Fig. 2.127).

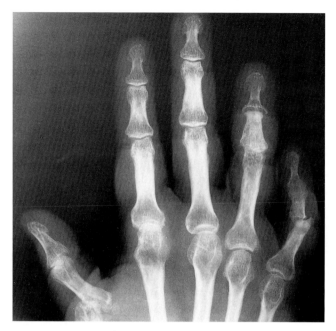

FIGURE 2.121. Psoriatic arthritis. Hand. There is involvement of the distal interphalangeal joint of the ring finger with widening and marginal spur formation. The proximal interphalangeal joint is uniformly narrowed. There is involvement of the proximal interphalangeal joint of the little finger with subluxation. There is subluxation at the metacarpophalangeal joint of the thumb. Periarticular osteoporosis and soft-tissue swelling are present.

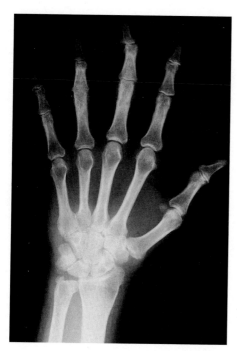

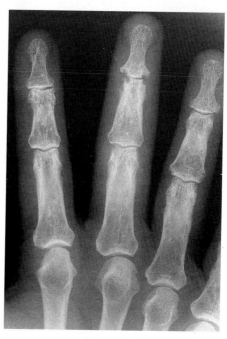

FIGURE 2.122. Psoriatic arthritis. Erosions at the distal interphalangeal joints of the middle and little fingers are seen with subluxation at the middle finger. There is joint space narrowing at the proximal interphalangeal joint of the ring finger. Erosion of the ulnar styloid process is also seen.

FIGURE 2.123. Psoriatic arthritis. Hand. Single ray involvement of the middle finger with marginal erosions at the distal interphalangeal joint and soft-tissue swelling of the entire digit.

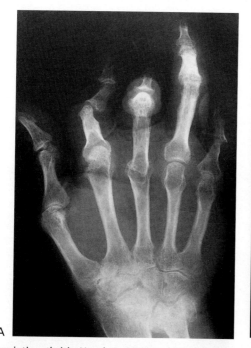

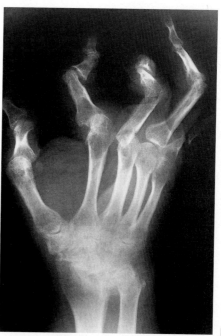

A   B

FIGURE 2.124. Psoriatic arthritis. Hand. **A:** AP view of the hand shows tapered appearances of the proximal phalanges of the index and ring fingers with a "pencil-in-cup" appearance at the proximal interphalangeal joints. There is a contracture of the middle finger with fusion across the proximal interphalangeal joint. Destructive changes in the wrist are seen as well as periarticular osteoporosis. **B:** Oblique view shows subluxation at the third metacarpophalangeal joint, and fusion across the interphalangeal joint of the middle finger in flexed position. Tapering of the proximal phalanx of the little finger is noted. Erosions at the metacarpophalangeal joint of the index finger are also seen.

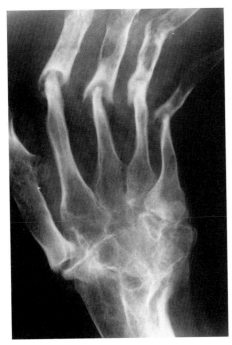

FIGURE 2.125. Psoriatic arthritis. Hand. Advanced disease. "Pencil-in-cup" appearance at the metacarpophalangeal joints is noted as well as fusion of the wrist and at the proximal interphalangeal joints.

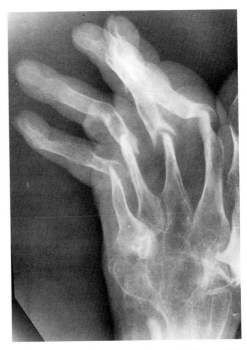

FIGURE 2.127. Psoriatic arthritis. Advanced disease. There is fusion of the carpus and compression erosions of the metacarpophalangeal joints, as well as fusion of the interphalangeal joints. This has resulted in shortening of the digits.

The *wrists* show pancarpal involvement, erosions, destruction (Fig. 2.128), and bony proliferation. This may proceed to complete carpal fusion.

In the *feet*, changes similar to those in the hands occur. The most destructive changes are at the metatarsophalangeal joints. Tapering of the bone ends and "pencil-in-cup" deformities are often seen.

Erosions at the interphalangeal joint of the great toe (Fig. 2.129), associated with irregular bony proliferation at the

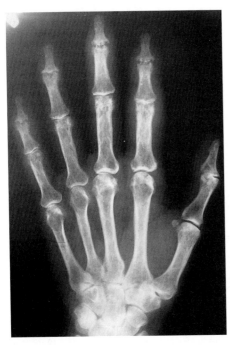

FIGURE 2.126. Psoriatic arthritis. Hand. "Sausage digit" of the ring and little finger are seen, as well as asymmetrical involvement of the distal interphalangeal joints. There is involvement of the proximal interphalangeal joints of the ring and little fingers. Extensive osteoporosis is present.

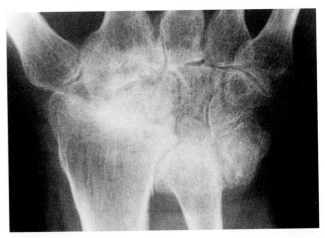

FIGURE 2.128. Psoriatic arthritis. Wrist. Extensive destruction of the proximal carpal row is seen with subluxation of the entire carpus and sclerotic change.

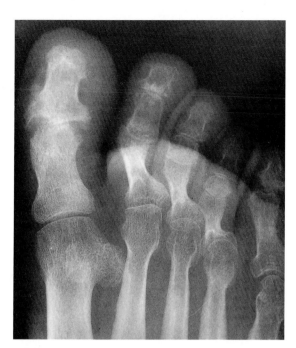

FIGURE 2.129. Psoriatic arthritis. Foot. There are marginal erosions at the interphalangeal joint of the great toe with proliferative bony reaction.

base of the distal phalanx, and resorption of the tufts of the distal phalanges of the toes, are seen. This may be associated with outward displacement of the nail, thickening, and deformity.

Symmetrical involvement of all of the distal interphalangeal joints is infrequent.

The calcaneus may show a picture similar to that of Reiter's disease, with erosions and fluffy sclerosis at the attachment of the Achilles tendon and at the inferior surface. A plantar calcaneal spur may also be present.

Asymmetrical or monarticular involvement of the *large joints* may occur (Fig. 2.130). Soft-tissue swelling and joint effusion are followed by marginal erosions, with progress to uniform joint space narrowing. Osteoporosis is not prominent. Proliferative enthesitis, periosteal new bone formation, and capsular ossification may be present.

Central Skeleton. In the *spine*, the characteristic finding is the presence of coarse, asymmetrical nonmarginal syndesmophytes, with skip areas of the spine (Figs. 2.131, 2.132, and 2.133). They differ in appearance from those seen in ankylosing spondylitis in that they do not originate from the vertebral margins, but rather from the midvertebral body. They are also more superficially situated. Their distribution is in the lumbar, dorsal, and less commonly in the cervical spine (Fig. 2.134). Paravertebral ossification may also be present.

Another not uncommon finding in the cervical spine is atlantoaxial subluxation. This can be demonstrated with careful flexion and extension lateral views. Bony proliferation at C1-2 also may be seen at times (Fig. 2.135).

Changes that rarely occur include "squaring" of vertebral bodies and apophyseal joint fusion.

Intersternal-costoclavicular ossification has been reported in this condition, as has involvement of the manubriosternal joint.[80]

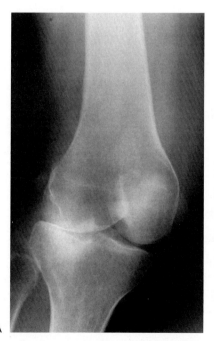
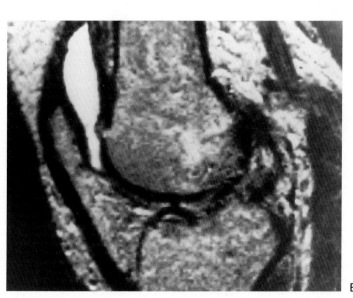

FIGURE 2.130. Psoriatic arthritis. AP view of the knee. **A:** Large joint effusion and soft-tissue swelling are seen as well as narrowing of the lateral compartment of the knee joint space with genu valgus. **B:** MRI T2-weighted image showing effusion in the suprapatellar recess.

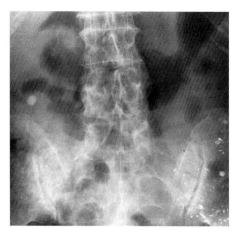

FIGURE 2.131. Psoriatic arthritis. Spine. Coarse, asymmetrical nonmarginal syndesmophytes are seen in the lower lumbar spine. There is also asymmetrical involvement of the sacroiliac joints.

The *sacroiliac joints* may show unilateral (Fig. 2.136) or bilateral involvement, which is bilaterally asymmetrical in most patients. Changes are first seen on the iliac side of the joint. The sequence of events is blurring of the subchondral margins, erosions narrowing the joint space, and reactive sclerosis (Fig. 2.137). This may proceed to bony ankylosis. The erosions may be more severe than those usually seen in AS.

Ligamentous calcifications in the upper third of the SI joints may also occur, as well as resorption at the *temporomandibular joints.*

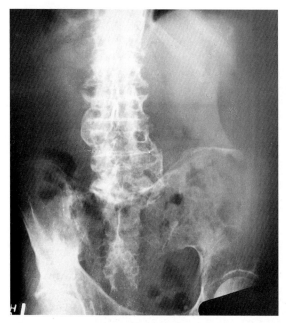

FIGURE 2.132. Psoriatic arthritis. Lumbar spine. Thick nonmarginal syndesmophytes are seen in the upper and in the lower lumbar spine. Sacroiliitis is also evident.

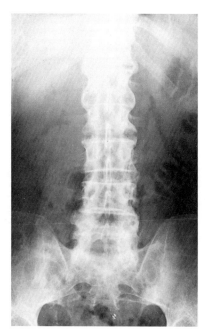

FIGURE 2.133. Psoriatic arthritis. Lumbar spine. Thick nonmarginal syndesmophytes are seen in the lumbar spine. Sacroiliitis is also present.

Case Report

Frank B. Vasey

A 30-year-old white woman developed scaling plaques in her scalp and swelling of her right knee in 1987. The skin disease spread to the groin. She was begun on UVB light treatment and naproxen. By 1990, she had developed a symmetrical swelling of hands and wrists. Marginal erosions were noted in the proximal phalangeal joints. She continued UVB and naproxen 375 mg twice daily. Vitamin D ointment (dovonex) was also helpful for her symptoms. Her joints were only intermittently swollen and she had no deformities. She was doing relatively well in March of 1998, when she slipped and fell on her right shoulder and elbow. Radiographs taken several days later showed erosions in the humeral head and in the distal humerus and olecranon (Fig. 2.138).

Reiter's Disease

Clinical Aspects

Frank B. Vasey

The classic Reiter's triad of conjunctivitis, urethritis, and arthritis is rarely seen. Most patients seen by rheumatologists have a pauciarticular asymmetric peripheral arthritis, which may or may not include spinal involvement at any level. Red eyes are noted historically, if at all. This variability has led to the concept of "incomplete Reiter's syndrome." Among the

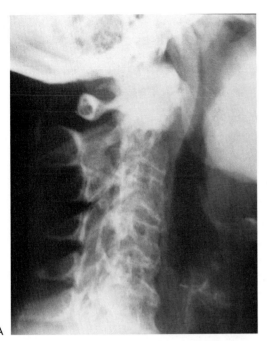
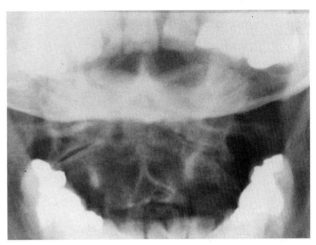

FIGURE 2.134. Psoriatic arthritis. Cervical spine. **A:** Lateral view shows bony proliferation at the C1-2 region. Fusion at the apophyseal joints is noted as well as syndesmophytes anteriorly at all of the intervertebral discs. **B:** Open mouth view showing narrowing and irregularity at the left interspace between C-1 and C-2.

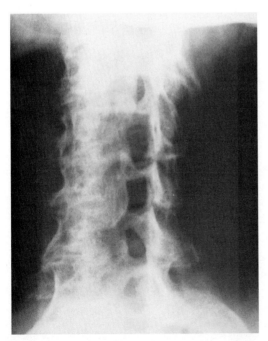
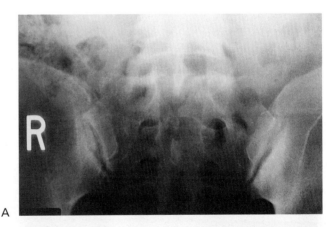
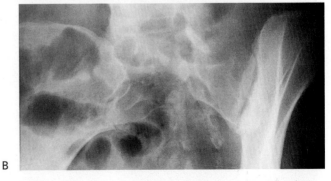

FIGURE 2.135. Psoriatic arthritis. Cervical spine. Oblique view shows nonmarginal syndesmophytes projected posteriorly.

FIGURE 2.136. Psoriatic arthritis. Sacroiliac joints. **A:** Ferguson's view. **B:** Oblique view. Unilateral sacroiliitis on the left side is seen as sclerosis on the iliac side with marginal irregularity. The right side shows no changes.

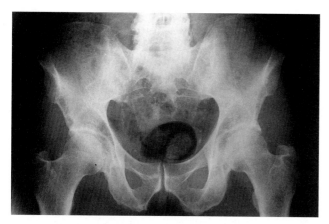

FIGURE 2.137. Psoriatic arthritis. Sacroiliac joints. There is sclerosis and partial obliteration of the sacroiliac joints, which is bilateral and symmetrical. Coarse syndesmophytes in the lower lumbar spine are also seen.

forms of spondylarthritis, the role of infectious agents is clearest for RS, now classed as reactive arthritis.

In the postchlamydial form, one expects the history of a sexually transmitted disease, which usually occurred in the distant past. Men may have an intermittent prostatitis or epididymitis. Women note a vaginal discharge, pain on sex, and an inflammatory pap smear.

In the postdysentery form, one looks for documentation of a severe enteric infection, which lasted days or weeks, with dehydration, usually requiring intravenous fluids. Actual documentation of the recognized causative organisms, including *Salmonella, Shigella, Yersinia,* or *Campylobacter* is helpful, but infrequently found. Still, there are few documented and well-studied epidemics such as that occurring aboard the USS Little Rock in the 1960s.[120]

Of the 600 men who developed *Shigella* dysentery, 10 developed postdysentery Reiter's syndrome. Six were found to have persistent problems 10 years later.[121]

Unfortunately, many patients have typical arthritis, but little clear documentation of sexually transmitted disease (STD) or dysentery. Some do have intermittent eye inflammation or a psoriaform scaly rash on the glans or shaft of the penis (circinate balanitis) or on the soles of the feet (keratoderma blennorrhagicum). In addition to skin disease, nails may also be affected in a similar fashion to psoriasis. Nails may be affected with pits and ridges. Ophthalmological evaluation when the eye is inflamed can clarify if the patient has an iritis associated with ankylosing spondylitis or the conjunctivitis of Reiter's syndrome.

The onset of arthritis may be either insidious or so fulminant as to suggest septic or infectious arthritis with a high fever. As in psoriatic arthritis, most patients have four or fewer peripheral joints involved. There is a greater tendency for the weight-bearing lower extremity joints to be affected. Back pain occurs in approximately 50% of patients. Diffuse swelling of the involved digits (fingers or toes) represents dactylitis, commonly called a "sausage digit". This is a very characteristic finding of spondyloarthritis and is distinctive from the fusiform swelling around the PIP joints in patients with rheumatoid arthritis. Enthesopathy is also a hallmark of this illness, especially in the feet, in the form of plantar fasciitis or Achillis tendinitis. This problem may occur widely in and around tendons, fasciae, and bursae.

Radiographic changes include marginal erosions and fluffy periostitis. Spinal disease is similar to psoriatic arthritis and may affect any part of the spine with nonmarginal syndesmophytes. Sacroiliitis, which occurs in 15% of patients, usually is asymmetrical.[122]

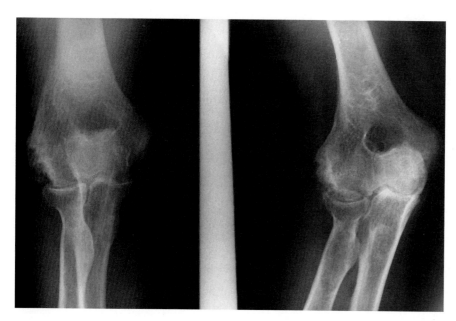

FIGURE 2.138. Psoriatic arthritis. Elbow. Large marginal erosions at the distal humerus are seen.

Crohn's disease, ulcerative colitis, and Whipple's disease are all associated with an inflammatory spondyloarthritis in which the inciting agent could be flora of the colon.

Radiologic Aspects

George B. Greenfield

Reiter's disease (Reiter's syndrome) is a reactive spondyloarthropathy associated with HLA-B27.[123,125] It is characterized by a triad of arthritis, urethritis, and conjunctivitis. Two additional consistent features are balanitis and a dermatitis, keratoderma blennorrhagicum. All symptoms are not always present simultaneously. Young adult men are chiefly affected. One type has a sexual transmission, following chlamydia urethritis. Reiter's original case followed severe diarrhea. This type occurs in susceptible individuals following infection with *Shigella, Salmonella,* and *Yersinia* organisms. The disease shows some similarity to psoriatic arthritis in skin lesions and radiologic features.

The feet, heels, sacroiliac joints, and knees are most frequently affected.

Peripheral Skeleton. Radiologically, the changes are similar to psoriatic arthritis, but their distribution is different. This disease characteristically predilects the lower extremities, including the foot, knee, and ankle. The typical distribution pattern is asymmetrical. Bone proliferation is prominent.

The *hand,* when the upper extremities are involved, is most often affected. A single joint or ray or several may show changes. The proximal interphalangeal joints are affected more commonly, followed by the distal interphalangeal joints. Metacarpophalangeal involvement is rare (Fig. 2.139). The initial change is fusiform or periarticular swelling. Soft-tissue swelling with a "sausage digit" configuration may occur, as in psoriasis. Uniform joint space narrowing and destruction follow. The *wrists* may show pancarpal involvement.

The elbows and hips are less frequently involved. Shoulder involvement is rare.

A case has been reported of massive synovial hypertrophy involving both upper and lower extremities, with invasion of tendons and destruction of the wrist joint.[126]

The *feet* are most commonly involved. One joint or several may show changes. The metatarsophalangeal joints, proximal interphalangeal joints of the toes, and interphalangeal joint of the great toe (Figs. 2.140, 2.141, and 2.142) are principal sites. Panarthritis is rare. Periarticular osteoporosis is commonly seen early, with later reossification. Uniform joint space narrowing and marginal erosions occur, followed by destruction and subluxation. Linear or fluffy periosteal new bone formation is frequent, particularly in the calcaneus, phalanges, metatarsals, and distal tibia and fibula, including the malleoli of the *ankle.* Soft-tissue

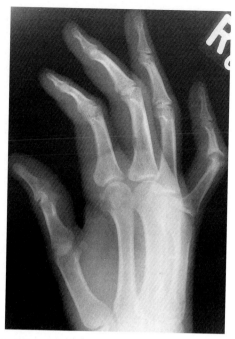

FIGURE 2.139. Reiter's disease. Hand. A "cup-in-saucer" erosion of the proximal interphalangeal joint of the little finger is seen associated with soft-tissue swelling. A small amount of reactive sclerosis is noted. There is no osteoporosis present.

swelling and erosions are also commonly seen in the ankle.

The calcaneus is involved in more than one-half of patients, and may show erosions and fluffy periosteal new bone formation and spurs, as well as increased density and size. The site of attachment of the Achilles tendon and the plantar surface are affected.

The disease may progress to a destructive picture termed *Launois' deformity.*

The *knee* is involved in a large percentage of patients, either unilaterally or bilaterally. There may be joint effusion, local osteoporosis, and, less commonly, uniform joint space narrowing. A Pellegrini-Stieda type of tendon calcification or ossification occasionally may be seen.

Central Skeleton. The *spine* is involved less frequently than the sacroiliac joints. It shows asymmetric involvement with coarse, nonmarginal syndesmophytes similar to those seen in psoriatic arthritis (Figs. 2.143 and 2.144). The distribution is discontinuous, with skipped segments. The thoracic and lumbar spine may show changes. Paravertebral ossifications with dense or fluffy bridging of vertebrae also occur.

Sacroiliac joint involvement occurs eventually in most patients. It may be unilateral or bilateral, usually asymmetric (Fig. 2.145). The changes are first seen on the iliac side. Joint effusion with loss of definition of the margins, erosions, narrowing, and reactive sclerosis are seen. Complete fusion does not typically occur.

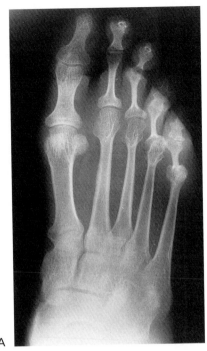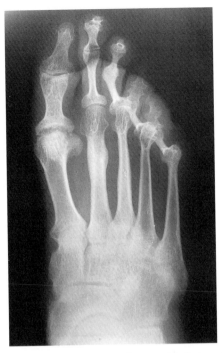

A   B

FIGURE 2.140. Reiter's disease. **A:** AP view of the foot showing erosion and soft-tissue swelling at the first metatarsophalangeal joint. Subluxations at the metatarsophalangeal joints of the fourth and fifth toes are also noted. **B:** Same patient 1 year later. The erosion of the first metatarsophalangeal joint has progressed to involve the articular surfaces. Subluxations of the fourth and fifth metatarsophalangeal joints are again noted, but there has been a new subluxation at the third metatarsophalangeal joint and ankylosis across the proximal interphalangeal joint of the third toe. There is also a healed fracture of the second metatarsal.

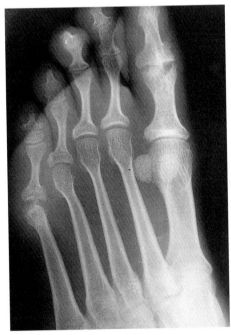

FIGURE 2.141. Reiter's disease. Foot. Erosive changes at the interphalangeal joint of the great toe are seen as well as at the metatarsophalangeal joint of the little toe, with associated soft-tissue swelling.

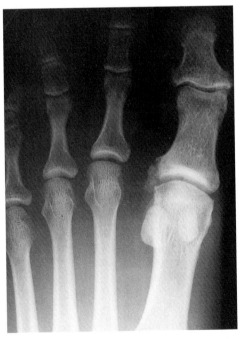

FIGURE 2.142. Reiter's disease. AP view of the foot shows bony proliferation at the metatarsophalangeal joint of the great toe as well at the interphalangeal joint.

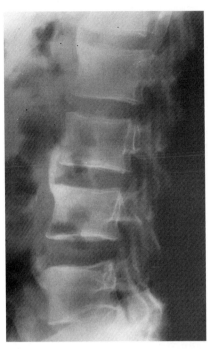

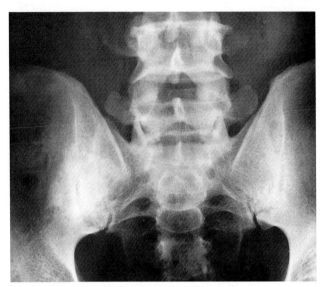

FIGURE 2.145. Reiter's disease. Sacroiliac joints. Bilateral changes are seen with asymmetrical involvement, more so on the right side.

FIGURE 2.143. Reiter's disease. Lateral view of the lumbar spine. A course syndesmophyte is seen in the upper lumbar spine, whereas dense bony bridges partially attached to the lumbar vertebral bodies are seen anteriorly in the mid and lower lumbar spine. The lower most formation has a fluffy appearance.

Case Reports

Frank B. Vasey

Case 1. A 43-year-old homosexual man developed diarrhea, fever to 100.5°F (38°C), and crampy abdominal pain that cultured positive for *Shigella*. He recalled a similar episode 5 years before that was not cultured, and he developed pain and swelling in the right wrist that persisted. Shortly after this episode of diarrhea, which responded to ciprofloxacin, his shoulders and right ankle became painful. ANA and rheumatoid factor were negative, and his sed rate was three. Radiographs of the foot showed degenerative changes in the midfoot but also marginal erosions in the second and third metatarsal heads.

He ultimately underwent a right midfoot arthrodesis. This was beneficial, but he continued to have variably swollen peripheral joints. He currently is benefiting from treatment with NSAIDs.

Case 2. A 30-year-old white man had an unprotected sexual contact with a prostitute. He developed urethral discharge, but did not seek medical attention. Several months later he wrenched his left knee and ankle in an industrial accident. This led to persistently swollen joints. He was seen by the rheumatology service several months later and treated with 3 months of doxycycline for postchlamydial Reiter's syndrome. Unfortunately, he experienced only modest benefit and ultimately went on to spinal fusion, including his neck, over the next decade.

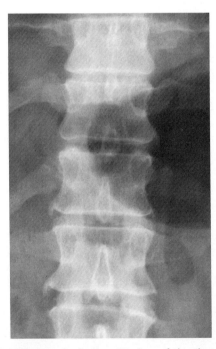

FIGURE 2.144. Reiter's disease. AP view of the thoracolumbar spine reveals nonmarginal syndesmophytes, which are thinner than those seen on the previous figure.

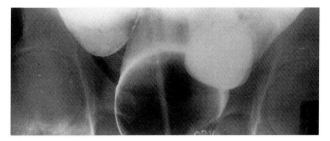

FIGURE 2.146. Enteropathic arthritis. A patient who has ulcerative colitis. Bilateral uniform narrowing of the hip joint spaces is seen.

Enteropathic Arthritis

George B. Greenfield

Clinically, up to 10% of patients with ulcerative colitis and regional enteritis have associated arthritis.[127,128] The arthritis may develop simultaneously with bowel disease, but usually follows it. In a significant number of patients who develop spondylitis, the spondylitis precedes the appearance of intestinal disease. Whipple's disease (intestinal lipodystrophy) may also be associated with arthritis. Migratory arthritis or arthralgia, sacroiliitis, erythema nodosum, and uveitis occur in some patients.

Radiologically, the disease manifests either as a central or peripheral type. The two types coexist only in a minority of patients.

The *hands, wrists,* and *feet* may be involved. Periarticular osteoporosis, followed by joint space narrowing, is seen, although it is less severe than in RA. Periosteal new bone also may be present. The *hip* may be involved with uniform joint space narrowing (Fig. 2.146).

Soft-tissue swelling also is seen, most commonly in the *knee* and *elbow.*

The most frequently affected site is the *sacroiliac joint,*

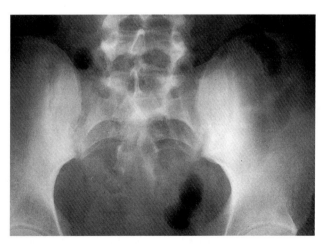

FIGURE 2.147. Enteropathic arthritis. The patient has ulcerative colitis. Bilateral sclerosis and erosions of the sacroiliac joints are seen.

usually with bilateral symmetrical involvement (Figs. 2.147 and 2.148). The most prominent finding is sclerosis; however, widening, erosions, and ankylosis also may occur.

The *spine* shows changes with syndesmophyte formation indistinguishable from that of ankylosing spondylitis in about 6% of patients with ulcerative colitis and regional enteritis.

Migratory polyarthritis and monarticular arthritis have been reported in patients with antibiotic-associated colitis.[129] Arthritis also has been reported to be associated with intestinal bypass procedures for morbid obesity.

Miscellaneous Conditions

George B. Greenfield

Acne Arthritis. Patients with severe acne rarely may develop syndesmophytes, erosive, and proliferative arthritis of the spine (Fig. 2.149), peripheral joints, and sacroiliac joints.[130] They may have acne fulminans, with ulcerating skin lesions and acute fever, or severe cicatricial acne. Coarse or fine syndesmophytes in the spine may be seen, as well as erosion, widening, and sclerosis of the sacroiliac joints and symphysis pubis. The joints of the upper and lower extremities may show periarticular osteoporosis, soft-tissue swelling, and erosive and proliferative changes that are indistinguishable from psoriatic arthritis or Reiter's disease.

Bowel-associated Dermatosis-arthritis Syndrome. Bowel-associated dermatosis-arthritis syndrome is well documented.[131,132] Changes include a pustular and purpuric dermatosis, nondeforming polyarthritis, fever, tenosynovitis, myalgias, joint effusions, Raynaud's phenomenon, paresthesias, pericarditis, and liver disease. The pathogenesis relates to circulating immune complexes derived from bacterial antigens from the bowel.

Behçet's Disease. Behçet's disease is characterized by a triad of aphthous and genital ulcerations and iritis.[133] It may be associated with arthritis. The joint manifestations are an intermittent peripheral arthritis similar to Reiter's disease. The small and large joints, especially the knees, may be involved. Erosive sacroiliitis and enthesopathy have also been described in this condition.

Axial Skeletal Changes in Paraplegics. Axial skeletal changes in paraplegics include sacroiliac joint marginal blurring, erosion, sclerosis, and narrowing of the joint space, which may progress to complete obliteration.[134] The thoracolumbar spine shows syndesmophytes, interspinous ossification, intervertebral disc calcification, and large osteophytes. These changes have no relation to age or paralysis level, but are related to the duration of paralysis. The changes mimic HLA-B27 arthropathy; however, negative HLA-B27 in paraplegics helps in the differential diagnosis.

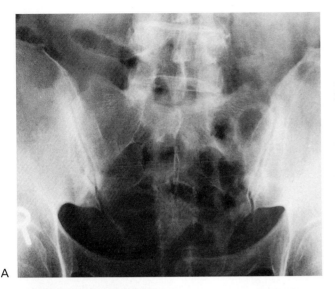

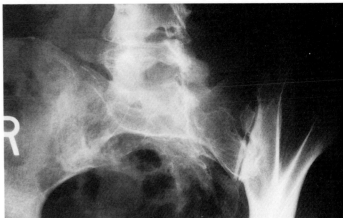

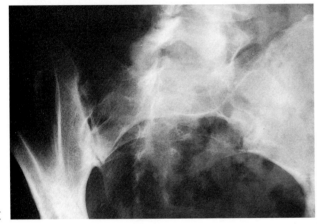

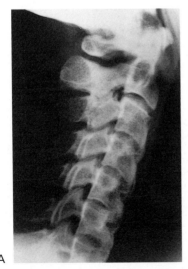

FIGURE 2.148. A,B,C: Enteropathic arthritis in a patient with Crohn's disease. Ferguson's view and oblique views of the sacroiliac joints reveal bilateral sacroiliitis with sclerosis and marginal irregularities.

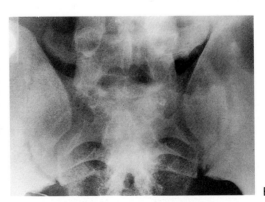

FIGURE 2.149. Patient with acne. **A:** Lateral view of the cervical spine shows extensive anterior syndesmophyte formation. **B:** Sacroiliac joints, bilateral sacroiliitis is seen.

REFERENCES

Rheumatoid Arthritis

1. Arnett FC, Edworthy SM, Bloch DA, et al. The American Rheumatology Association 1987 revised criteria for the classification of rheumatoid arthritis. *Arthritis Rheum* 1988;31:315–324.
2. Hochberg MC. Adult and juvenile rheumatoid arthritis, current epidemiologic concepts. *Epidemiol Rev* 1981;3:27–44.
3. Aho K, Koskenvuo M, Tuominen J, et al. Occurrence of rheumatoid arthritis in a nationwide series of twins. *J Rheumatol* 1986;3:899–902.
4. Steen-Hansen E, Hove B, Andresen J. Bone mass in patients with rheumatoid arthritis. *Skeletal Radiol* 1987;16:556–559.
5. Renner WR, Weinstein AS. Early changes of rheumatoid arthritis in the hand and wrist. *Radiol Clin North Am* 1988;6:1185–1193.
6. Martel W, Hayes JT, Duff IF. The pattern of bone erosion in the hand and wrist in rheumatoid arthritis. *Radiology* 1965;84:204–214.
7. Forrester DM, Brown JC, Nesson JW. *The radiology of joint disease,* 2nd ed. Philadelphia: WB Saunders, 1978.
8. Resnick D, Gmelich JT. Bone fragmentation in the rheumatoid wrist: radiographic and pathologic consideration. *Radiology* 1975;114:315–321.
9. Collins LC, Lidsky LD, Sharp JT, et al. Malposition of carpal bones in rheumatoid arthritis. *Radiology* 1972;103:95–98.
10. Hendrix RW, Urban MA, Shroeder JL, et al. Carpal predominance in rheumatoid arthritis. *Radiology* 1987;164:219–222.
11. Resnick D, Niwayama G. Resorption of the undersurface of the distal clavicle in rheumatoid arthritis. *Radiology* 1976;120:75–77.
12. Jackman RJ, Pugh DG. The positive elbow fat pad sign in rheumatoidarthritis. *AJR* 1970;108:812–818.
13. Murphy WA, Siegel MJ. Elbow fat pads with new signs and extended differential diagnosis. *Radiology* 1977;124:659–665.
14. Anderson J, Stewart AM. The significance of the magnitude of the medial hip joint space. *Br J Radiol* 1970;43:238–239.
15. Hermodsson I. Roentgen appearances of arthritis of the hip. *Acta Radiol [Diagn]* 1972;12:865–881.
16. Armstrong P, Saxton H. Iliopsoas bursa. *Br J Radiol* 1972;45:493–495.
17. Staple TW. Arthrographic demonstration of iliopsoas bursa extension of the hip joint. *Radiology* 1972;102:515–516.
18. Peh WCG, Reinus WR. Piriform bursitis causing sciatic neuropathy. *Skeletal Radiol* 1995;24:474–476.
19. Harris RD, Hecht HL. Suprapatellar effusions: a new diagnostic sign. *Radiology* 1970;97:1–4.
20. Pastershank SP, Mitchell DM. Knee joint bursal abnormalities in rheumatoid arthritis. *J Can Assoc Radiol* 1977;28:199–203.
21. Carter AR, Liyanage SP. Large subarticular cysts—geodes adjacent to the knee joint in rheumatoid arthritis. *Clin Radiol* 1975;26:353–538.
22. Resnick D, Newell JD, Guerra J Jr, et al. Proximal tibiofibular joint: anatomic pathologic-radiographic correlation. *AJR* 1978;131:133–138.
23. Pastershank SP. Mid-foot disassociation in rheumatoid arthritis. *J Can Assoc Radiol* 1981;32:166–167.
24. Resnick D, Feingold ML, Curd J, et al. Calcaneal abnormalities in articular disorders. *Radiology* 1977;125:355–366.
25. Resnick D. Roentgen features of the rheumatoid mid and hind foot. *J Can Assoc Radiol* 1976;27:99–107.
26. Resnick D. The interphalangeal joint of the great toe in rheumatoid arthritis. *J Can Assoc Radiol* 1975;26:255–262.
27. Linquist PR, McDonnell DE. Rheumatoid cyst causing extradural compression. *J Bone Joint Surg [Am]* 1970;52:1235–1240.
28. Glay A, Rona G. Nodular rheumatoid vertebral lesions versus ankylosing spondylitis. *AJR* 1965;94:631–638.
29. Bunton RW, Grennan DM, Palmer DG. Lateral subluxation of the atlas in rheumatoid arthritis. *Br J Radiol* 1978;51:963–967.
30. Crellin RQ, Maccabe JJ, Hamilton EBD. Severe subluxation of the cervical spine in rheumatoid arthritis. *J Bone Joint Surg [Br]* 1970;52:244–251.
31. Rana NA, Hancock DO, Taylor AR, et al. Atlantoaxial subluxation in rheumatoid arthritis. *J Bone Joint Surg [Br]* 1973;55:458–470.
32. Chevrot A, Correas G, Pallardy G. Atteinte cervicale de la polyarthrite rhumatoide. *J Radiol* 1978;59:545–550.
33. Rana NA, Hancock DO, Taylor AR, et al. Upward translocation of the dens in rheumatoid arthritis. *J Bone Joint Surg [Br]* 1973;55:471–477.
34. El-Khoury GY, Wner MH, Menezes AH, et al. Cranial settling in rheumatoid arthritis. *Radiology* 1980;137:637–642.
35. Weissman BNW, Aliabadi P, Seinfeld M, et al. Prognostic features of atlantoaxial subluxation in rheumatoid arthritis patients. *Radiology* 1982;144:745–751.
36. Reynolds H, Carter SW, Murtagh FR, et al. Cervical rheumatoid arthritis: value of flexion and extension views in imaging. *Radiology* 1987;164:215–218.
37. Stevens JM, Barter S, Kendall BE, et al. Case reports: massive intracranial pannus and a pseudomeningocoele in the atlantodental interval in rheumatoid arthritis. *Br J Radiol* 1987;60:185–188.
38. Heywood AWB, Meyers OL. Rheumatoid arthritis of the thoracic and lumbar spine. *J Bone Joint Surg* 1986;68B:362–368.
39. DeCarvalho A, Graudal H. Sacroiliac joint involvement in classical or definite rheumatoid arthritis. *Acta Radiol [Diagn]* 1980;21:417–423.
40. Cummings JK, Taleisnik J. Peripheral gangrene as a complication of rheumatoid arthritis: report of a case and review of the literature. *J Bone Joint Surg [Am]* 1971;53:1001–1006.
41. Sandusky WR, Rudolf LE, Leavell BS. Splenectomy for control of neutropenia in Felty's syndrome. *Ann Surg* 1968;167:744–751.
42. Gelman MI, Ward JR. Septic arthritis: a complication of rheumatoid arthritis. *Radiology* 1977;122:17–23.
43. Resnick D. Pyarthrois complicating rheumatoid arthritis. *Radiology* 1975;114:581–586.
44. Schneider R, Kaye JJ. Insufficiency and stress fractures of the long bones occurring in patients with rheumatoid arthritis. *Radiology* 1975;116:595–599.
45. Hamilton S. Unilateral rheumatoid arthritis in hemiplegia. *J Can Assoc Radiol* 1983;34:49–50.
46. Yaghmai I, Rooholamini SM, Faunce HF. Unilateral rheumatoid arthritis: protective effect of neurologic deficits. *AJR* 1977;128:299–301.
47. Resnick D, Niwayama G. *Diagnosis of bone and joint disorders,* vol 3. Philadelphia: WB Saunders, 1981.
48. Bohndorf K. MRI of synovial arthritis. Lecture at meeting of the International Skeletal Society, Dublin, 1998.
49. Pavlov H, Heneghan MA, Hersh A, et al. The Haglund syndrome: initial and differential diagnosis. *Radiology* 1982;144:83–88.

Juvenile Arthritis

50. Towner SR, Michet CJ Jr, O'Fallon WM, et al. The epidemiology of juvenile arthritis in Rochester, Minnesota 1960–1979. *Arthritis Rheum* 1983;26:1208–1213.

51. Ansell BM, Fink C, Wood PHN. Juvenile arthritis in England: a long-term follow-up. *Arthritis Rheum* 1980;23:673.

52. Brewer EJ, Bass JC, Cassidy JT, et al. Current proposed revision of JRA criteria. *Arthritis Rheum* 1977;20:195–199.

53. Wood PHN. Special meeting on nomenclature and classification of arthritis in children. 1978. In Munther EP, ed. *The care of rheumatic children.* Basel: EULAR, 1978:47.

54. Oen K, Wood S, Anderson S, et al. Remission rates and disease duration in patients with JRA. Park City IV, American Academy of Pediatrics (AAP), Park City, Utah, March 14–18, 1998. See *J Rheumatol* 2000;27:69

55. Cassidy JT, Brody GL, Martel W. Monarticular juvenile rheumatoid arthritis. *J Pediatr* 1967;70:867–875.

56. Bywaters EGL, Ansell BM. Monoarticular arthritis in children. *Ann Rheum Dis* 1965;24:116.

57. Watanabe KN, Polomeno R, Gibbon M, et al. Prevalence and severity of chronic uveitis in children with juvenile arthritis. Park City IV, American Academy of Pediatrics (AAP), Park City, Utah, March 14–18, 1998. See *J Rheumatol* 2000;27:70

58. Singsen BH. Rheumatic diseases of childhood. *Rheum Dis Clin North Am* 1990;16(3):581–599.

59. Sullivan DB, Cassidy JT, Petty RE. Pathogenic implications of age of onset in juvenile rheumatoid arthritis. *Arthritis Rheum* 1975;18(3):251–255.

60. White PH. Growth abnormalities in children with juvenile rheumatoid arthritis. *Clin Orthop Rel Res* 1990;259:46–50.

61. Davies U, Rooney M, Preece MA, et al. Treatment of growth retardation in juvenile chronic arthritis with recombinant human growth hormone. *J Rheumatol* 1994;21:153–158.

62. Chipman JJ, Boyar RM, Fink CW. Anterior pituitary adrenal function of gold-treated patients with juvenile rheumatoid arthritis. *J Rheumatol* 1982;9:63–68.

63. Allen RC, Jimenez M, Cowell CT. Insulin-like growth factor and growth hormone secretion in juvenile chronic arthritis. *Ann Rheum Dis* 1991;50:602–606.

64. Motil KJ, Grand RJ, Maletskos CJ, et al. The effect of disease, drug, and diet on whole body protein metabolism in adolescents with Crohn disease and growth failure. *J Pediatr* 1982;101: 345–351.

65. Falcini F, Taccetti G, Trapani S, et al. Growth retardation in juvenile chronic arthritis patients treated with steroids. *Clin Exp Rheumatol* 1991;9(Suppl 6):37–40.

66. Lovell DJ, Gregg D, Heubi J, et al. Bone mineralization in juvenile rheumatoid arthritis patients [abstract]. *Arthritis Rheum* 1986;29(Suppl):S67.

67. Reed AM, Haugen MS, Pachman LM, et al. Osteopenia in children with chronic rheumatic diseases correlates with disease activity [abstract]. *Arthritis Rheum* 1991;34(Suppl 9):B158.

68. Hillman L, Cassidy JT, Johnson L, et al. Vitamin D metabolism and bone mineralization in children with juvenile rheumatoid arthritis. *J Pediatr* 1994;124:910–916.

69. Hickman PL, Johnson L, Lorrens C, et al. Skeletal maturation and bone mineral metabolism in children with juvenile rheumatoid arthritis. *Arthritis Rheum* 1992;35:S189.

70. Warady BD, Lindsley CB, Robinson FG, et al. The effects of nutritional supplementation on bone mineral status of children with rheumatic diseases on corticosteroid therapy. *J Rheumatol* 1994;21:530–535.

71. Reed A, Haugen M, Pachman LM, et al. Abnormalities in serum osteocalcin values in children with chronic rheumatic diseases. *J Pediatr* 1990;116:574–580.

72. Davies UM, Green JR, Reeve J. Serum osteocalcin levels in children with juvenile chronic arthritis with impaired linear growth [abstract]. *Br J Rheumatol* 1989;28(2Suppl):84S.

73. Reed A, Haugen M, Pachman LM, et al. 25-Hydroxyvitamin D therapy in children with active juvenile rheumatoid arthritis: short-term effects on serum osteocalcin levels and bone mineral density. *J Pediatr* 1991;119(4):657–660.

74. Bywaters EGL. Still's disease in the adult. *Ann Rheum Dis* 1971; 30:138–148.

75. Fabricant MS, Chandor SB, Friou GJ. Still disease in adults: a cause of prolonged undiagnosed fever. *JAMA* 1973;225: 273–276.

76. Martel W, Holt JF, Cassidy JT. Roentgenologic manifestations of juvenile rheumatoid arthritis. *AJR* 1962;88:400–423.

77. Ansell BM, Kent PA. Radiological changes in juvenile chronic polyarthritis. *Skeletal Radiol* 1977;1:129–144.

78. Mitnick JS, Mitnick HJ, Genieser NB. Proliferative changes of the hip in juvenile rheumatoid arthritis. *Radiology* 1980;136:369–371.

79. Chlosta EM, Kuhns LR, Holt JF. The "patellar ratio" in hemophilia and juvenile rheumatoid arthritis. *Radiology* 1975; 116:137–138.

80. Gilsanz V, Bernstein BH. Joint calcification following intraarticular corticosteroid therapy. *Radiology* 1984;151:647–649.

81. Rombouts JJ, Rombouts-Lindemans C. Scoliosis in juvenile rheumatoid arthritis. *J Bone Joint Surg [Br]* 1974;56:478–483.

82. Azouz EM, Duffy CM. Juvenile spondylarthropathies: clinical manifestations and medical imaging. *Skeletal Radiol* 1995; 24:399–408.

Juvenile Spondylarthropathies

83. Kleinman P, Rivelis M, Schneider R, et al. Juvenile ankylosing spondylitis. *Radiology* 1977;125:775–780.

84. Riley MJ, Ansell BM, Bywaters EGL. Radiologic manifestations of ankylosing spondylitis according to age at onset. *Ann Rheum Dis* 1971;30:138–148.

Ankylosing Spondylitis

85. Asim Khan Muhammad. Ankylosing spondylitis. In Schumacher R, ed. *Primer on rheumatic diseases,* 10th ed. Atlanta: Arthritis Foundation, 1993:154.

86. Kinsella TD, Espinoza LR, Vasey FB. Serum complement and immunoglobulin levels in sporadic and familial ankylosing spondylitis. *J Rheumatol* 1975;2:308–313.

87. Khan MA, Khan MK. Diagnostic value of HLA-B27 testing in ankylosing spondylitis and Reiter's syndrome. *Ann Intern Med* 1982;96:70–76.

88. Steinberg GG, Akins CM, Baran DT. Shoulder and upper arm. In Steinberg GG, Akins CM, eds. *Orthopedics in primary care,* 2nd ed. Baltimore: Williams & Wilkins, 1992: 26–61.

89. Fam AG, Rubenstein JD, Chin-Sang H, et al. Computed tomography in the diagnosis of early ankylosing spondylitis. *Arthritis Rheum* 1985;930–937.

90. Beren DL. Roentgen features of ankylosing spondylitis. *Clin Orthop* 1971;74:20–33.

91. Patton JT. Differential diagnosis of inflammatory spondylitis. *Skeletal Radiol* 1976;1:77–85.

92. Rodnan GP, ed. Primer on the rheumatic diseases, 7th ed. *JAMA* 1973;224:662–812.

93. Resnick D. Temporomandibular joint involvement in ankylosing spondylitis: comparison with rheumatoid arthritis and psoriasis. *Radiology* 1974;112:587–591.

94. Ginsburg WW, Cohen MD. Peripheral arthritis in ankylosing spondylitis. *Mayo Clin Proc* 1983;58:593–596.

95. Pritchett JW. Ossification of the coracoclavicular ligaments in ankylosing spondylitis. *J Bone Joint Surg [Am]* 1983;65: 1017–1018.

96. Karasick D, Schweitzer ME, Abidi NA, et al. Fractures of the vertebrae with spinal cord injuries in patients with ankylosing spondylitis: imaging findings. *AJR* 1995;165:1205–1208.
97. Harding RJ, McCall IW, Park WM, et al. Fracture of the cervical spine in ankylosing spondylitis. *Br J Radiol* 1985;58:3–7.
98. Bachynski JE. An expanding lesion of the intervertebral disc in a case of ankylosing spondylitis. *J Can Assoc Radiol* 1970; 21:110–112.
99. Dihlmann W, Dwelling G. Discovertebral destructive lesions (so-called Anderson lesions) associated with ankylosing spondylitis. *Skeletal Radiol* 1978;3:10–16.
100. Gelman MI, Umber JS. Fractures of the thoracolumbar spine in ankylosing spondylitis. *AJR* 1978;130:485–491.
101. Rivelis M, Freiberger RH. Vertebral destruction at unfused segments in late ankylosing spondylitis. *Radiology* 1969;93: 251–256.
102. Pastershank SP, Resnick D. Pseudoarthrosis in ankylosing spondylitis. *J Can Assoc Radiol* 1980;31:234–235.
103. Bonvoism B, Bouvier M, Perrin G, et al. Discopathies erosives mutifocales au cours d'une spondylarthrite ankylosante. *J Radiol* 1981;62:463–466.
104. Chan FL, Ho EK, Chau EM, et al. Spinal pseudarthrosis complicating ankylosing spondylitis: comparison on CT and conventional tomography. *AJR* 1988;150:611–614.
105. Yu W, Feng F, Dion E, et al. Comparison of radiography, computed tomography and magnetic resonance imaging in the detection of sacroiliitis accompanying ankylosing spondylitis. *Skeletal Radiol* 1998;27:311–320.
106. Lindsley HB, De Smet AA, Neff JR, et al. Ankylosing spondylitis presenting as juxta-articular masses in females. *Skeletal Radiol* 1987;16:142–145.
107. Bunch TW, Hunder GG. Ankylosing spondylitis and primary hyperparathyroidism. *JAMA* 1973;225:1108–1109.
108. Jimenea CV, Frame B, Chaykin LB, et al. Spondylitis of hypoparathyroidism. *Clin Orthop* 1971;74:84–89.
109. Sage MR, Gordon TP. Muscle atrophy in ankylosing spondylitis: CT demonstration. *Radiology* 1983;149:780.
110. Colhoun EN, Hayward C, Evans KT, et al. Inter-sterno-costo-clavicular ossification. *Clin Radiol* 1987;38:33–38.

Psoriatic Arthritis

111. Vasey FB. Psoriatic arthritis. In Schumacher R, ed. *Primer on the rheumatic diseases,* 10th ed. Atlanta: Arthritis Foundation, 1993:161–163.
112. Vasey FB, Dietz CB, Fenske NA, et al. Possible involvement of group A streptococci in the pathogenesis of psoriatic arthritis—PsA). *J Rheumatol* 1982;9:556–560.
113. Wang Q, Vasey FB, Mahfood JP, et al. V2 regions of 16S ribosomal RNA used as a molecular marker for the species identification of streptococci in peripheral blood and synovial fluid from patients with psoriatic arthritis. *Arthritis Rheum* 1999;42:10:2055–2059.
114. Gladman DD, Stafford-Brady F, Chi-Hsing C. Longitudinal study of clinical and radiological progression in psoriatic arthritis. *J Rheumatol* 1990;17:809–812.
115. Martel W, Stuck KJ, Dworin AM, et al. Erosive osteoarthritis and psoriatic arthritis: radiologic comparison in the hand, wrist and foot. *Am J Rosentgenol* 1976;127:579–584.
116. Lambert JR, Wright V. Psoriatic spondylitis: a clinical and radiological description of the spine in psoriatic arthritis. *Q J Med* 1979;184:411–425.

117. Killebrew K, Gold RH, Sholkoff SD. Psoriatic spondylitis. *Radiology* 1973;108:9–16.
118. Resnick D, Broderick TW. Bony proliferation of terminal toe phalanges in psoriasis: the "ivory" phalanx. *J Can Assoc Radiol* 1977;28:187–189.
119. Sundaram M, Patton JT. Paravertebral ossification in psoriasis and Reiter's disease. *Br J Radiol* 1975;48:628–633.

Reiter's Disease

120. Noer-Rolf CH. An experimental epidemic of Reiter's syndrome. *JAMA* 1966;197(7):693–698.
121. Calin A, Fries JF. An experimental epidemic of Reiter's syndrome revisited. Follow-up evidence on genetic and environmental factors. *Ann Int Med* 1976;84:564–566.
122. Resnick D. Reiter's syndrome. In Resnick D, Niwayama G, eds. *Diagnosis of bone and joint disorders,* 2nd ed. Philadelphia: WB Saunders 1988:1199–1217.
123. Martel W, Brannstein EM, Borlaza G, et al. Radiologic features of Reiter disease. *Radiology* 1979;132:1–10.
124. Sholkoff SD, Glickman MG, Steinback HL. Roentgenology of Reiter's syndrome. *Radiology* 1970;97:497–503.
125. Mongey AB, Hess EV. Advances in rheumatology. *Radiol Clin North Am* 1988;6:1157–1164.
126. Finder JG, Ellman MH, Jablon M. Massive synovial hypertrophy in Reiter's syndrome. *J Bone Joint Surg [Am]* 1983;65: 555–557.

Enteropathic Arthritis

127. Clark RL, Muhletaler CA, Margulies SI. Colitic arthritis: clinical and radiographic manifestations. *Radiology* 1971;101: 585–594.
128. Mueller CE, Seeger JF, Martel W. Ankylosing spondylitis and regional enteritis. *Radiology* 1974;112:579–581.
129. Rothchild BM, Masi AL, June PI. Arthritis associated with ampicillin colitis. *Arch Intern Med* 1977;137:1605–1607.

Acne Arthritis

130. Ellis BI, Shier CK, Leisen JJC, et al. Acne-associated spondylarthropathy: radiographic features. *Radiology* 1987;162: 541–545.

Bowel-associated Dermatitis-arthritis Syndrome

131. Dicken CH. Bowel-associated dermatosis-arthritis syndrome: bowel bypass syndrome without bowel bypass. *Mayo Clin Proc* 1984;59:43–46.
132. Jorizzo JL, Schmalstieg FC, Dinehart SM, et al. Bowel-associated dermatosis-arthritis syndrome. *Arch Intern Med* 1984; 144:738–740.

Behçet's Syndrome

133. Caporn N, Higgs ER, Dieppe PA, et al. Arthritis in Behçet's syndrome. *Br J Radiol* 1983;56:87–91.

Axial Skeletal Changes

134. Bhate DV, Pizarro AJ, Seitam A, et al. Axial skeletal changes in paraplegics. *Radiology* 1979;133:55–58.

POLYARTHRITIS ASSOCIATED WITH OTHER DISEASES

Synovial inflammatory arthritis and involvement of ligaments and tendons may be associated with the various collagen diseases, particularly systemic lupus erythematosus (SLE) and scleroderma. Pulmonary hypertrophic osteoarthropathy (PHO) also has a synovial inflammatory component. Hemophilic arthropathy results from posttraumatic bleeding into joints. Rare diseases such as multicentric reticulohistiocytosis, Jaccoud's arthritis, and SAPHO syndrome also involve the joints.

SYSTEMIC LUPUS ERYTHEMATOSUS

Clinical Aspects

Keith Kanik

Systemic lupus erythematosus (lupus) is a systemic autoimmune disease characterized by the production of antibodies directed against the cell nucleus and/or its components. The diagnosis of lupus is based on the presence of four out of 11 clinical or laboratory criteria.[1] One of the criteria is the presence of arthritis. Lupus arthritis is typically nonerosive and it affects the hands, wrists, and knees in a symmetric fashion. Effusions are uncommon. Chronic arthritis may lead to deformities involving ulnar deviation, subluxation, and contractures. X-ray findings may reveal soft-tissue swelling and periarticular osteopenia.

Jaccoud's arthropathy may affect some patients with SLE. Joint deformities typically are reversible (unlike RA) and radiologic examination is most remarkable for ulnar deviation with minimal joint damage. Jaccoud's arthropathy can be seen in postrheumatic fever, Parkinson's disease, and other connective tissue disorders.

Bone infarcts and avascular necrosis are common in patients with SLE and may be secondary to high-dose or long-term steroids, or simply may be a feature of SLE. Central nervous system (CNS) lupus is one of the 11 criteria used in the diagnosis of lupus. It can take many forms and may present with seizures, psychosis, strokes, and other neurologic symptoms. Magnetic resonance imaging (MRI) sometimes can detect changes consistent with cerebritis or myelitis.

Radiologic Aspects

George B. Greenfield

Systemic lupus erythematosus may involve the joints.[2–4] The changes are typically bilateral and symmetrical nonerosive arthritis.

Peripheral Skeleton. Characteristic findings are seen in the *hands*. Soft-tissue atrophy is severe, with concave rather than convex margins to the thenar and hypothenar borders. Osteoporosis is present with a periarticular or diffuse pattern. Joint effusion and soft-tissue swelling may be seen. Changes include subluxations and malalignment, effusion, osteoporosis, and soft-tissue atrophy. Erosion is typically absent, and joint space narrowing appears only minimally.

The hallmark is ulnar deviation at the metacarpophalangeal joints with the absence of erosions and ease of reversibility (Fig. 3.1). A "boutonniere" or "swan neck" deformity may be present as well as multiple subluxations (Fig. 3.2). Subluxation of the interphalangeal joints of the thumb often is seen. Severe ulnar deviation may exist (Fig. 3.3), resulting in pressure erosion of adjacent bone ends. The de-

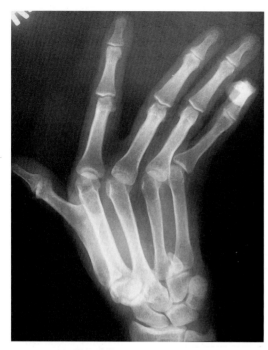

FIGURE 3.1 Systemic lupus erythematosus. Hand. Ulnar deviation at metacarpophalangeal joints is noted. There is atrophy of both thenar and hypothenar musculature giving a concave appearance. Fusion at the first metacarpophalangeal joint from an unrelated cause is also present.

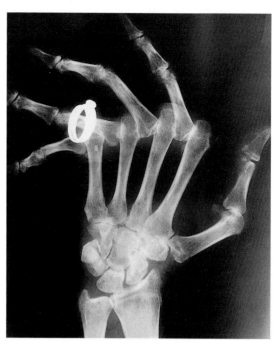

FIGURE 3.3 Systemic lupus erythematosus. Hand. Severe ulnar deviation and subluxation at the metacarpophalangeal joints are seen. No well-defined erosions are present. Osteoporosis is also noted.

formities are caused by neuromuscular weakness, muscle wasting, and contractures (Fig. 3.4), rather than bony erosion and destruction. Sclerosis of the terminal phalanges may also be seen. Resorption of the terminal phalanges may occur in patients with Raynaud's phenomenon.

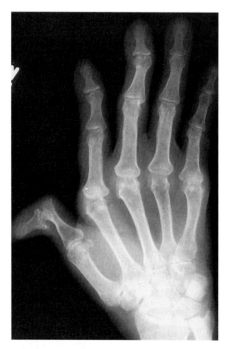

FIGURE 3.2 Systemic lupus erythematosus. AP view of the hand shows subluxation of the thumb. There is also subluxation at the metacarpophalangeal joints.

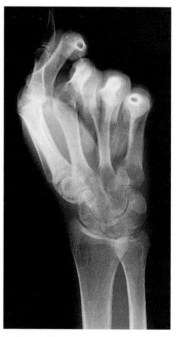

FIGURE 3.4 Systemic lupus erythematosus. Hand. Contractures of all of the fingers are seen.

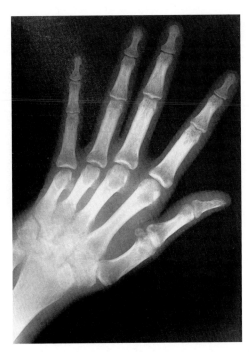

FIGURE 3.5 Systemic lupus erythematosus. Hand and wrist. There has been avascular necrosis of all of the carpal bones. Soft-tissue swelling about the ulnar styloid is present as well as hypothenar atrophy. Periarticular osteoporosis is also seen.

Subchondral cystic lesions in the small joints of the *hands and feet* are thought to be caused by vasculitis.[5] Paraarticular calcification may be seen rarely.

In the *wrist,* avascular necrosis of the scaphoid and metacarpals, as well as in the entire carpus (Fig. 3.5) may occur. This process may be accelerated by steroid therapy.

Ischemic necrosis in the *humeral* and *femoral heads* may be caused by steroid therapy or the primary disease process (Fig. 3.6).[6] This also has been reported in the foot.[6] Periosteal reaction also may occur.[7]

Bilateral spontaneous patellar tendon rupture has been reported as an unusual complication. It can be demonstrated by MRI.[8]

Central Skeleton. The *spine* may show osteoporosis and compression fractures of the vertebral bodies. This may be accelerated by steroid therapy. Atlantoaxial subluxation without erosions may also be present.

Sacroiliitis, both unilateral and bilateral, with increased activity on radionuclide bone scans, has been reported in the active phase of this disease.[9]

Case Reports

Keith Kanik

Case 1. A 36-year-old woman with a history of SLE and Raynaud's phenomenon for 22 years presented for treatment. SLE was diagnosed on the basis of discoid lupus, arthritis, pleurisy, photosensitivity, +ANA and anti-DNA. The patient's radiographs revealed periauticular demineralization and soft tissue calcifications of the right elbow, as well as flexion contractures of the second through fifth MCP joints (Fig. 3.7). Note the marked erosion noted on the distal phalanx of the index finger of the right hand with absorption of the distal tuft.

Case 2. A 59-year-old woman presented with a history of discoid lupus, a positive ANA and recurrent urticaria, who developed rapidly progressive weakness of the right upper and lower extremities. Hyperesthesia was present over dermatomes C-2, C-3, and the mandibular division of the trigeminal nerve. MRI found a cervical cord intramedullary lesion (Fig. 3.8), which responded to intravenous bolus methylprednisolone. Steroids were tapered slowly and discontinued over a 1-month period. Serial MRIs showed improvement of the lesion. The patient had a relapse 1 year later, and MRI showed recurrence in the same area. The pa-

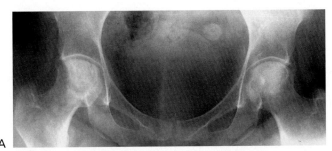
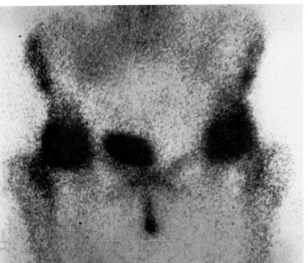

FIGURE 3.6 Systemic lupus erythematosus. **A:** AP view of both hips shows avascular necrosis. **B:** Radionuclide bone scan shows increased activity in both hips.

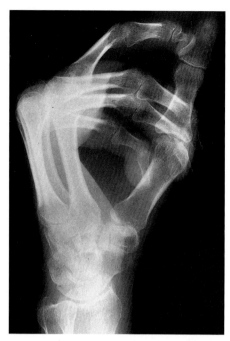

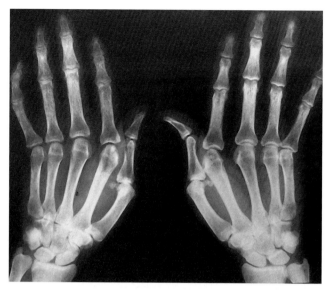

FIGURE 3.9. Jaccoud's arthritis. Ulnar deviation of the fingers bilaterally in seen.

FIGURE 3.7. Systemic lupus erythematosus. Hand. Flexion contractures at the metacarpophalangeal joints 2–5 are noted. There is marked resorption of the distal tuft of the right index finger.

tient was restarted on steroids, and 1 month later Plaquenil and Imuran. The symptoms resolved, and follow-up MRI showed resolution of the lesion. The patient has been tapered off steroids, and is currently asymptomatic on azathioprine and hydroxychloroquine.

JACCOUD'S ARTHRITIS

George B. Greenfield

Jaccoud's arthritis uncommonly follows rheumatic fever during the subsiding stage, resulting in deformity of the hands.[10,11] Periarticular swelling may be seen, most frequently at the metacarpophalangeal joints and occasionally the proximal interphalangeal joints. Ulnar deviation at the metacarpophalangeal joints follows, along with subluxation and flexion deformities (Fig. 3.9). The ulnar deviation is easily reversible in the early stages. Hyperextension at the interphalangeal joints may also be present. The bone is typically not involved, although erosions may follow in some cases. "Hooklike" projections and pseudocysts at the radiopalmar aspects of metacarpal heads may occur rarely.[12] These would have to be differentiated from calcium pyrophosphate deposition disease (CPPD) and hemochromatosis.

SCLERODERMA (PROGRESSIVE SYSTEMIC SCLEROSIS)

Clinical Aspects

Keith Kanik

Scleroderma (progressive systemic sclerosis) is a systemic connective tissue disease that can result in fibrosis of the skin, as well as internal organs. An erosive arthritis with telescoping of digits has been reported. Scleroderma can overlap with other connective tissue diseases such as SLE. When such a patient has a positive Anti-RNP autoantibody, the condition is often labeled mixed connective tissue disease (MCTD).[13]

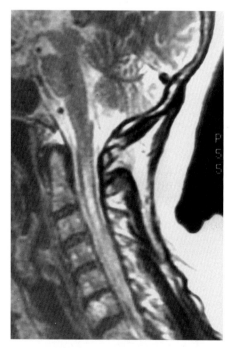

FIGURE 3.8. Systemic lupus erythematosus. MRI. T2-weighted image. High signal intensity is seen in the upper cervical spinal cord indicating transverse myelitis.

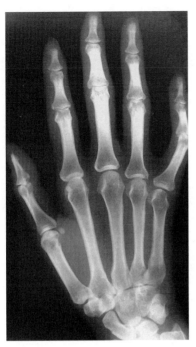

FIGURE 3.10. Scleroderma. Hand. There is resorption of the terminal tufts of the thumb and the index finger, as well as periarticular osteoporosis.

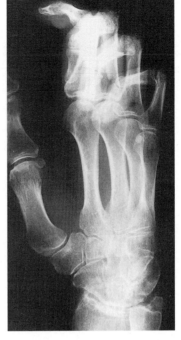

FIGURE 3.12. Scleroderma. Hand. Contractures of the fingers are present.

Radiologic Aspects

George B. Greenfield

Scleroderma is characterized radiologically in the hands by terminal phalangeal resorption (Fig. 3.10) and soft-tissue calcification[14] (Fig. 3.11). Contractures may be present

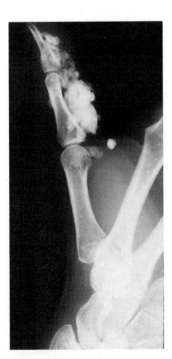

FIGURE 3.11. Scleroderma. Thumb. Extensive soft-tissue calcification along the thumb is noted. The bone is not involved.

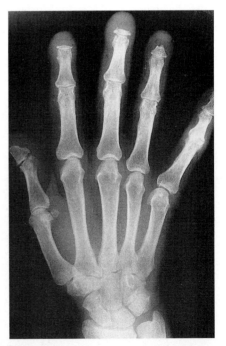

FIGURE 3.13. Scleroderma. Hand. There is resorption of the major portions of the distal phalanges of digits 1–4. Erosive changes and soft-tissue swelling at the proximal interphalangeal joint of the little finger is seen as well as marginal erosions at the proximal interphalangeal joint of the ring finger. The bone density is maintained.

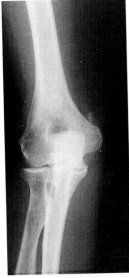
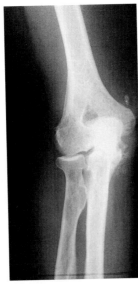
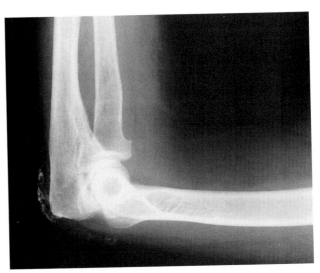

A   B

FIGURE 3.14. Scleroderma. **A,B:** AP, lateral, and oblique views of the left elbow show subcutaneous calcifications at the extensor surface along the ulna.

(Fig. 3.12). In addition, erosive arthritis may rarely be seen. "Pencil-in-cup" deformities of the distal interphalangeal joints have been described, as well as joint space narrowing with bone resorption at the proximal interphalangeal joints (Fig. 3.13). Osteoporosis or bone proliferation may be present. Selective involvement of the first carpometacarpal joint occurs, with erosions and radial subluxation of the metacarpal base.[15] Erosions at the distal ulna and radius may also be seen.[16] Subcutaneous (Fig. 3.14), intraarticular, lig-

amentous, and periarticular calcifications may occur. Osteolysis of the toes, superior margins of the ribs, and mandible is common. Flexion deformities and soft-tissue atrophy also occur.[17] Extensive soft tissue calcifications sometimes may be seen.

Variations include CRST syndrome, which is a combination of calcinosis, Raynaud's phenomenon, sclerodactyly, and telangiectasia; CREST syndrome, which also has esophageal abnormalities in addition to CRST; and

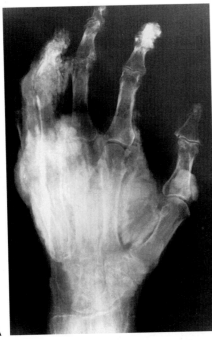
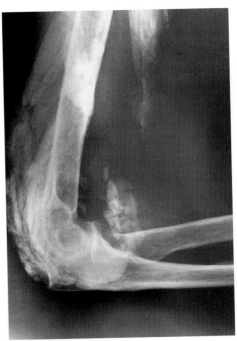

A   B

FIGURE 3.15. CRST syndrome. **A:** Hand showing extensive subcutaneous calcifications. There is also resorption of several terminal tufts. **B:** Elbow showing extensive subcutaneous calcifications.

Thibierge-Weissenbach syndrome, which is calcinosis and digital ischemia.

Case Reports

Kieth Kanik

Case 1. A 20-year-old woman presented with a chief complaint of painful fingertips for several years. Physical examination of the hands revealed loss of distal tufts, sclerodactyly, and color changes consistent with Raynaud's phenomenon. Serological markers showed a high titer ANA, a positive anti-RNP, negative anti-SCL-70 antibody, and negative anticentromere antibody. Radiographs of the hands revealed resorption of distal phalanges consistent with scleroderma (Fig. 3.16).

Calcinosis. Systemic calcinosis is found in CREST syndrome, dermatomyositis (usually only in childhood onset disease), mixed connective tissue disease, and SLE. The typical radiological findings include subcutaneous calcium deposits in areas of frequent friction, trauma, or at sites of inflammation. Treatment of the underlying inflammation can sometimes decrease the calcium buildup.

Case 2: Systemic Calcinosis. A 79-year-old woman presented with painful digits and grotesque nodular calcium deposits throughout her left hand and elbows. Radiographs of the left hand and bilateral elbows revealed extensive soft-tissue calcification, some of which were directed longitudinally and some grouped. Note that patients with such extensive calcifications are prone to false-positive bone scans (Fig. 3.15).

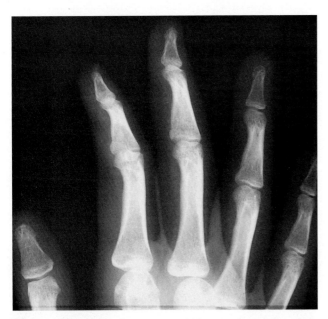

FIGURE 3.16. Hand. Resorption of the terminal tufts of the distal phalanges is seen.

MIXED CONNECTIVE TISSUE DISEASE

George B. Greenfield

Mixed connective tissue disease is considered to be a definitive syndrome with a combination of features of scleroderma, systemic lupus erythematosus, polymyositis, and rheumatoid arthritis.[18–20] Patients possess an antinuclear antibody that reacts with a ribonuclease-sensitive extractable nuclear antigen.

Arthritis has been reported in over 75% of patients. Involvement of the hands show osteoporosis, both periarticular and diffuse. Periarticular soft-tissue swelling, narrowing of the joint spaces, and marginal erosions may be seen. Flexion deformities, subluxation, and marked ulnar deviation of the phalanges also may occur, as well as resorption of the terminal tufts, soft-tissue atrophy, and calcification. "Sausagelike" swelling of one or a few fingers may be seen. The large joints are not involved often. Avascular necrosis of the femoral head has been reported.

PULMONARY HYPERTROPHIC OSTEOARTHROPATHY

Clinical Aspects

George B. Greenfield

Pulmonary hypertrophic osteoarthropathy, is a triad of periosteal new bone formation, clubbing of the fingers, and synovitis.[21] It is associated with a wide variety of pulmonary and pleural diseases, which may be inflammatory or neoplastic.

In adults, the condition is most commonly caused by carcinoma of the lung. In infants and children, it commonly results from cystic fibrosis, and has been reported to be present in 5% of patients. Also, it has been reported as a rare complication of congenital cyanotic heart disease.

Hypertrophic osteoarthropathy has also been reported in aortic graft infection, and unilateral changes have been seen in infected vascular grafts.[22] This entity is different from simple clubbing of the fingers without periostitis or arthritis, which has a much broader range of etiologies. An international workshop has defined this overall condition as hypertrophic osteoarthropathy. The etiologies are primary and secondary, and the grading of severity was delineated.[23]

The triad of clubbing, periostitis, and arthralgia may all be present or may occur in various combinations and in various orders of appearance. The tubular bones show periosteal new bone formation and cortical thickening, most marked at the diaphysis. The bone ends are not involved. At first, the new bone is sharply demarcated from the cortex. As the deposit thickens, the deeper part can merge with the cortex. There is no endosteal deposition of bone. The joints show synovial inflammatory changes and effusion.

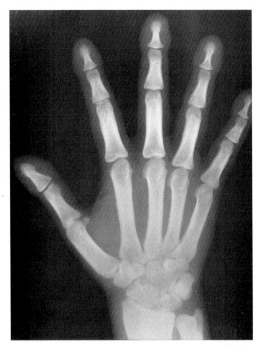

FIGURE 3.17. Pulmonary hypertrophic osteoarthropathy. Clubbing of the fingers is noted.

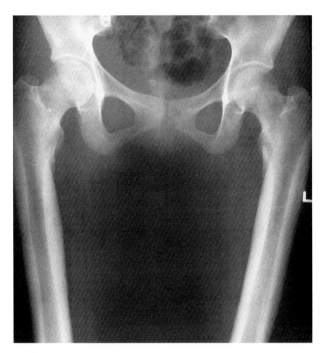

FIGURE 3.19. Long-standing periostitis has resulted in cortical thickening.

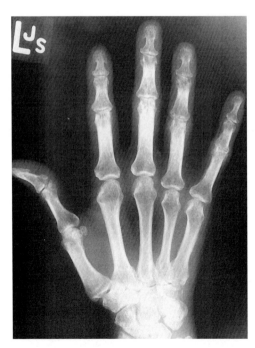

FIGURE 3.18. Pulmonary hypertrophic osteoarthropathy. Hand. This patient had carcinoma of the lung. Marked periarticular osteoporosis is seen, and there are several erosions at the proximal and distal interphalangeal joints. A "spadelike" configuration of the terminal tufts is noted, which would make differentiation from acromegaly difficult. The hand, however, is not enlarged, and the joint spaces are not widened, as would be seen in acromegaly.

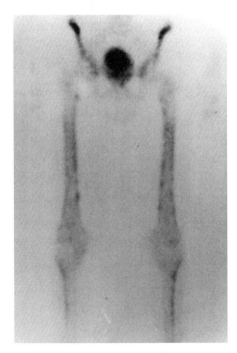

FIGURE 3.20. Pulmonary hypertrophic osteoarthropathy. Radionuclide bone scan showing bilateral increased activity in both medial and lateral aspects of the bony cortex. This is the "double rail" sign.

Radiologic Aspects

Radiologically, soft-tissue signs are clubbing of the fingers with soft-tissue prominence at the terminal tufts (Fig. 3.17). There are most often no bone changes in the distal phalanges; specifically, there is no periosteal new bone and usually not a spadelike configuration as seen in acromegaly; however, this can be seen rarely (Fig. 3.18). Periosteal changes are evident in the diaphyses of the tubular bones, sparing the ends. In decreasing order, the following structures are most frequently involved: the radius and ulna, the tibia and fibula, the humerus and femur, the metacarpals and metatarsals, and the proximal and middle phalanges. Long-standing periostitis results in cortical thickening (Fig. 3.19).

Joint effusions may be seen. No erosions or cartilage destruction occur. Occasionally massive distention of the knee joint can be seen. Acroosteolysis has been reported. The axial skeleton is spared. Radioscintigraphy shows symmetrical distribution of increased activity in the diaphyses of the long bones, with uptake on both sides of the cortex, called the "double rail" sign (Fig. 3.20). These changes can be seen earlier on MRI than on conventional radiography.

HEMOPHILIC ARTHROPATHY

Clinical Aspects

George B. Greenfield

Hemophilia causes intraarticular, intraosseous, and subperiosteal hemorrhages with growth disturbances.[24,25]

This disease is caused by deficiency of a clotting factor. Hemophilia A has a deficiency of factor VIII, and hemophilia B (Christmas disease) has a deficiency of factor IX. Hemophilia A and B are sex-linked recessives and can occur only in males, transmitted by female carriers. Hemophilia C is autosomal dominant and can affect both males and females. It is less severe, and only rarely has bone and joint involvement.[26]

Severe hemarthrosis is unusual in hemorrhagic diseases other than hemophilia. The bleeding is always caused by trauma, unless the plasma clotting factor is at the 1% level. Subcutaneous, intramuscular, intraosseous, intraarticular, and internal hemorrhages occur.[27] Arthropathy is almost always present in adulthood.

Radiologic Aspects

Radiologic changes are most common in the knee, elbow, ankle, hip, and shoulder. These are the joints involved with intraarticular hemorrhages. The small peripheral joints are only rarely involved. Osteoporosis may be periarticular or diffuse. The appearance is similar to JRA, except without ankylosis and periosteal new bone, and with dense surrounding soft tissue. The affected joints tend to hemorrhage recurrently; therefore, the involvement of the various joints is not uniform or symmetric.

Increased radiopacity of the periarticular soft tissue as

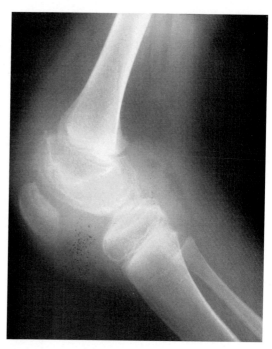

FIGURE 3.21. Hemophilia. A large hemorrhage into the knee capsule is noted, which combined with synovial thickening, causes a marked amount of soft-tissue swelling. There is irregularity at the patellofemoral joint.

well as distension of the joint (Figs. 3.21 and 3.22) is common to all involved joints. The increased density of soft tissue results from deposition of hemosiderin.

Epiphyseal overgrowth is present. Limitation of motion causes disuse osteoporosis. The thickened synovia causes erosions of the articular surface. The cartilage is destroyed

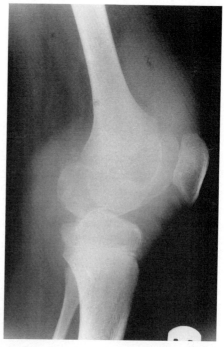

FIGURE 3.22. Knee. Lateral view. Hemophilia. Marked synovial thickening is seen in the suprapatellar and popliteal areas.

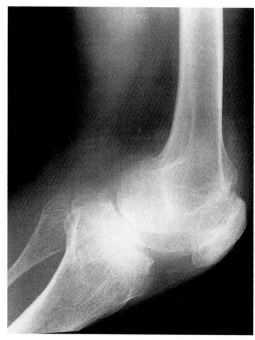

FIGURE 3.23. Hemophilia. Lateral view of the knee showing secondary osteoarthritic changes with narrowing of the patellofemoral joint as well as hypotrophic changes throughout.

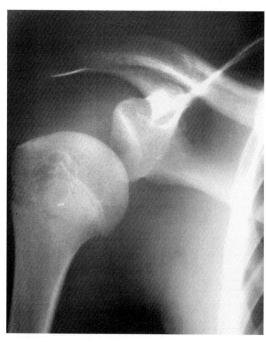

FIGURE 3.24. Hemophilia. Shoulder. Hemorrhage into the shoulder joint has caused widening and a lower position of the humerus. A cyst in the humeral head and neck is noted.

and the joint space narrows. Secondary osteoarthritic changes may develop (Fig. 3.23). Erosions and subchondral cysts may be seen, although hemophilia may exist without subchondral cyst formation. There is accelerated maturation of the epiphyses owing to chronic hyperemia. There is also enlargement of the epiphyses with prominent trabeculae-oriented parallel to the shaft of the bone.

In the *shoulder,* there may be widening of the glenohumeral joint (Fig. 3.24). The humeral epiphysis may be enlarged. Humerus varus is commonly seen because of premature fusion of the physis (Fig. 3.25). Subluxation may occur secondary to hemorrhage.

In the *elbow,* intraarticular hemorrhage is seen as a positive "fat pad" sign, with displacement of fat planes away from the elbow joint, particularly posteriorly. This is followed by chronic synovitis from repeated hemorrhage (Fig. 3.26). Widening of the olecranon fossa and the radial notch of the ulna has been described.[28] The head of the radius may be flattened.

Severe degenerative arthritis of the *hip* also develops in this condition.[29] Hemorrhage may occur into the epiphyseal cartilage, causing slipped epiphyses, premature fusion, and deformity.

In the *knee,* widening of the intercondylar notch caused by hemorrhage at the insertions of the cruciate ligaments and enlargement of the femoral condyles is almost pathognomonic. Erosions caused by hemorrhage at other locations also can be seen (Figs. 3.27 and 3.28). Flattening of the inferior apex of the patella may also occur if the onset of bleed-

ing in the joint was at an early age (Fig. 3.29). The latter finding also can be seen in juvenile rheumatoid arthritis.

In the *ankle,* tibiotalar slant is common (Fig. 3.30). The talus may be flattened. *Intraosseous hemorrhage* causes cystic lesions in bone, which may be large and can mimic neo-

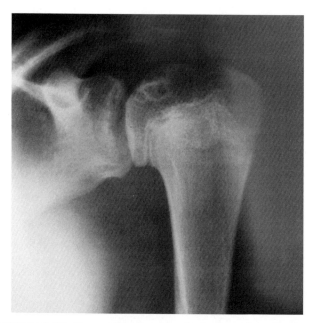

FIGURE 3.25. Hemophilia. Shoulder. Deformity of the humeral head from premature fusion resulting in humerus varus is seen. Cyst formation and erosions of the articular surface are also seen.

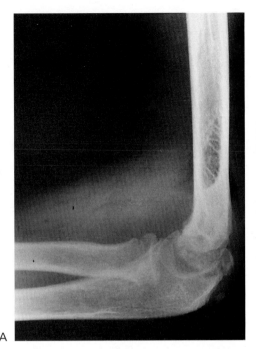
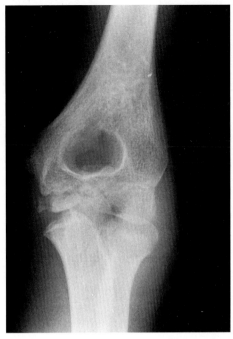

A

B

FIGURE 3.26. Hemophilia. Elbow. **A:** Lateral view shows a positive "fat pad" sign secondary to chronic hemarthrosis. There is also irregularity of the olecranon. **B:** AP view shows widening of the olecranon fossa, irregularity of the trochlea, and enlargement of the capitellum.

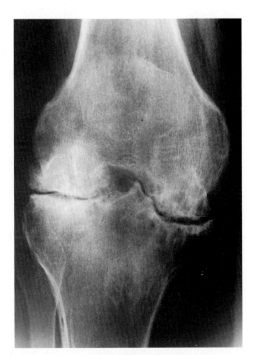

FIGURE 3.27. Hemophilia. Knee. There is marked widening of the intercondylar notch and narrowing of the joint space. Subchondral cyst formation on both sides of the knee joint is also noted.

plasms. This is the hemophilic pseudotumor.[30] Hemophilic pseudotumors may extend from a hemarthrosis under pressure, form from pressure necrosis following intraosseous hemorrhage, or develop from soft-tissue or subperiosteal bleeding with cyst formation. A picture similar to that of avascular necrosis may result if the hemorrhage occurs in an epiphysis.

Subperiosteal hemorrhages are uncommon. If present, a large subperiosteal hematoma causes pressure erosion of the cortex. A Codman's triangle, bone spiculation, and calcification may be seen. This type of hemophilic pseudotumor is most common in the femur and the iliac bone.[31–33] A large area of expansion and destruction with an associated soft-tissue mass is sometimes present. Hemophilic pseudotumors also occur in other long bones, and the hands and feet. It is estimated that 1% to 2% of severe hemophiliacs are affected.

MRI can show early effusion (Fig. 3.31) and details of destruction of cartilage and the synovium. The thickened and irregular synovium with fibrosis and hemosiderin deposition shows low-signal intensity foci on both T1W and T2W images. Hemorrhages and pseudotumors may be evaluated by ultrasound or MRI.[34] The latter has the ability to characterize blood clots and can display multiplanar images.[35]

Chondrocalcinosis has been reported to be associated with hemophilia.[36] Patients with synovial hemangiomas of the knee have been described as showing changes that simulate hemophilic arthropathy.[37] Phleboliths characterize the hemangiomas. Septic arthritis has been reported as a rare complication of hemophilia.[38]

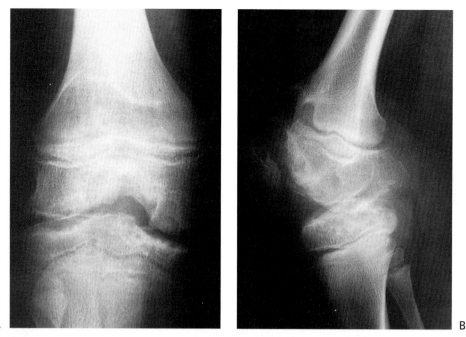

A   B

FIGURE 3.28. Hemophilic arthropathy. Knee. **A:** AP view shows marked erosion at the intercondylar notch and subchondral cyst formation. **B:** Lateral view shows erosions at the distal femoral metaphysis, articular surface of the patella, and cyst formation in the distal femoral and proximal tibial epiphyses. The metaphyseal erosion is seen on AP view as a well-demarcated radiolucency with a superior sclerotic margin involving the entire width of the bone.

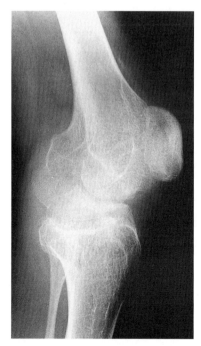

FIGURE 3.29. Hemophilia. The patella has a more squarish appearance at its inferior margin than is normally seen. Irregularities of the articular surfaces of the knee joint are also seen.

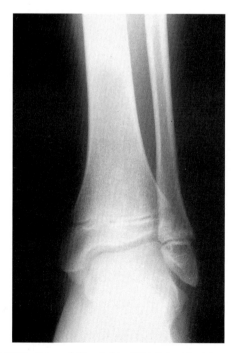

FIGURE 3.30. Hemophilia. Ankle. Tibiotalar slant is noted. This finding may also be seen in juvenile rheumatoid arthritis.

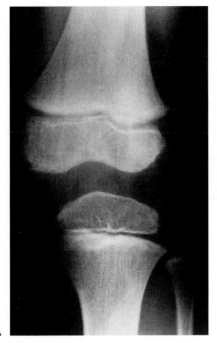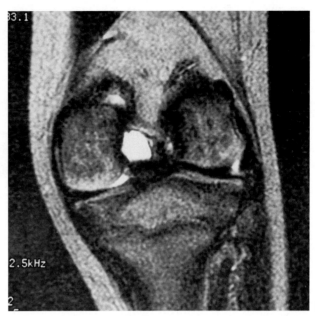

FIGURE 3.31. Hemophilia. **A:** AP view of the knee shows enlargement of the epiphyseal ossification centers. **B:** MRI. T2-weighted image shows knee joint effusion in the intercondylar notch.

MULTICENTRIC RETICULOHISTIOCYTOSIS

George B. Greenfield

Multicentric reticulohistiocytosis (reticulohistiocytoma, lipoid dermatoarthritis) is a rare condition of unknown etiology in which cutaneous xanthomas are associated with erosive arthritis leading to severe deformities.[39–41] Arthritis usually precedes cutaneous changes. *Radiologically,* marginal erosions with articular cartilage and subchondral bone destruction are seen. These are sharply defined with little accompanying osteoporosis. They are bilaterally symmetrical. The distal interphalangeal joints of the hands and feet show early involvement, with proximal interphalangeal joint involvement later. Severe resorption of the digits may follow. The distal clavicle may also show resorption. Other joints may be involved, including the shoulders, elbows, wrists, and hips. The cervical spine may be involved with destruction, resulting in atlantoaxial subluxation. Sacroiliac fusion and ischial erosion also have been described. Soft-tissue masses without calcification are seen also.

SAPHO SYNDROME

George B. Greenfield

SAPHO syndrome represents a combination of synovitis, acne, pustulosis, hyperostosis, and osteitis.[42] It is considered to be a type of seronegative spondyloarthropathy, encompassing several overlapping conditions. The cause is poorly understood. Synovitis in the joints of the upper anterior chest wall is most often seen, including the sternocostoclav-

icular and manubriosternal joints. Unilateral sacroiliitis also may occur. Bony proliferation is most often manifest by sternocostoclavicular hyperostosis, which is characterized by hyperostosis and soft-tissue ossification between the clavicle and anterior part of the upper ribs.[43,44] Radiologically, the clavicles, sternum, and first ribs are enlarged and increased in density. There is ossification of the sternoclavicular and sternocostal junctions.

Phlebography may show subclavian vein occlusion. Histological findings are hyperostosis without osteoclast inclusions. The chief differential diagnosis is Paget's disease. Other ligamentous ossification may be present. Osteitis is also present, with pain, tenderness, and infiltration of bone with inflammatory cells, usually without causative agents found. Chronic recurrent multifocal osteomyelitis may be within this spectrum. The skin manifestations include palmoplantar pustulosis, acne, and pustular psoriasis.

SARCOIDOSIS

Clinical Aspects

George B. Greenfield

Sarcoidosis is a generalized systemic granulomatous disease of unknown etiology involving principally the skin, lungs, lymph nodes, and viscera.[45] Bone involvement occurs in about 10% or more of patients at some time during the course of the disease. The bone lesions have a tendency to regress. Blacks are more frequently affected than whites in the United States. The diagnosis is usually made when a routine chest radiograph of a young asymptomatic adult discloses bilateral hilar and right paratracheal lymphadenopathy associated with pulmonary fibrosis. Children are rarely affected. Hypercalcemia, which regresses to normal values after cortisone administration, may be present. The serum alkaline phosphatase and globulin levels are frequently elevated. The albumin to globulin ratio may be reversed. The osseous lesions of sarcoidosis are characteristically painless. Bone involvement usually occurs in patients with generalized chronic disease and irreversible sarcoidosis in all systems. Bone and chronic skin lesions often are associated. Pseudoclubbing of the fingertips caused by sarcoid dactylitis, as well as true clubbing, may exist.

Radiologic Aspects

Radiologically, the bones most often involved are the middle and distal phalanges of the fingers (Figs. 3.32 and 3.33) and toes; the metacarpals and metatarsals are involved less frequently. Rarely, a lytic lesion may be seen in the epiphysis of a long bone. A diffuse, coarsened trabecular pattern of long bones or the scapula may be present less commonly. The disease may take three forms in the short tubular bones.

Diffuse Sarcoidosis. The contour of the bone is widened with a reticular or honeycomb structure of the spongiosa. There is loss of definition between cortex and medulla.

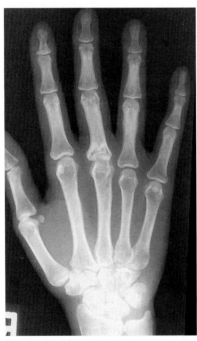

FIGURE 3.32. Sarcoidosis. Hand. There is involvement of the proximal phalanx of the middle finger and the distal phalanx of the index finger. A coarsened trabecular pattern is seen. Resorption of bone at the base of the proximal phalanx of the middle finger is seen involving the metacarpophalangeal joint.

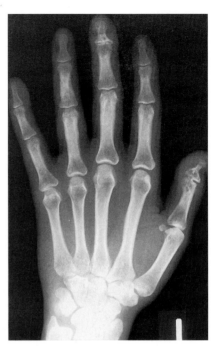

FIGURE 3.33. Sarcoidosis. There is resorption of bone at the distal interphalangeal joint and the distal phalanx of the middle finger as well as resorption of bone at the interphalangeal joint of the thumb with resorption of the terminal tuft of the distal phalanx of the thumb.

Resorption of the terminal tuft also has been observed in rare cases. Very rarely, resorption of the cortex reminiscent of hyperparathyroidism may be seen.

Circumscribed Sarcoidosis. "Punched-out," cystlike lesions up to 5 mm in diameter with a narrow sclerotic rim, as well as small multilocular expanded areas may be seen.

Mutilating Sarcoidosis. The "punched-out" areas may coalesce, forming larger areas of destruction. The cortex may be destroyed. No periosteal reaction, new bone formation, or sequestration is present. The three forms may coexist. Areas of sclerosis in the terminal phalanges may be seen, as may small nodular densities in the medulla of the phalanges and metacarpals. Destructive changes rarely may be found in the nasal bones, calvarium, spine, and pelvis. A small number of cases have been reported involving the spine. One or more vertebrae may be involved. The lesions may be destructive, destructive with collapse, destructive with a sclerotic margin, or sclerotic. The bodies with or without the pedicles may be affected. If more than one vertebral body is involved, the lesions may or may not be adjacent. The disk space is usually preserved, although narrowing has been reported. A paraspinal soft-tissue mass may be associated. This picture may mimic tuberculosis.

Lesions in the skull may occur in association with, or independent of, other bony lesions. The destruction may involve both tables and may be progressive. The lesions may be single or multiple, are characteristically small in size, and show no sclerotic reaction. Diffuse widening of the cervical spinal cord has been reported. Isolated reports of disseminated osteosclerotic lesions of sarcoidosis in the pelvis, femora, vertebrae, ribs, sphenoid, and a terminal phalanx have been published. These changes are rare. Osteosclerosis may be combined with osteolysis. Asymptomatic joint swellings in a child and joint disease in an adult have been reported. Also reported are pathological fracture of the elbow, sarcoid arthritis of the knees with marginal destructive changes, and sarcoid arthritis of the ankle. Involvement of the large joints is very rare.

REFERENCES

Systemic Lupus Erythematosus

1. Tan EM, Cohen AS, Fries JF, et al. The 1982 revised criteria for the classification of systemic lupus erythematosus (SLE). *Arthritis Rheum* 1982;25:1271–1277.
2. Bleifeld CJ, Inglis AE. The hand in systemic lupus erythematosus. *J Bone Joint Surg [Am]* 1974;56:1207–1215.
3. Noonan CD, Odone DT, Engelman EP, et al. Roentgen manifestations of joint disease in systemic lupus erythematosus. *Radiology* 1963;80:837–843.
4. Weissman BN, Rappaport AS, Sossman JL, et al. Radiographic findings in the hands in patients with systemic lupus erythematosus. *Radiology* 1978;126:313–317.
5. Leskinen SH, Skrifvars V, Laasonen LS, et al. Bone lesions in systemic lupus erthematosus. *Radiology* 1984;153:349–352.
6. Resnick D, Pineda C, Trudell D, et al. Widespread osteonecrosis of the foot in systemic lupus erythematosus: radiographic and gross pathologic correlation. *Skeletal Radiol* 1985;13:33–38.
7. Glickstein M, Neustadter L, et al. Periosteal reaction in systemic lupus erythematosus. *Skeletal Radiol* 1986;15:610–612.
8. Gould ES, Taylor S, Naidich JB, et al. MR appearance of bilateral, spontaneous patellar tendon rupture in systemic lupus erythematosus. *J Comput Assist Tomogr* 1987;11:1096–1097.
9. DeSmet AA, Mahmood T, Gobinson RG, et al. Elevated sacroiliac joint uptake ratios in systemic lupus erythematosus. *AJR* 1984;143:351–354.

Jaccoud's Arthritis

10. Murphy WA, Staple TW. Jaccoud's arthropathy reviewed. *AJR* 1973;118:300–307.
11. Twigg HL, Smith BF. Jaccoud's arthritis. *Radiology* 1963;80:417–421.
12. Pastershank SP, Resnick D. "Hook" erosions in Jaccoud's arthropathy. *J Can Assoc Radiol* 1980;31:174–175.

Scleroderma

13. Sharp GC, Irwin WS, May CM, et al. Association of antibodies to ribonucleoprotein and SM antigens with mixed connective tissue disease, systemic lupus erythematosus and other rheumatic disease. *N Engl J Med* 1976;29:1149–1154.
14. Resnick D, Scavulli JF, Goergen TG, et al. Intra-articular calcification in scleroderma. *Radiology* 1977;124:685–688.
15. Resnick D, Greenway G, Vint VC, et al. Selective involvement of

the first carpometacarpal joint in scleroderma. *AJR* 1978;131:283–286.
16. Wild W, Beetham WP. Erosive arthropathy in systemic scleroderma. *JAMA* 1975;232:511–512.
17. Bassett LW, Blocka KLN, Clements PJ, et al. Skeletal findings in progressive systemic sclerosis (scleroderma). *AJR* 1981;136:1121–1126.

Mixed Connective Tissue Disease

18. Lacombe P, Zenny JC, Benhamou L, et al. Memoires originaux. *J Radiol* 1981;62:417–423.
19. O'Connell DJ, Bennett RM. Mixed connective tissue disease: clinical and radiological aspects of 20 cases. *Br J Radiol* 1977;50:620–625.
20. Udoff EJ, Genant HK, Kozin F, et al. Mixed connective tissue disease: the spectrum of radiographic manifestations. *Radiology* 1977;124:613–618.

Pulmonary Hypertrophic Osteoarthropathy

21. Greenfield GB. *Radiology of bone diseases,* 5th ed. Philadelphia: JB Lippincott, 1990.
22. Stevens M, Helms C, El-Khoury G, et al. Unilateral hypertrophic osteoarthropathy associated with aortobifemoral graft infection. *AJR* 1998;170:1584–1586.
23. Martinez-Lavin M, Matucci-Cerinic M, Jajic I, et al. Hypertrophic osteoarthropathy: consensus on its definition, classification, assessment and diagnostic criteria. *J Rheumatol* 1993;20:1396–1397.

Hemophilic Arthropathy

24. Brant EE, Jordan HH. Radiologic aspects of hemophilic pseudotumors in bone. *AJR* 1972;115:525–539.
25. Steel WM, Duthie RB, O'Connor BT. Haemophilic cysts. *J Bone Joint Surg [Br]* 1969;51:614–626.
26. Heller RM, Roloff JS, Kirchner SG, et al. Hemophilia and the female: considerations for the radiologist. *Radiology* 1979;133:601–603.
27. Railton GT, Aronstam A. Early bleeding into upper limb muscles in severe haemophilia. *J Bone Joint Surg* 1987;69:100–102.
28. Perri G. Widening of the radial notch of the ulna: a new articular change in haemophilia. *Clin Radiol* 1978;29:61–62.
29. Gilchrist GS, Hajedory AB, Stauffer RN. Severe degenerative joint disease, mild and moderately severe hemophilia. *JAMA* 1977;238:2383–2385.
30. Gaary E, Gorlin JB, Jamarillo D. Pseudotumor and arthropathy in the knees of a hemophiliac. *Skeletal Radiol* 1996;25:85–87.
31. Brant EE, Jordan HH. Radiologic aspects of hemophilic pseudotumors in bone. *AJR* 1972;115:525–539.
32. Forbes CD, Moule B, Grant H, et al. Bilateral pseudotumors of the pelvis in a patient with Christmas disease: with notes on localization by radioactive scanning and ultrasonography. *AJR Radium Ther Nucl Med* 1974;121:173–176.
33. Grauthoff H, Hoffmann P, Lackner K, et al. Haemophilic pseudotumours and iliac haematomas: radiological and clinical findings. *Fortschritte a/d Gebeit Röntgenstrahlen* 1978;129:614–620.
34. Wilson DJ, Smith-McLardy PD, et al. Diagnostic ultrasound in haemophilia. *J Bone Joint Surg* 1987;69:103–107.
35. Wilson DA, Prince JR. MR imaging of hemophilic pseudotumors. *AJR* 1988;150:349–350.
36. Jensen PS, Putman CE. Chondrocalcinosis and haemophilia. *Clin Radiol* 1977;28:401–405.
37. Resnick D, Oliphant M. Hemophilialike arthropathy of the knee

associated with cutaneous and synovial hemangiomas: report of 3 cases and review. *Radiology* 1975;114:323–326.

38. Wilkins RM, Wiedel JD. Septic arthritis of the knee in a hemophiliac. *J Bone Joint Surg [Am]* 1983;65:267–268.

Multicentric Reticulohistiocytosis

39. Brodey PA. Multicentric reticulohistiocytosis: a rare cause of destructive polyarthritis. *Radiology* 1975;114:327–328.
40. Gold RH, Metzger AL, Mirra JN, et al. Multicentric reticulohistiocytosis (lipoid dermatoarthritis): an erosive polyarthritis with distinctive clinical, roentgenographic, and pathological features. *AJR* 1975;124:610–624.
41. Martel W, Abell MR, Duff IF. Cervical spine involvement in lipoid-dermato-arthritis. *Radiology* 1961;77:613–617.

SAPHO Syndrome

42. Boutin RD, Resnick D. The SAPHO syndrome: an evolving concept for unifying several idiopathic disorders of bone and skin. *AJR* 1998;170:585–591.
43. Prost A, Dupas B, Rymer R, et al. Hyperostose sterno costo claviculaire. *J Radiol* 1980;61:807–812.
44. Resnick D. Sternocostoclavicular hyperostosis. *AJR* 1980;135:1278–1280.

Sarcoidosis

45. Greenfield GB. *Radiology of bone diseases,* 5th ed. Philadelphia: JB Lippincott, 1990, pp. 161–166.

CRYSTAL DEPOSITION AND METABOLIC ERROR DISEASE

The major crystal deposition diseases are gout and pseudogout. Chondrocalcinosis refers to deposition of calcium pyrophosphate in cartilage (CPPD). If this is symptomatic, it is called pseudogout. Calcific deposits also occur in hydroxyapatite deposition disease (HADD), dialysis arthropathy, and certain inborn errors of metabolism.

GOUT

Clinical Aspects

Joanne Valeriano-Marcet

Gout is a disease in which tissue deposition of crystals of monosodium urate occurs. Articular manifestations include recurrent attacks of severe acute or chronic articular and periarticular inflammation. The four stages in the evolution of gouty arthritis include asymptomatic hyperuricemia, acute gouty arthritis, intercritical gout, and chronic tophaceous gout.

Acute arthritis is the most common early clinical manifestation. The first metatarsophalangeal joint is involved most frequently. Other commonly affected joints include the ankle, tarsal area, and knee.[1]

The first attack is most commonly monarticular. The affected joint is warm, red, tender, and extremely painful. Early attacks tend to subside over 3 to 10 days even when untreated. Patients are usually symptom-free following the acute attack. Subsequent episodes may increase in frequency, last longer, and may be polyarticular.

Intercritical Gout. The intercritical periods are those between attacks. Early in the course of disease the intercritical periods are symptom-free and may last months to years. With recurring attacks, the intercritical periods become shorter, and eventually the recovery between acute attacks becomes incomplete.

Chronic Tophaceous Gout. Tophi containing deposits of monosodium urate crystals occur in fairly advanced gout. They appear an average of about 10 years after the first episode of arthritis.[2] Deforming arthritis can develop as a result of erosion of cartilage and subchondral bone caused by the chronic inflammatory reaction and crystal deposition. The chronic arthritis may mimic RA, although it tends to be less symmetric.

Laboratory Findings. The diagnosis of acute gouty arthritis depends on the detection of intracellular monosodium urate crystals. Serum urate levels may be misleading because they can be normal during the face of an acute attack. The crystals are needle-shaped and visible with the light microscope. Definitive diagnosis relies on the use of the polarizing microscope. Monosodium urate crystals are highly negatively birefringent. Synovial fluid leukocytes are elevated from 20,000 to 100,000 cells/mm^3 in acute gouty arthritis with a predominance of neutrophils.

In almost all cases, a serum uric acid level will be elevated at some time. Measurements are important in following treatment. A 24-hour urine uric acid measurement helps to determine the risk of renal stones, to elucidate underlying predisposing factors, as well as to determine types of treatment. Laboratory tests also help to rule out other gout-associated diseases, including renal insufficiency, hyperlipidemia, and diabetes.

Radiologic Aspects

George B. Greenfield

Gout (podagra) is a condition of hyperuricemia with deposition of monosodium urate crystals.[3,4] It can be caused by

**TABLE 4.1. DISEASES ASSOCIATED WITH
SECONDARY GOUT CAUSED BY EXCESSIVE
BREAKDOWN OF NUCLEOPROTEINS**

Anemia
Glycogen storage disease[5]
Hemoglobin E disease[6]
Leukemia
Lymphoma
Multiple myeloma
Myelofibrosis
Polycythemia
Psoriasis
Renal failure

overproduction of uric acid or a failure of renal excretion of uric acid. If overproduction of uric acid is caused by an inherited enzyme defect or has an unknown etiology, the process is referred to as *primary gout.*

If overproduction can be explained on the basis of excessive breakdown of nucleoproteins in diseases such as those listed in Table 4.1, the process is termed *secondary gout.*

Decreased renal excretion of uric acid may result from the diseases listed in Table 4.2, and is also termed secondary gout.[7] Secondary gout produces radiographic changes less often than primary.

Uric acid is a purine. All known uric acid in the body is derived from the oxidation of xanthine. Humans lack hepatic uricase, which catalyzes the production of soluble allantoin from relatively insoluble uric acid. The major portion of uric acid must be excreted by way of the kidneys. The principal organs affected are the joints, kidneys, and heart.

In the joints, monosodium urate crystals are deposited in cartilage and the synovia. They can be identified in synovial fluid microscopically as needle-shaped, 2 to 10 microns in length, and strongly negatively birefringent on polarized microscopy. These crystals cause an inflammatory reaction forming tophi, which range up to several centimeters in size, and are deposited in cartilage, synovia, bone, ligaments,

**TABLE 4.2. DISEASES ASSOCIATED WITH
SECONDARY GOUT CAUSED BY DECREASED
RENAL EXCRETION OF URIC ACID**

Alcoholism
Chronic renal disease
Diuretics
Glycogen storage disease type 1
Hyperparathyroidism
Hypoparathyroidism
Lead nephropathy (saturnine gout)
Low-dose salycilates
Myxedema
Pyrazinamide
Starvation

bursa, and subcutaneous tissues. They cause extensive erosion in joints and destruction of bone. They may become calcified.

Primary gout is transmitted as an autosomal dominant with low penetrance in women. Only 5% to 10% of cases occur in women, where it occurs postmenopausally. Gout is less common in Blacks than in whites.

The clinical stages of primary gout are: asymptomatic hyperuricemia, which usually occurs during puberty; acute gouty arthritis, which occurs 20 to 30 years later; then chronic tophaceous gout, which occurs about another decade later.[8,9] Juvenile gout is rare.

Radiologically, the joints most often involved are the foot, ankle, hand, wrist, elbow, and knee. Destructive changes are seen in only about one-half of patients. They can be extremely destructive. They occur late in the course of the disease, usually 6 to 8 years after the onset of symptoms. The distribution is asymmetrical.

Common to all joints, early acute changes are joint effusion and swelling. Soft-tissue swelling is usually localized, but may involve an entire digit. Osteoporosis does not usually occur, but gout may occur in a patient with osteoporosis (Fig. 4.1). A lacelike erosion may be seen as an early change, with a fine striated or spiculated pattern of periosteal reaction along the cortex adjacent to a soft-tissue tophus, which abuts the bone. The joint space may be normal, osteoarthritic, or there may be uniform narrowing of the joint. There may be paraarticular, marginal, and sub-

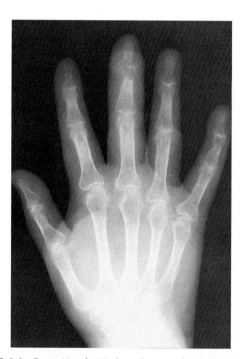

FIGURE 4.1. Gout. Hand. AP view shows a destructive lesion at the distal interphalangeal joint of the middle finger and a destructive intraosseous lesion at the base of the fifth metacarpal. Uniform osteoporosis is present. There is also soft-tissue swelling of the entire middle finger.

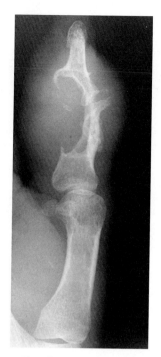

chondral erosions. These lesions are cystlike or "punched-out"; they have a sharp margin with a thin sclerotic rim, usually with little surrounding reactive sclerosis, and are associated with little regional osteoporosis until late stages. They show sharp overhanging margins (Fig. 4.2). A large expansile tophus, or a subchondral cyst, may at times also be seen.[10]

Periosteal reaction also may be present. One important feature distinguishing gout from other arthritides is the presence of destructive lesions in bone that are remote from the articular surface. The margins are well defined, in contrast to RA, where they are usually less well demarcated. Calcification within tophi may occur at times. Calcifications are usually in the soft tissues (Fig 4.3), but may also be intraosseous.[11] Severe bony destructive lesions follow. Bony ankylosis may occur. Secondary osteoarthritis may develop.

The lesions are usually asymmetrical; however, a bilateral symmetrical distribution may be seen on rare occasion (Fig. 4.4).

FIGURE 4.2. Gout. Thumb. A large lytic lesion is seen on both sides of the interphalangeal joint with sharp overhanging margins. A large amount of soft-tissue swelling representing a tophus is seen.

Peripheral Skeleton. The *hand* is involved with a random distribution of lesions (Figs. 4.5, 4.6, and 4.7). There may or may not be narrowing of the joint spaces. Local osteoporosis does occur in later stages. There is no ulnar deviation of the fingers. Terminal phalangeal resorption and flexion

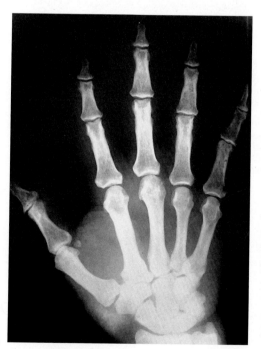

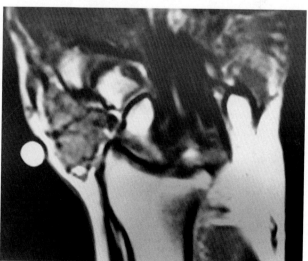

A   B

FIGURE 4.3. Gout. **A:** AP view of the hand shows a soft-tissue tophus adjacent to the first carpometacarpal joint containing a large amount of calcification. There is no evidence of bony involvement. **B:** MRI. T1-weighted image shows the gouty tophus as an inhomogeneous mixed signal intensity soft-tissue mass. The irregular signal void corresponds to the calcification.

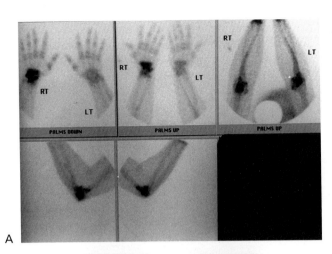

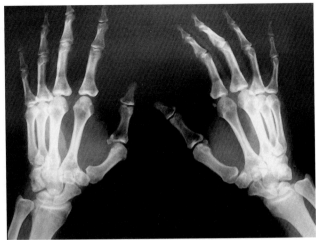

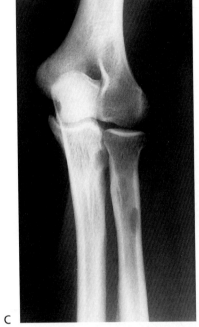

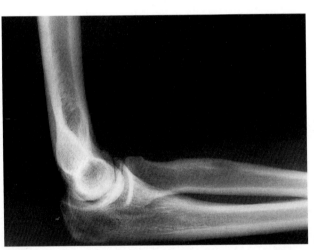

FIGURE 4.4. Gout with symmetrical distribution. **A:** Radionuclide bone scan showing increased activity in both wrists, the right greater than the left, and both elbows. **B:** Oblique views of both wrists show bilateral "punched-out" lesions in the carpal bones, more on the right than on the left. **C:** AP view of the right elbow shows radiolucencies in the proximal radius and ulna. **D:** Lateral view of the elbow shows a destructive area at the olecranon as well as a radiolucency in the proximal radius.

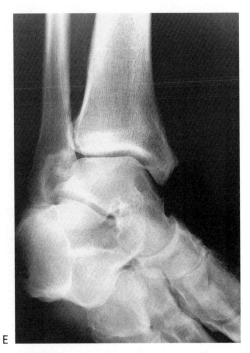
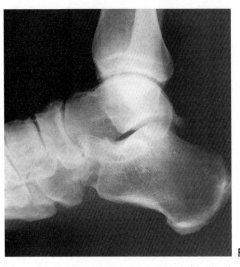

E

F

FIGURE 4.4. *(continued)* **E:** Mortise view of the right ankle shows a destructive area at the distal fibula. **F:** Lateral view of the right ankle shows a destructive area at the distal calcaneus.

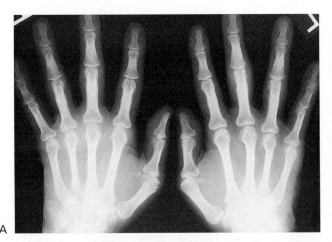
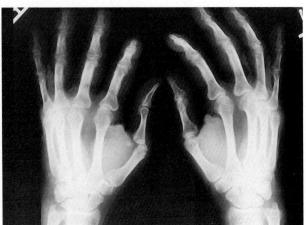

A

B

FIGURE 4.5. Gout. Hands. **A,B:** AP and oblique views of both hands. On the right side, erosions at the distal first metacarpal are seen. Periarticular osteoporosis of fingers at other than the involved site is noted. On the left side, erosions and soft-tissue swelling at the proximal interphalangeal joint of the left middle finger are noted, as well as a sharply marginated erosion at the fifth metacarpal head. Soft-tissue swelling around the wrists bilaterally is also seen.

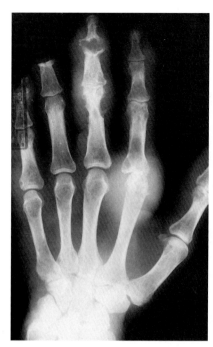

FIGURE 4.6. Gout. Hand. Extensive destructive changes of the middle finger are seen as well as multiple soft-tissue tophi. There has been an amputation of the distal phalanx of the ring finger from an unrelated cause.

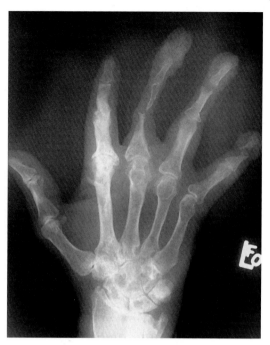

FIGURE 4.8. Gout. Hand and wrist. There has been resorption of the distal phalanx of the middle finger and a neurotrophic-like appearance of the middle finger. Resorption at the distal interphalangeal joints of the ring and little fingers is seen. Soft-tissue tophi are present. There is sclerosis of the index finger with fusion of the proximal interphalangeal joint, and osteoarthritis at the first metacarpophalangeal joint. Lytic lesions in the wrist are seen and there is a lytic lesion in the ulnar notch.

deformities also may occur (Fig. 4.8). Severe deformities of the hands with telescoping of the digits may occur during treatment, owing to rapid resorption of osseous tophi that are not replaced by bone matrix.[12]

The *wrist* shows a tendency to involve the carpometacarpal compartment (Figs. 4.9, 4.10), although pan-

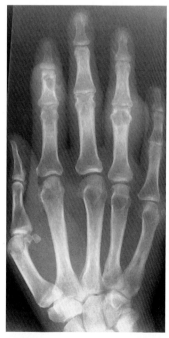

FIGURE 4.7. Gout. Hand. Lytic lesions with thin sclerotic margins are seen associated with soft-tissue tophi. The lesion in the middle phalanx of the index finger is not at the articular surface. Periosteal new bone formation at that site is noted.

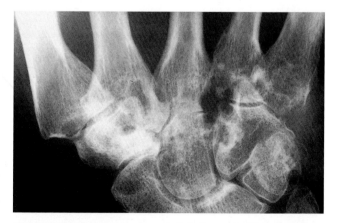

FIGURE 4.9. Gout. Wrist. Osteolytic lesions principally in the carpometacarpal region are seen. Some have no margin, some have a sclerotic margin, and dense reactive sclerosis in the trapezium is noted. A small amount of periosteal new bone formation at the base of the third metacarpal is seen.

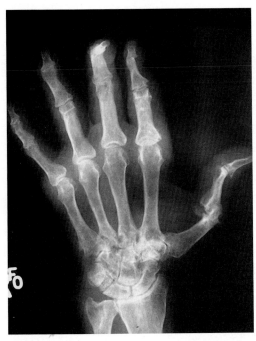

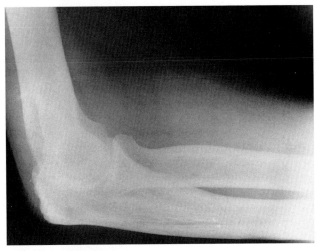

FIGURE 4.12. Gout. Elbow. Erosion at the olecranon is seen. The bony density is maintained.

FIGURE 4.10. Gout. There is carpometacarpal involvement of the wrist as well as a lytic lesion in the distal ulna. Changes in the hand include marginal erosions, secondary osteoarthritis in the thumb, and contractures of the distal phalanges of the index and middle fingers.

carpal involvement also may occur. The distal radius and ulnar styloid may also be affected. Erosions and soft-tissue swelling are seen. If the ulnar styloid is involved, the sharp margination of the erosion will help to differentiate this condition from RA (Fig. 4.11).

The *shoulder* is rarely involved, possibly because of lack of pressure in the glenohumeral joint.

In the *elbow,* a tophus is not uncommonly seen posterior to the olecranon process, where erosion or spur formation may occur (Figs. 4.12 and 4.13). Unilateral or bilateral olecranon bursitis may be present.

In the *hips,* avascular necrosis of the femoral heads and medullary bone infarcts may occur.

The *knees* may show tophi and effusion, but more often show a picture of osteoarthritis. At times, chondrocalcinosis is present, which is a concurrent or resultant manifestation of CPPD. Rupture of the quadriceps tendon with

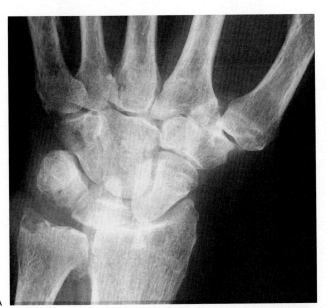

A

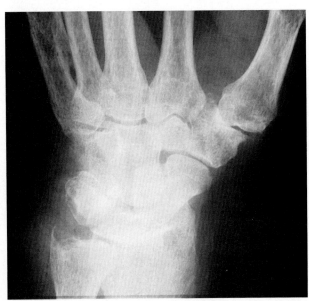

B

FIGURE 4.11. Gout. Wrist. **A,B:** AP and oblique views of the wrist shows an erosion at the ulnar styloid process as well as an erosion at the distal radius. Soft-tissue swelling representing a tophus is seen adjacent to the ulnar styloid process. The erosion is sharply marginated with an overhanging edge. An adjacent erosion of the triquetrum is also seen. The fifth metacarpal is also involved.

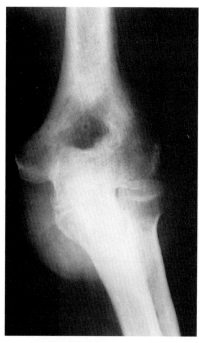

FIGURE 4.13. Gout. Elbow. A large tophus is seen and there is erosion at the radial side. Periarticular osteoporosis is noted as well as periosteal new bone formation at the distal humeral metaphysis on the radial side.

downward displacement of the patella has been reported.[13] A synovial popliteal cyst may develop, similar to that seen in RA.[14] It may dissect down the leg and clinically simulate deep vein thrombosis.[15]

The *ankles* are commonly affected and show tophi and erosions. The tarsal bones, and especially the tarsometatarsal joints, are typically involved. Destruction at the latter site may be severe.

The hallmark location of gout is in the *foot* at the metatarsophalangeal joint of the great toe (Fig. 4.14). In the acute stage, it is exquisitely tender. The interphalangeal joint of the great toe follows, but all joints may be involved (Figs. 4.15, 4.16, and 4.17). At the first metatarsophalangeal and interphalangeal joints, the tophus is usually dorsally situated, causing erosions or bony reaction on those surfaces (Fig. 4.18). Hallux valgus is usually present. A large destructive area with an overhanging margin may be present, or a large expansile calcified lesion. Considerable reactive sclerosis around the tophus may be seen. Osteoporosis occurs at this stage. Osteoarthritis also may be present. Erosion of a terminal tuft may occur (Fig. 4.19).

Central Skeleton. Rarely, the *spine* may be involved. Narrowing of the intervertebral disc and end plate erosion, as well as erosion of the odontoid process and atlantoaxial subluxation, may rarely occur.

Changes in the *sacroiliac joints* are not uncommon.[16] They include sclerosis, marginal irregularity, erosions (Fig. 4.20) and cystlike lesions with sclerotic margins. Obliteration of the

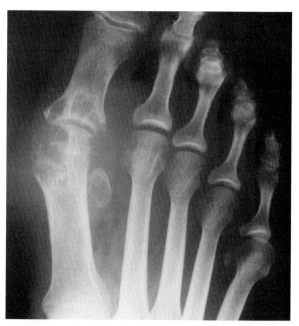

FIGURE 4.14. Gout. Advanced changes in the first metatarsophalangeal joint with marked destruction and soft-tissue swelling are noted. A cyst in the sesamoid bone is also seen.

joint space has been described. Osteoarthritis may also be present. The *symphysis pubis* may also be involved.

A series of patients was reported with onset of gout in adolescence. In the rare cases of juvenile gout, growth disturbances of the long bones owing to epiphyseal injury have

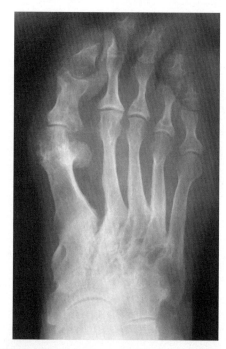

FIGURE 4.15. Gout. Foot. Erosions, hallux valgus, and subluxation at the first metatarsophalangeal joint are seen. Erosions at the second and third metatarsophalangeal joints are also noted. Erosions and fusion in the tarsus are present. There is marked osteoporosis.

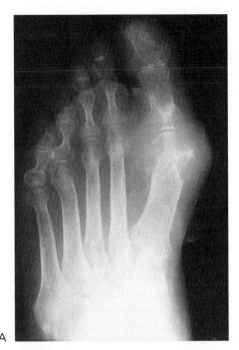
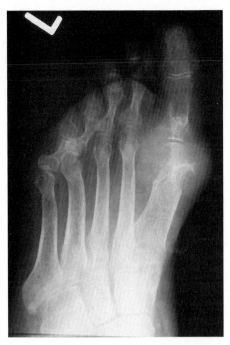

A   B

FIGURE 4.16. Gout. Foot. **A,B:** AP and oblique views of the foot show advanced destructive changes at the first metatarsophalangeal joint with sharply marginated lesions and overhanging edges. A large soft-tissue tophus and soft-tissue swelling are also present. Diffuse osteoporosis is seen. This is an 87-year-old woman with uric acid level of 10.7 mg %.

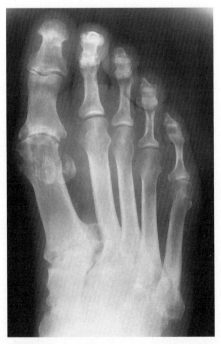

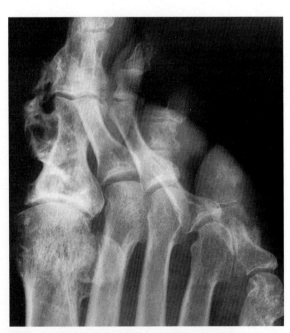

FIGURE 4.17. Gout. Foot. Erosions at the first metatarsophalangeal joint are seen with hallux valgus. Erosions also at the fifth metatarsophalangeal joint are seen. Osteoarthritic changes and erosions at the articular surfaces at the first tarsometatarsal joint are seen, as well as involvement with joint space narrowing of the joints of the tarsus.

FIGURE 4.18. Gout. Oblique view of the toes shows that there is a tophus at the dorsum of the interphalangeal joint of the great toe and a large amount of bony reaction that has resulted in bridging within the tophus. There is also erosion at the distal first metatarsal.

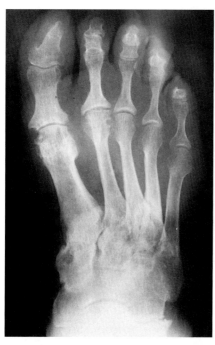

FIGURE 4.19. Gout. Foot. Extensive involvement of the distal tarsal bones and the tarsometatarsal joints are seen as well as erosions at the first and second tarsometatarsal joints. There is resorption of the terminal phalanx of the great toe.

been described. Chronic synovitis rather than tophus deposition may rarely predominate in gout. RA is then simulated with joint space narrowing.[17] The coexistence of gout and rheumatoid arthritis in the same patient is extremely rare.[18] Quadriceps tendoyrupture, as well as gouty tophi have been

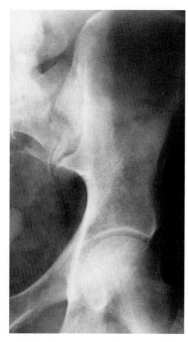

FIGURE 4.20. Gout with chronic renal failure. Sacroiliac joint. Erosions and calcification within the sacroiliac joint are seen.

reported in the periosteum overlying a compression plate in the tibia.[19,20] A radiologic appearance of the hands with erosions similar to those of gout has been described in lymphoma cutis.[21]

Lesch-Nyhan syndrome, a rare syndrome of hyperuricemia and mental retardation in children, is caused by total deficiency of the enzyme hypoxanthine-guanine phosphoribosyltransferase. It is transmitted by a recessive gene on the X chromosome, and thus only occurs in male children. There is a characteristic pattern of mental retardation and abnormal aggressive behavior, with self-mutilation by biting of the fingers and lips, choreoathetosis, hyperuricemia, and uric acid nephrolithiasis. *Saturnine gout* is a form of secondary gout caused by decreased renal urate clearance owing to lead nephropathy.[22] It usually affects patients with chronic lead toxicity owing to the ingestion of illegal alcohol. The radiological features of saturnine gout are similar to those of primary gout. Radioopaque material within several joints that resembles milk of calcium has been reported in this condition. Aspiration revealed a combination of monosodium urate and calcium pyrophosphate dihydrate.

Case Reports

Joanne Valeriano-Marcet

Case 1 (Gout Presenting as RA). In a patient with an acute presentation of monarthritis, synovial fluid aspiration and visualization under polarized microscopy will differentiate crystal versus septic arthritis. In a patient who presents with chronic arthritis, aspiration of a tophus with the demonstration of urate crystals will confirm the diagnosis of gouty arthritis. In situations where joint or tophus aspiration is not possible, routine radiographs may support the diagnosis of gout over RA or another chronic arthritis. Gout can be seen to progress, particularly in a patient with neglected treatment (Fig. 4.21).

Case 2. A 52-year-old man with a history of gout for 15 years was admitted with 3 weeks of swelling in multiple joints. His left knee had been severely swollen for several months. The patient was noncompliant with allopurinol and colchicine.

Physical Examination. Multiple soft tissue masses over the olecranon, first metatarsophalangeal (MTP) joints bilaterally, and marked swelling and warmth of the left knee were present. Swelling and tenderness of both ankles, first and several other MTP joints, and wrists bilaterally were also seen.

Laboratory Findings. Left knee aspiration revealed many WBCs with intracellular uric A crystals. The patient was treated with corticosteroid for his acute polyarticular gout with some improvement.

Imaging. Radiographs of the hands were obtained (Fig. 4.22).

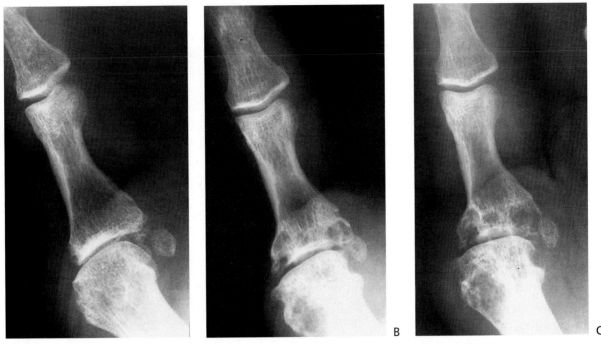

A   B   C

FIGURE 4.21. Gout. **A,B,C:** Progress of erosions at the first metacarpophalangeal joint is seen.

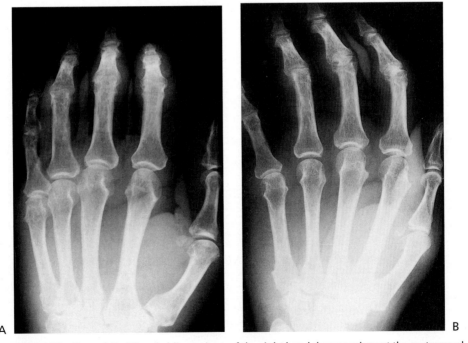

A   B

FIGURE 4.22. Gout. **A,B:** AP and oblique views of the right hand show erosions at the metacarpal heads.

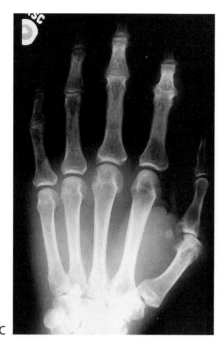
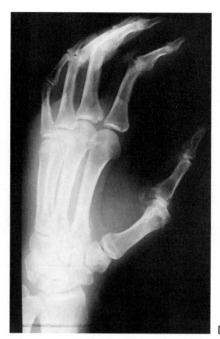

FIGURE 4.22. *(continued)* **C,D:** AP and oblique views of the left hand show irregular erosions around the metacarpophalangeal joint of the thumb.

MRI of the knee was obtained for evaluation of persistent pain and swelling in the left knee (Fig. 4.23).

CHONDROCALCINOSIS

Clinical Aspects

Joanne Valeriano-Marcet
Calcium pyrophosphate deposition disease (CPPD) is a disease state associated with calcium pyrophosphate dihydrate crystal deposition. Chondrocalcinosis refers to the abnormal calcifications in or around joints, and calcification of articular hyaline cartilage and fibrocartilage. Cases of CPPD can be classified as sporadic (idiopathic), hereditary, or secondary. A number of secondary associations exist. CPPD has varied clinical presentations that have been classified by McCarty into six patterns (Table 4.3). For classification of CPPD cases see Table 4.4.

Laboratory Findings. Routine blood chemistries and urine determination are normal in the sporadic or familial forms of the disease. It is important to exclude underlying metabolic disease at the time of initial diagnosis. Serum calcium, phosphorus, alkaline phosphatase, iron, iron binding capacity/saturation, and magnesium determinations help to exclude hyperparathyroidism, hemochromatosis, hypophosphatasia, and hypomagnesium. Definitive diagnosis of CPPD is on the basis of synovial fluid analysis with the demonstration of intracellular CPPD crystals using polarized microscopy (Table 4.5). Synovial fluid findings vary depending on the degree of

TABLE 4.3. PATTERN OF PRESENTATION OF CPPD CRYSTAL DEPOSITION DISEASE

Pattern	Presentation
Type A (pseudogout)	Acute or subacute arthritis attacks, duration 1–2 days, or several weeks Knees most commonly affected. Monarticular or polyarticular
Type B (pseudorheumatoid)	Subacute or chronic synovitis of large joints, especially knees, wrists, and elbows
Type C and D (pseudoosteoarthritis)	C: Low-grade arthralgias and degenerative changes are associated with superimposed acute attacks D: Chronic symptoms without acute exacerbations
Type E (lanthnic form)	Most common form. Calcium deposition is noted as a coincidental observation on radiograph involving asymptomatic joints
Type F (pseudoneurotrophic)	Severely destructive disease similar to changes described in Charcot's joints

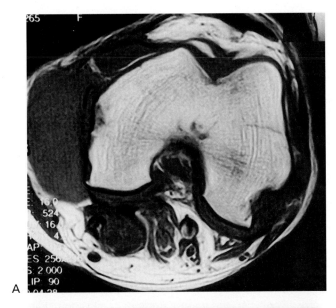

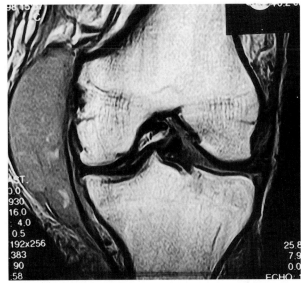

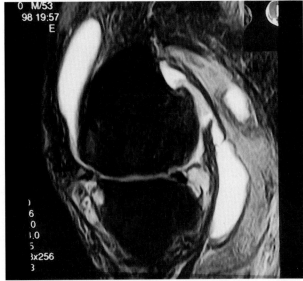

FIGURE 4.23. Gout. Knee. MRI. **A:** T1-weighted axial image shows a large tophus medially eroding the cortex to a slight degree. **B:** Protein density coronal image shows the extent of the tophus along with a small amount of cortical erosion in the medial femoral epiphysis. **C:** T2-weighted sagittal image showing knee joint effusion as high signal intensity.

TABLE 4.4. CLASSIFICATION OF CPPD AND POSSIBLE DISEASE ASSOCIATIONS

Sporadic (idiopathic)
Hereditary
Secondary
  Strong association: hyperparathyroidism, hemochromatosis, hypomagnesemia, aging
  Likely association: OA, amyloid, Barter's syndrome, hypocalciuric hypercalcemia

TABLE 4.5. DIFFERENTIATION OF CALCIUM PYROPHOSPATE DIHYDRATE CPPD AND MONOSODIUM URATE (MSU)

	CPPD	MSU
Shape	Rhomboid	Needle shaped
Birefringence	**Weak or absent**	**Strong**
(Direction)	Positive	Negative

inflammation. White blood cell (WBC) count may approach that seen in septic arthritis, 100,000.

The radiographic finding of chondrocalcinosis in a patient with chronic inflammatory polyarthritis or a more acute polyarthritis or monarthritis may raise the possible diagnosis of CPPD, but synovial fluid aspiration is required for definitive diagnosis. The differential diagnosis of patients presenting with the Type A form of CPPD disease includes septic arthritis, thus making synovial fluid analysis obligatory to rule out an infectious process

Radiologic Aspects

George B. Greenfield

Chondrocalcinosis refers to the deposition and presence of calcification in hyaline articular cartilage or fibrocartilage in the form of calcium pyrophosphate.[23] Chondrocalcinosis may be associated with several different conditions, summarized in Table 4.6. One or several joints may be involved. It may be asymptomatic or there may be a crystal-induced synovitis called pseudogout. The symptoms may simulate other arthritides.

Pseudogout Syndrome. Pseudogout is a common crystal-induced acute or chronic synovitis and arthritis.[26–30] The crystals in the synovial fluid are calcium pyrophosphate dihydrate, which can be identified under polarized light microscopy. They show weak positive birefringence, are rhombic or rod-shaped, and are shorter than urate crystals. Effusions contain both extracellular and intracellular crystals. The middle and older age groups are usually affected.

Pseudogout syndrome is a metabolic disturbance consisting of excessive production or impaired degradation of pyrophosphate. A low concentration of pyrophosphate is normally present in plasma. Pyrophosphatase rapidly transforms pyrophosphate to orthophosphate. Inhibition of

the activity of this enzyme by divalent ions of calcium, iron, or copper leads to crystal deposition. Pseudogout may be clinically confused with rheumatoid arthritis or gout.[31] It may be present without radiographically visible calcifications.

Radiologically, chondrocalcinosis is characterized by the presence of calcification in intraarticular fibrocartilage, hyaline cartilage, articular capsule, and periarticular soft tissues, including tendons, ligaments, and bursae. The triceps, quadriceps, and Achilles are the tendons more commonly involved. More than one joint is usually involved, and the distribution is often bilaterally symmetric. The knees are very frequently involved. The wrists, metacarpophalangeal joints, hips, symphysis pubis, sacroiliac joints, and lumbar intervertebral discs are commonly involved, and any joint may be affected, including the shoulder, elbow, and ankles.[32,33]

Common to all joints, the fibrocartilage shows a characteristic punctate and linear pattern of calcification. This includes the menisci of the knee, the triangular cartilage of the wrist (Fig. 4.24), fibrocartilage of the acetabular and glenoid labra, and the symphysis pubis. Hyaline articular cartilage appears as a delicate radiopaque line paralleling the articular cortex (Fig. 4.25).

In the early stages, there is relatively little osteoporosis; however, in the predelicted age group, an underlying osteoporosis may be present.

A distinctive type of associated osteoarthritis occurs with uniform narrowing of the joint space. There is subchondral sclerosis, cyst formation, and osteophytes, with a bilateral distribution. Giant cysts and pathological fractures also may occur.[34,35]

The process may progress to extensive collapse and fragmentation of subchondral bone, resulting in fragmentation

TABLE 4.6. CONDITIONS ASSOCIATED WITH CHONDROCALCINOSIS

Significant for CPPD crystal deposition
    Hemochromatosis
    Hyperparathyroidism[24]
Incidental to CPPD crystal deposition
    Acromegaly
    Diabetes mellitus
    Gout
    Hemophilia
    Hypomagnesemia[25]
    Hypophosphatasia
    Ochronosis
    Osteoarthritis
    Rheumatoid arthritis
    Senescence
    Systemic lupus erythematosus
    Wilson's disease

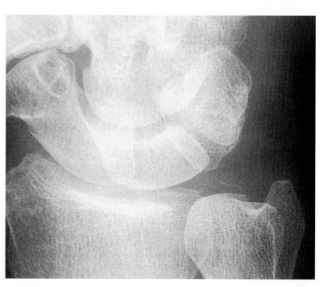

FIGURE 4.24. CPPD. Wrist. A fine thin line in the triangular fibrocartilage distal to the ulna.

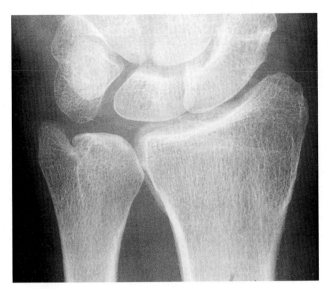

FIGURE 4.25. CPPD. Wrist. A fine thin calcific line in the hyaline articular cartilage is seen in the proximal carpal row.

and joint disintegration, with multiple intraarticular loose bodies. This is seen most often in the knees, hips, talocalcaneal joints, glenohumeral joints, and cervical spine.

Periarticular calcific deposits, which may be large and often associated with erosions, may occur and are termed tumorous or tophaceous pseudogout.[36,37]

Peripheral Skeleton. In the *hands,* flattening of the metacarpal heads, with sclerosis, cyst formation, and narrowing of the joint space can be seen. Capsular calcification is common. Hooklike osteophytes at the radial side of the metacarpal heads are characteristic (Fig. 4.26). An identical

picture in the metacarpophalangeal joints may be present in hemochromatosis. The interphalangeal joints are usually spared, except for possible joint space narrowing and periarticular calcification. (Fig. 4.27).

In the *wrist,* there is a tendency toward involvement of the radiocarpal compartment. The radial articular surface has a characteristic erosion with a "reverse 3" contour (Fig 4.28). Large cysts in the distal radius and ulna may also occur. Calcification in the triangular fibrocartilage (Fig. 4.29) and the lunatotriquetral ligament and cartilage are commonly seen, as well as between the scaphoid and lunate.[38]

Calcification in the first carpometacarpal joint may also occur (Fig. 4.30). Destructive arthritis with carpal bone separation and osteonecrosis simulating neuropathic arthropathy may occur, particularly in the wrists.[39]

The *shoulder* can show chondrocalcinosis. The disease may progress to marked osteoarthritis, with joint space narrowing, subchondral sclerosis, and osteophyte formation. Acromioclavicular arthritis may also be present.

The *elbow* may also develop chondrocalcinosis and osteoarthritis.

The *hip* is frequently involved. Early signs are calcification of the hyalin cartilage paralleling the articular surface. The glenoid labrum and the capsule may also show calcification. There is uniform loss of articular cartilage with resultant medial migration of the femoral head, as in RA

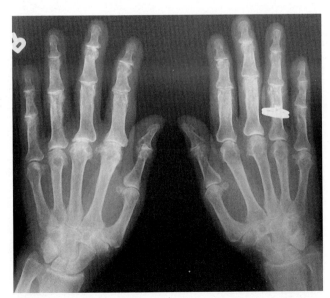

FIGURE 4.26. Pseudogout. Hands. "Hooklike" osteophytes present at the metacarpal heads bilaterally. Osteoarthritic changes are also seen.

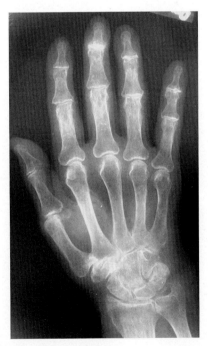

FIGURE 4.27. Pseudogout. Hand and wrist. There is calcification in the triangular fibrocartilage distal to the ulna. Narrowing of the interphalangeal joints is present, and there is osteoarthritis at the distal interphalangeal joint of the middle finger. Diffuse osteoporosis is also seen.

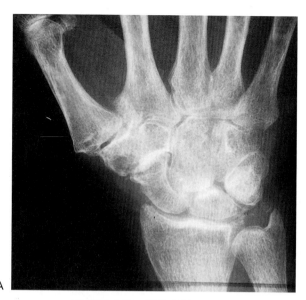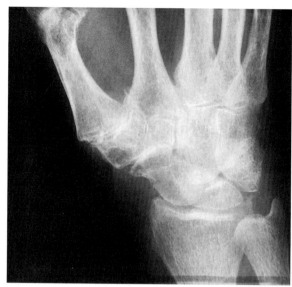

FIGURE 4.28. CPPD. Wrist. **A,B:** AP and oblique views of the wrist reveal involvement of the radiocarpal joint with erosion of the articular surface in a "reverse 3" appearance. Erosions at the trapezium is also seen.

(Fig. 4.31). Osteoarthritis follows with subchondral sclerosis and cyst formation.

This disease shows a predilection for the *knees,* where chondrocalcinosis in the articular cartilage and the menisci is present. The latter are seen as coarser triangular deposits (Figs. 4.32, 4.33, 4.34, and 4.35).

Osteoarthritis occurs, with narrowing often of the medial compartment (Fig. 4.36), but eventually the lateral compartment as well.

Only the patellofemoral joint may be initially narrowed,

and is a clue to suggest CPPD. This joint may show complete cartilage loss and dense subchondral sclerosis (Fig. 4.37). In cases with advanced cartilage loss, calcification may be difficult to visualize. Calcification of the gastrocnemius tendon is then an accurate marker of chondrocalcinosis.[40] Subchondral cysts, particularly in the knee, can attain large size. Medial femoral condyle necrosis may also occur.[30]

The *ankle* and *foot* also may show changes of chondrocalcinosis and osteoarthritis. The talonavicular joint may be involved.

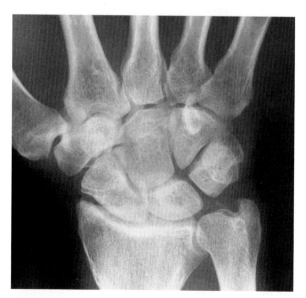

FIGURE 4.29. Pseudogout. Wrist. Calcification in the triangular fibrocartilage is seen as well as erosion and subchondral sclerosis of the radial articular surface.

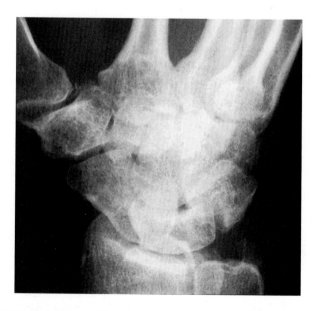

FIGURE 4.30. Calcification in the first carpometacarpal joint is seen.

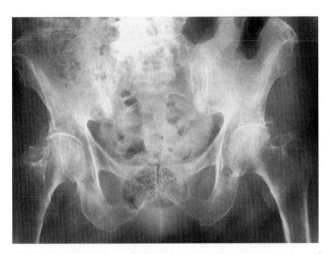

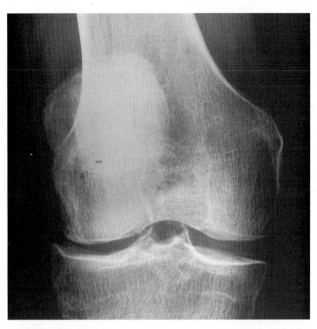

FIGURE 4.31. AP view of the pelvis. Pseudogout. Narrowing of the medial aspects of both hip joint spaces are seen with medial drift of the femoral heads. There is chondrocalcinosis in both hip joints. The symphysis pubis shows a thin vertical line of calcification. Osteoarthritis in both sacroiliac joints is seen. Degenerative changes in the lower lumbar spine and in the lumbosacral region are also noted. There is also calcification in Cooper's ligament.

FIGURE 4.32. Chondrocalcinosis. Knee. Hyaline cartilage calcification is noted principally in the medial compartment. Osteoarthritis is also seen.

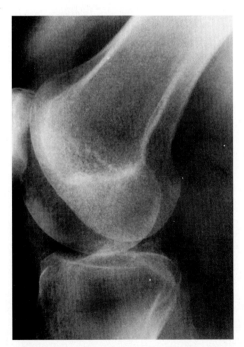

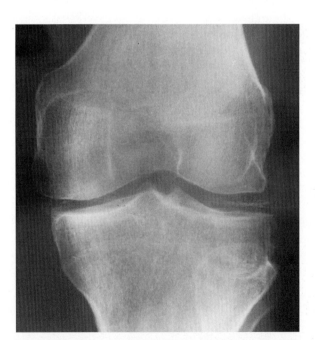

FIGURE 4.33. Chondrocalcinosis. Knee. Lateral view. Calcification in the posterior horn of the meniscus is seen as a punctate and linear pattern.

FIGURE 4.34. Pseudogout. Knee. Linear calcification in the lateral compartment of the knee joint is noted, and triangular calcification of the meniscus in the medial compartment is also seen.

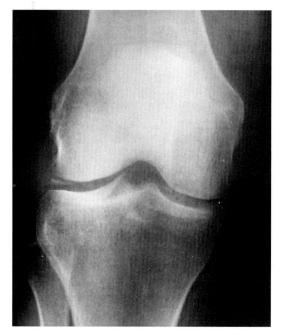

FIGURE 4.35. Pseudogout. AP view of the knee shows triangular calcifications within the menisci.

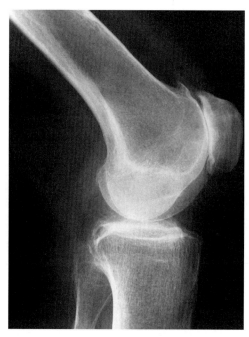

FIGURE 4.37. Pseudogout. Marked narrowing of the patellofemoral joint with subchondral sclerosis and spur formation is noted. Chondrocalcinosis in the posterior aspect of the knee joint is seen with meniscal calcification.

Central Skeleton. In the spine, particularly the cervical spine, involvement may be severe with intervertebral disc calcification and vertebral body and intervertebral space destruction. Calcification in the syndesmoodontoid region may be seen.[41] Atlantoaxial subluxation, anterior osseous

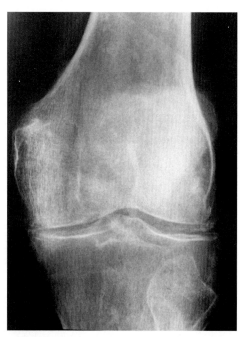

FIGURE 4.36. Pseudogout. AP view of the knee shows calcification in the menisci and in the hyaline articular cartilage. There has been narrowing of the medial compartment of the knee joint space consistent with osteoarthritis.

fragmentation, and apophyseal joint changes may also occur. Calcification of the transverse ligament may be seen.[42] A calcified mass with spinal cord displacement at the craniovertebral junction has also been reported in this condition.[43] Tophaceous pseudogout in the atlantoaxial joint with progressive cervical cord compression has been reported.[44] Odontoid fractures may occur.[45] Multiple levels of intervertebral disc degeneration associated with vacuum signs and calcifications around the disc and annulus fibrosus, end plate sclerosis, and osteophytes may occur throughout the spine. Intervertebral disc calcification is often seen in the annulus fibrosus.

The *sacroiliac joints* may show osteoarthritis.

The *symphysis pubis* may show a thin vertical linear calcification.

Calcification may also be present in the pinna of the ear. Chondrocalcinosis may be seen following surgery or trauma to the involved joint in a younger age group.[46]

Case Report

Joanne Valeriano-Marcet

A 74-year-old woman presented for treatment. She had been well until 7 months prior, when she developed right shoulder discomfort and pain in the MCPs (metacarpophalangeal joints). One month later a diagnosis of rheumatoid arthritis was made, and the patient was given prednisone 20 mg daily. Over the ensuing 5 months the patient noted pain and swelling in the wrists, dorsum of the hands, and knees. She denied any other significant joint complaints. Her symptoms would flare with a decrease in prednisone to 15 mg or lower. Methotrexate had been added to her regimen, without improvement of symptoms.

Physical Examination. The physical examination was remarkable for marked erythema, warmth and swelling of both wrists, and puffiness over the dorsum of the hands.

Laboratory Findings. WBC 9.2, Hgb 12, plt 469k, nl SGOT, SGPT, GGTP, alkaline phosphatase, Ca 9.7 nL, phosphorous 3.8 (nl), RF 66 (20), and ESR 81 (30).

Radiograph of the wrist revealed chondrocalcinosis. Aspiration of the wrist was performed and examination under polarized microscopy showed intracellular CPPD crystals.

The patient was tapered off the prednisone and started on a nonsteroidal antiinflammatory drug (NSAID) with improvement of symptoms. In this situation, the definitive diagnosis of pseudogout (CPPD), allowed more appropriate treatment of the patient.

CALCIUM HYDROXYAPATITE AND BASIC CALCIUM PHOSPHATE DEPOSITION DISEASE

Clinical Aspects

Joanne Valeriano-Marcet

***Basic Calcium Phosphate Crystal Deposition Disease.*[47–51]** Basic calcium phosphate crystal deposition disease (BCP) crystals include hydroxyapatite (HA) octacalcium phosphate, and tricalcium phosphate. Several articular and periarticular syndromes have been described in association with BCP crystals (Table 4.7).

In the shoulder, the rotator cuff may develop primary or secondary calcifications owing to degenerative enthesopathy. The deposits tend to be reabsorbed over time. Periarticular calcifications are found most commonly around the shoulder, but have been described near many other joints. Most cases of acute calcific periarthritis occur as a single attack, in a single joint with localized warmth, erythema, swelling, and pain for up to a few weeks. Hydroxyapatite pseudopodagra presents as acute inflammation in the first MTP joint, usually in young women. Radiographs usually show periarticular calcific deposits that later disappear. Familial occurrences of calcific arthritis and periarthritis have been described.

BCP crystals may be found in cartilage and synovium and have been associated with chronic and acute arthritis. Recurrent episodes of pain and swelling may be associated with gradual erosion and destructive changes in MCP, PIP, and wrist joints.

Milwaukee shoulder syndrome is a progressive destructive shoulder arthropathy, usually bilateral, in elderly wo-

TABLE 4.7. BASIC CALCIUM PHOSPHATE CRYSTAL ASSOCIATED JOINT DISEASE

Calcific periarthritis
    Unifocal
    Multifocal
    Familial
Calcific tendinitis and bursitis, Intraarticular BCP, arthropathies
    Acute goutlike attacks
    Milwaukee shoulder/knee syndrome
    Erosive polyarticular disease
    Mixed crystal deposition disease (BCP and CPPD)
Secondary BCP crystal arthropathies/Periarthropathies
    Chronic renal failure
    "Collagen" disease (calcinosis)
    Sequel to severe neurologic injury
    Postlocal corticosteroid injection
    Other
Tumoral calcinosis
    Hyperphosphatemic
    Nonhyperphosphatemic

From McCarty DJ, Halverson PB. Basic calcium phosphate (apatite, octacalcium phosphate, tricalcium phosphate) crystal deposition diseases in arthritis and allied conditions, 12th ed. Philadelphia. Lea & Febiger, 1993: 1857–1872, with permission.

men. Symptoms are variable but range from asymptomatic to severe pain. Radiographic features include glenohumeral joint degeneration, soft tissue calcification, and upward subluxation of the humeral head. Synovial fluid findings include low leukocyte counts and BCP crystal aggregates. The knee joint may also be involved with preferentially lateral compartment narrowing.

Radiographically, BCP crystal deposits are rounded or fluffy calcifications varying from a few millimeters to several centimeters in diameter. They may occur in solitary or multiple deposits.

Alizarin red staining of synovial fluid pellets may help as a screening tool for diagnosis of BCP crystals. Phase contrast polarized light microscopy is not useful in identifying BCP crystals, because their size is below the limits of resolution of optical microscopy. Electron diffraction, high resolution, TEM, and FTIRM spectroscopy are useful research tools but are not practical for daily clinical use.

Radiological Aspects

George B. Greenfield

Hydroxyapatite deposition disease (HADD) is a common cause of periarticular disease, such as in the rotator cuff tendon or the trochanteric bursa. The symptoms include acute pain and swelling. Hydroxyapatite may also be deposited intraarticularly, but without the typical appearance of chondrocalcinosis, unless there is associated CPPD. Osteoarthritis is often associated. The disease may be either primary or secondary. Conditions associated with secondary HADD include collagen vascular disease, renal failure, and osteoarthritis.

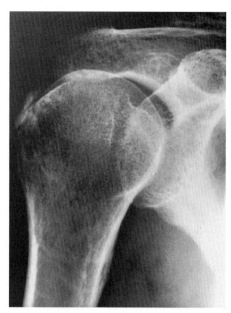

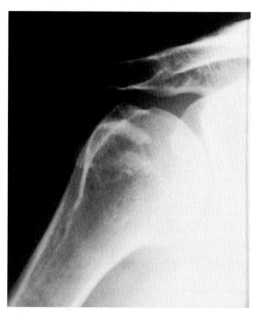

FIGURE 4.38. Hydroxyapatite deposition disease. Shoulder. Calcification in the rotator cuff tendon is noted.

FIGURE 4.40. Hydroxyapatite deposition disease. Shoulder. Calcifications adjacent to the humeral head are seen.

The picture may range from monarticular periarthritis to destruction. The shoulder is primarily affected. Other joints that may be involved include the hip, knees, wrists, hands, ankles, and feet, as well as the longus colli muscle. There may be simultaneous HADD and CPPD in the same joint.

Radiologically, amorphous calcifications around or within joints, tendons (Figs. 4.38, 4.39, and 4.40), or bursae may be seen, and may change in size over time. Synovial and

capsular calcification may occur. The joint space becomes narrowed, followed by subchondral sclerosis and destructive changes. Osteophytes and subchondral cysts are not prominent unless there is associated osteoarthritis. There may be polyarticular disease with joint erosions and destruction.

In the *shoulder,* there can be destruction of the rotator cuff tendon with subsequent elevation of the humeral head and erosion of the acromioclavicular area. This can progress

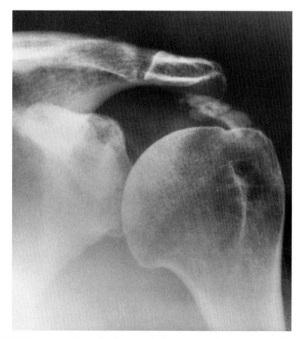

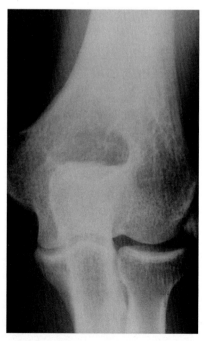

FIGURE 4.39. Hydroxyapatite deposition disease. Shoulder. Calcification of the rotator cuff tendon as it inserts onto the greater tuberosity is seen.

FIGURE 4.41. Hydroxyapatite deposition disease. Elbow. Amorphous dense calcification adjacent to the lateral epicondyle of the humerus is noted.

to rapid destruction with bloody effusion and calcium deposition, known as Milwaukee shoulder syndrome. Rapid destruction of the shoulder chiefly affects elderly women.[52]

The metacarpophalangeal joints may be involved. Calcifications about the elbow may occur (Fig. 4.41).

Destructive arthropathy may also occur in the knees.

Reports suggest that repeated intraarticular injections of steroids in osteoarthritic patients possibly induce or accelerate the deposition of hydroxyapatite. Periarticular calcifications have been reported following these injections.[53]

HEMOCHROMATOSIS

George B. Greenfield

Hemochromatosis is a rare chronic disease of iron overload in which excess iron is deposited in parenchymal tissues.[54–58] It may be inherited or acquired. It may be owing to a deficiency of hepatic xanthine oxidase. It is associated with HLA-A3, HLA-B7, and HLA-B14. The male to female ratio is 10 to 1, and it usually occurs in the 40- to 60-year age group. The classic findings are liver cirrhosis and "bronze diabetes."

The mechanism of joint involvement is that synovial deposition of iron inhibits pyrophosphatase activity, and the deposition of calcium pyrophosphate dihydrate in cartilage follows.

Twenty to 50 percent of patients show radiologically detectable bone and joint changes.

Radiologically, the joint findings are osteoporosis, chondrocalcinosis, and a distinctive arthropathy.

Diffuse osteoporosis occurs, not periarticular as seen in RA. Chondrocalcinosis owing to deposits of calcium pyrophosphate dihydrate in hyaline cartilage and fibrocartilage is a frequent finding.

Hyaline cartilage calcification in the shoulders, elbows, hips, knees, and ankles may be present. The calcification in articular cartilage is seen as a thin radiopacity paralleling the articular surface. Fibrocartilage calcification in the menisci of the knees, the triangular ligament of the wrist, and the pubic symphysis is seen. Calcification in hyaline cartilage is said to be more marked in patients with hemochromatosis than in patients with chondrocalcinosis.

In the *hands,* arthritic changes are frequently seen in the metacarpophalangeal joints, typically symmetrically distributed in the second and third rays. The findings are joint space narrowing, subarticular cysts and erosions, "hooklike" osteophytes from the medial aspects of the heads of the metacarpals, sclerosis and irregularity of the articular surface, subluxations, and flattening and widening of the metacarpal heads (Fig. 4.42).

Initially, a subarticular cyst 1 to 3 mm in diameter appears in a metacarpal head, bounded by a sclerotic rim. Small marginal osteophytes may develop. The width of the joint space may be reduced, usually but not necessarily, in a uniform manner.

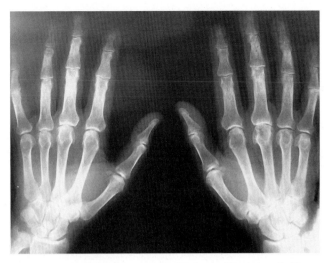

FIGURE 4.42. Hemochromatosis. AP view of both hands. There is narrowing of several metacarpophalangeal joint spaces. Flattening of several metacarpal heads is also seen bilaterally. Bilateral "hooklike" osteophytes are noted throughout. Narrowing of several interphalangeal joint spaces is also seen. No cartilage calcifications are noted.

CPPD would be difficult radiologically to differentiate from hemochromatosis, because similar metacarpophalangeal arthritis and cartilage calcification may be seen. The destruction and neuropathic appearance that may occur in pseudogout does not occur in this condition.

In the *wrist,* cysts may also be present in the carpal bones and the ulnar styloid. Any compartment may show joint space narrowing and sclerosis.

The *hips* and *shoulders,* in addition to chondrocalcinosis, may rarely show avascular necrosis of the femoral and humeral heads. In the shoulder, a medial osteophyte may also be seen (Fig. 4.43).

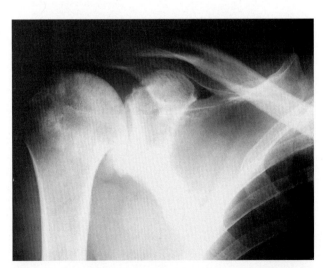

FIGURE 4.43. Hemochromatosis. AP view of the shoulder shows sclerosis of the humeral head indicating avascular necrosis. There is narrowing of the joint space and a large inferior osteophyte of the humeral head as well as a smaller osteophyte at the inferior aspect of the glenoid.

In the *hips,* uniform joint space narrowing is seen with cyst formation, marginal spurs, and chondrocalcinosis.

In the *knee,* narrowing of the medial compartment and the patellofemoral joint may occur, along with cartilage calcification. Synovial iron deposits have also been described.

In the *spine,* syndesmophytes and calcification in the longitudinal ligaments of the lumbar spine, and in the soft tissues around the heel have been reported.[59]

OCHRONOSIS

George B. Greenfield

Ochronosis is a rare inborn error of metabolism in which pigmentation of connective tissue occurs along with alkaptonuria.[60,61] It is caused by complete deficiency of the enzyme homogentisic acid oxidase, which converts homogentisic acid to malylacetoacetic acid, in the metabolic pathways of phenylalanine and tyrosine. All patients do not develop ochronotic arthropathy. In some patients, a dark yellow pigment is deposited in cartilage and connective tissue, causing pigmentation, degeneration, and calcification. The peak incidence of arthropathy is in the fifth decade, with a ratio of 2 to 1 men to women. Ochronotic spondylosis and intervertebral disc involvement is more common than peripheral arthropathy.

In the *peripheral joints,* osteoarthritis occurs. The most commonly involved joints are those of the knees, shoulders, and hips (Fig. 4.44). Joint effusion precedes osteoarthritis.

In the *knee,* there is uniform loss of joint space with secondary osteoarthritic changes. Calcification of the menisci may rarely be present.

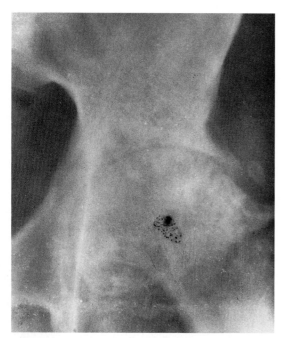

FIGURE 4.44. Ochronosis. Hip. Uniform narrowing of the joint space, flattening of the femoral head, hypertrophic spurring at the acetabular margin, and dense sclerosis are seen.

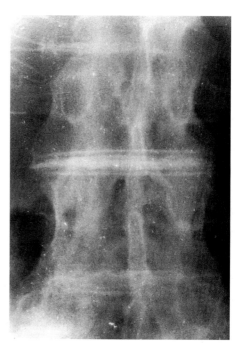

FIGURE 4.45. Ochronosis. Lumbar spine. There is narrowing of the intervertebral discs with dense calcification within.

In the *hip,* joint space narrowing, femoral head erosions, flattening, fragmentation, osteophyte formation, and remodeling of the acetabulum may occur.[62] Calcified loose bodies and ligamentous ossifications also may occur.

In the *shoulder,* narrowing of the glenohumeral joint space occurs. There may be flattening and fragmentation of the humeral head.

Rupture of the Achilles tendon has been reported.

The *hands* and *feet* are not usually involved.

In the *spine* the lumbar region is often initially affected, followed by the thoracic and cervical spine. Intervertebral space narrowing occurs with dense calcification from deposition of calcium hydroxyapatite (Fig. 4.45). Vacuum signs at multiple intervertebral discs may be present, as well as end plate sclerosis. Osteoporosis is diffuse. Osteophytes are mild, but may be prominent in late stages. Calcification of the interspinous ligament has also been described. Kyphosis and scoliosis may occur. The apophyseal joints are not involved.

The *sacroiliac joints* show osteoarthritis with sclerosis on both sides of the joint, bilaterally and symmetrically.

AMYLOID ARTHROPATHY AND DIALYSIS ARTHRITIS; ARTHROPATHIES IN CHRONIC RENAL FAILURE

Clinical Aspects

Joanne Valeriano-Marcet

Uremia and hemodialysis predispose to osteodystrophy, tendinitis, tendon rupture, carpal tunnel syndrome, and several forms of arthritis and periarthritis (Table 4.8). Erosive arthropathy occurs in the small joints of the hands

TABLE 4.8. ARTHROPATHIES ASSOCIATED WITH CHRONIC RENAL FAILURE

Erosive arthropathy
  Hands (Z [secondary] hyperparathyroidism)
  Large joints (especially shoulders)
  Axial skeletal
  Erosive azotemia arthropathy (large and small joints and renal osteodystrophy)
Crystal deposition
  Monosodium urate monohydrate
  Calcium pyrophosphate dihydrate
  Calcium oxalate
  Aluminum phosphate
B2 Microglobulin amyloid
  Carpal tunnel syndrome
  Bone cysts

From McCarty DJ, Halverson PB. Basic calcium phosphate (apatite, octacalcium phosphate, thricalcium phosphate crystal deposition diseases in arthritis and allied conditions, 12th ed. Philadelphia. Lea & Febiger, 1993: 1857–1872, with permission.

and has been ascribed to secondary hyperparathyroidism. The axial and large joints, and especially the shoulder, may also develop erosive changes.[63] An erosive arthritis of large and small joints with noninflammatory synovial fluid has been described in association with renal osteodystrophy, and has been termed erosive azotemia arthropathy.[64]

Amyloid. B2 microglobulin amyloid deposits in the articular and periarticular tissues of dialysis patients.[65] Carpal tunnel syndrome, which is the most frequent presentation of B2 microglobulin amyloidosis, occurs with an excessive frequency in patients with end stage renal disease (ESRD).[66] Many of these cases result from deposition of B2 microglobulin into the flexor tendon sheath with a resultant compressive neuropathy. Deposition in the flexor tendon sheath may result in a permanent flexion deformity of the digits, and may become palpable. This usually becomes clinically apparent after only 5 years of dialysis, and occurs with increasing frequency as the time on dialysis increases.

Chronic arthropathy owing to B2 microglobulin amyloid deposition may present deposit as chronic arthralgias (especially shoulders), chronic joint swelling, finger tenosynovitis, large subchondral bone erosions (particularly hand and wrist), and destructive arthropathy. The frequency of dialysis arthropathy increases with the length of patient survival. Deposition of amyloid in and around the rotator cuff results in a progressive limitation of shoulder abduction and pain. A "shoulder pad" sign may develop as these deposits continue to enlarge. These often accompany amyloid filled bone cysts in the humeral heads.[67]

The skeletal manifestations of B2 microglobulin amyloidosis are typically cysts that occur in the knees, hips, shoulders, elbows, ankles, and digits. The cysts can become sufficiently large to compromise the bone structure and result in pathologic fractures. This is especially common in the hip.[68]

Renal transplantation may be beneficial in patients with the B2 microglobulin amyloid arthropathy. Therapeutic op-

tions include surgical removal of amyloid deposits or the use of NSAIDs.[69–71]

Crystal Induced Arthritis. Crystal induced arthritis is common in uremia. Hyperuricemia predisposes to gout. Basic calcium phosphate (BCP) crystals form in or around joints and in other tissue in the face of excess calcium and phosphates. Hyperparathyroidism has been associated with CPPD crystal deposition.[72] Patients receiving chronic hemodialysis have been found to have calcium oxalate in synovial fluid.[73] Patients taking aluminum compounds (phosphate binders) have been found to have aluminum phosphate in the synovium.[74,75]

Radiologic Aspects

George B. Greenfield

The types of amyloid that most often cause joint disease are amyloid associated with light chain (AL) and with beta 2-microglobulin (Abeta2M). AL is related to primary amyloidosis and plasma cell dyscrasias. Abeta2M is related to chronic hemodialysis.

The radiologic findings are periarticular osteoporosis and nodular soft tissue masses. Multiple erosions and subchondral intraosseous cysts are seen, which may lead to pathological fracture. Joint space narrowing is not a prominent feature. The involvement is usually bilaterally symmetric. It most frequently involves the shoulders, hips, wrists, and knees. Radionuclide bone scan shows increased activity.[76] The radiolucent foci may be owing to amyloid deposits or brown tumors of hyperparathyroidism.

Patients on long-term hemodialysis have joint changes related to renal osteodystrophy.[77,78] Chondrocalcinosis and capsular and periarticular calcifications may occur (Figs. 4.46, 4.47, 4.48, and 4.49). Erosive arthropathy at

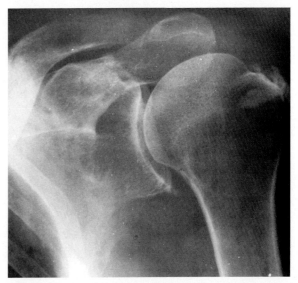

FIGURE 4.46. Dialysis arthritis. Shoulder. Calcifications around the greater tuberosity and at the inferior aspect of the glenoid fossa are seen.

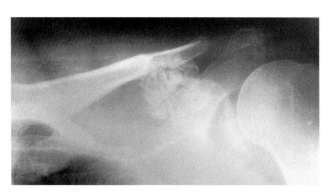

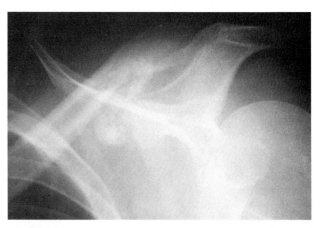

FIGURE 4.47. Dialysis patient. A large calcification at the under-surface of the clavicle is seen with subperiosteal resorption and erosion, and widening of the acromioclavicular joint.

FIGURE 4.48. Patient on dialysis. Calcification inferior to the distal clavicle is noted. There is no resorption of the distal clavicle in this case.

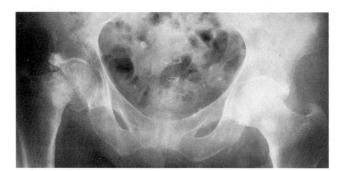

FIGURE 4.49. Dialysis arthritis. Hips. Bilateral calcifications at the acetabular margins are seen. There is a fracture of the right femoral neck.

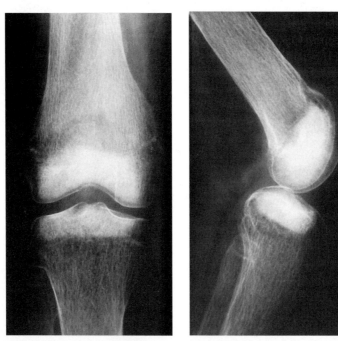

FIGURE 4.50. Renal osteodystrophy. The patient is on dialysis. Knee. **A,B:** AP and lateral views show marked osteopenia and an increased trabecular pattern with dense epiphyseal sclerosis. A subchondral radiolucent band is also noted.

the joint margins and subchondrally may occur, which can lead to bony collapse in weight-bearing joints. Epiphyseal sclerosis without calcifications may be seen rarely (Fig. 4.50).

Erosive arthropathy of the *hands* with a predilection for the distal interphalangeal joints as well as the carpal joints may occur. Subperiosteal resorption and resorption of the terminal tufts are characteristic of hyperparathyroidism (Fig. 4.51). Paraarticular calcification may also occur (Fig. 4.52).

In the *wrist*, chondrocalcinosis, erosions, cysts, resorption, and subluxations may be seen (Fig. 4.53).

Large erosions of the *humeral head* may be seen.

The *elbows* and *knees* may be involved with effusion, subchondral cysts, and erosions.

Spontaneous tendon ruptures occur in a minority of patients, particularly the quadriceps.

The *spine* may show erosive spondylarthropathy and reactive sclerosis, which can simulate discitis, although without a paraspinal mass.

The *sacroiliac joints* and *symphysis pubis* may also be involved with subchondral resorption, widening, and irregularity.

Erosive and destructive changes in the *sternoclavicular joint* in a patient on hemodialysis has been reported.[79]

Wilson's disease is a rare disease of copper deposition causing hepatolenticular degeneration.[80,81] It has skeletal manifestations of osteoarthritis, osteochondritis dissecans, marginal bone fragmentation, and subchondral cystic changes, as well as cysts in areas of tendon and ligament in-

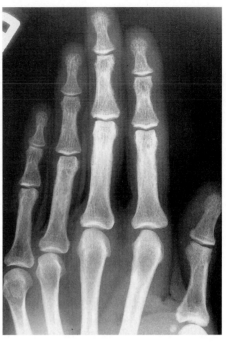

FIGURE 4.51. Renal osteodystrophy with hyperparathyroidism. Subperiosteal bone resorption is noted in the middle phalanges and erosions at the terminal tufts are seen. There are marginal erosions at the distal interphalangeal joint of the middle finger.

sertions. Schmorl's nodes and bone fragmentation are seen in the spine. Renal failure leads to rickets, osteomalacia, pseudofractures, pathological fractures, osteopenia, and paraarticular calcifications.

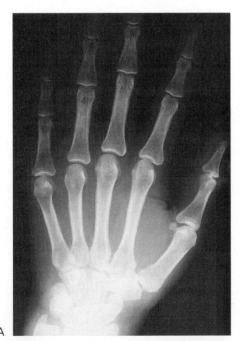
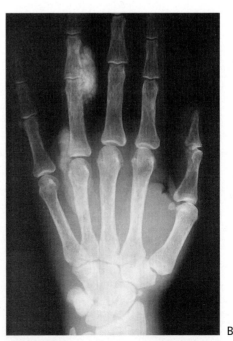

A   B

FIGURE 4.52. Patient on dialysis. **A:** Hand. Subperiosteal bone resorption is noted indicating hyperparathyroidism. **B:** One year later. There is extensive paraarticular calcification.

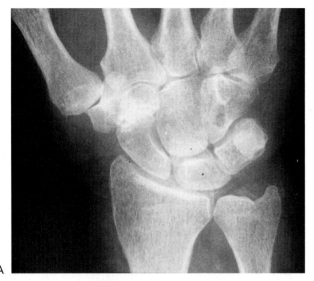
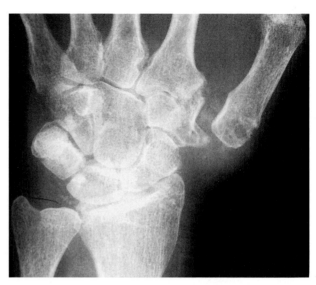

FIGURE 4.53. Patient on dialysis. **A:** Right wrist. Chondrocalcinosis in the triangular fibrocartilage and along the proximal carpal row is noted as well as osteosclerosis in the joint between the scaphoid and lesser multangular bones. A cyst in the hamate is also seen. **B:** Left wrist. There is marked resorption and subluxation of the first metacarpophalangeal joint with calcifications. Chondrocalcinosis of the proximal carpal row is also seen. There are erosions at the base of the first metacarpal, fifth metacarpal, and hamate bones.

Case Report

Joanne Valeriano-Marcet

A 36-year-old Black woman presented for treatment. She had a history of sickle trait and ESRD owing to hypertension and had been on hemodialysis for 3 1/2 years. She presented with 1 week of pain and swelling of the left fourth finger. She had had a previous episode of swelling in this area several months ago, which resolved spontaneously over the course of 2 weeks. The patient had also been having progressive pain and limitation of motion in both shoulders for several months. The patient denied fever, sweats, skin rashes, any other joint complaints or history of podagra. She had been noncompliant with her calcium supplements and phosphate binders.

Physical Examination. The physical examination revealed tenderness and swelling of the soft tissues surrounding the left fourth PIP joint. There was a 2-cm nodule over the lateral aspect of the PIP joint. Aspiration of the area of soft tissue swelling yielded a few drops of thick yellow fluid. Crystal analysis of the fluid included examination under polarized microscopy, which demonstrated no birefringent crystals. Alizarin red stain was positive for calcium, and electromicroscopy confirmed the presence of calcium hydroxyapatite crystals.

Laboratory Findings. Uric acid 8.6 mg/dL (1–7), Ca 10.4 mg/dL (8.5–10), PTH N terminal 160 pg/nL (4–9), PO4 8.8 mg/dL (2.7–4), and alkaline phosphatase 213 Iu/l (37–110).

REFERENCES

Gout

1. Grahame R, Scott JT. Clinical survey of 354 patients with gout. *Am Rheum Dis* 1970;29:461–468.
2. Herich PS. Diagnosis of gout and gouty arthritis. *J Lab Clin Med* 1936;22:48–55.
3. Gutman AB. Views on the pathogenesis and management of primary gout:1971. *J Bone Joint Surg [Am]* 1972;54:357–372.
4. Watt I, Middlemiss H. The radiology of gout. *Clin Radiol* 1975; 26:27–36.
5. Smith EE, Kurlander GJ, Powell RC. Two rare causes of secondary gouty arthritis. *AJR* 1967;100:550–553.
6. Lambeth JT, Burns-Cox CJ, MacLean R. Sacroiliac gout associated with hemoglobin E and hypersplenism. *Radiology* 1970; 95:413–415.
7. Cornelius R, Schneider HJ. Gouty arthritis in the adult. *Radiol Clin North Am* 1988;26:1267–1276.
8. Resnick D, Reinke RT, Taketa RM. Early-onset gouty arthritis. *Radiology* 1975;114:67–73.
9. Chaoui A, Garcia J, Kurt AM. Gouty tophus simulating soft tissue tumor in a heart transplant recipient. *Skeletal Radiol* 1997; 26:626–628.
10. Foucar E, Buckwalter J, El-Khoury GY. Gout presenting as a femoral cyst. *J Bone Joint Surg [Am]* 1984;66:294(297.
11. Resnick D, Broderick TW. Intraosseous calcifications in tophaceous gout. *AJR* 1981;137:1157–1161.
12. Gottlieb NL, Gray RG. Allopurinol-associated hand and foot deformities in chronic tophaceous gout. *JAMA* 1977;238: 1663–1664; Schabel SI, et al. Bone infarction in gout. *Skeletal Radiol* 1978;3:42–47.
13. Levy M, Seelenfreund M, Maur P, et al. Bilateral spontaneous and simultaneous rupture of the quadriceps tendon in gout. *J Bone Joint Surg [Br]* 1971;53:510–513.

14. Peavy PW, Franco DJ. Gout: presentation as a popliteal cyst. *Radiology* 1974;111:103–104.
15. Levitin PM, Keats TE. Dissecting synovial cyst of the popliteal space in gout. *AJR* 1975;124:32–33.
16. Alarcon-Segovia D, Cetina JA, Diaz-Jovanen E: Sacroiliac joints in primary gout: clinical and roentgenographic study of 143 patients. *AJR* 1973;118:438–443.
17. Trentham DE, Masi AT. Chronic synovitis in gout simulating rheumatoid arthritis. *JAMA* 1976;235:1358–1360.
18. Schwartzberg M, et al. Rheumatoid arthritis and chronic gouty arthropathy. *JAMA* 1978;240:2658–2659.
19. Levy M, Seelenfreund M, Maur P, et al. Bilateral spontaneous and simultaneous rupture of the quadriceps tendon in gout. *J Bone Joint Surg [Br]* 1971;53:510–513.
20. Shuhaibar H, Friedman L. Periosteal gouty tophi of the anterior mid tibia. *Skeletal Radiol* 1997;26:260–262.
21. Campbell JB, Reeder MM, Sewell J. Lymphoma cutis with osseous involvement. *Radiology* 1972;103:99–100.
22. Daniel WW, Wees SJ. Intra-articular milk of calcium in saturine gout. *Radiology* 1983;137:389–392.

Calcium Pyrophosphate Deposition Disease
23. Hollander JL, McCarty DJ. *Arthritis and allied conditions,* 8th ed. Philadelphia: Lea & Febiger, 1972.
24. Dodds WJ, Steinback HL. Primary hyperparathyroidism and articular cartilage calcification. *AJR* 1968;104:884–892.
25. Jensen PS. Chondrocalcinosis and other calcifications. *Radiol Clin North Am* 1988;26:1315–1325.

Pseudogout Syndrome/CPD Deposition Disease
26. Helms CA, Chapman GS, Wild JH. Charcot-like joints in calcium pyrophosphate dihydrate deposition disease. *Skeletal Radiol* 1981;7:55–58.
27. Hollander JL, McCarty DJ. *Arthritis and allied conditions,* 8th ed. Philadelphia: Lea & Febiger, 1972.
28. Martel W, McCarter DK, Solsky MA, et al. Further observations of the arthropathy of calcium pyrophosphate crystal deposition disease. *Radiology* 1981;141:1–15.
29. Resnick D, et al. Clinical, radiographic, and pathologic abnormalities in calcium pyrophosphate dihydrate deposition disease (CPPD): pseudogout. *Radiology* 1977;122:1–15.
30. Watt I, Dieppe PA. Medial femoral condyle necrosis and chondrocalcinosis: a causal relationship. *Br J Radiol* 1983;56:7–11.
31. Martin W, Klein A. Chondrocalcinosis and tophaceous erosions: gout or pseudogout? *J Can Assoc Radiol* 1982;33:260–263.
32. Atkins CJ, McIvor J, Smith PM. Chondrocalcinosis and arthropathy: studies in haemochromatosis and in idiopathic chondrocalcinosis. *Q J Med* 1970;39:71–82.
33. Martel W, Champion CK, Thompson GR, et al. A roentgenologically distinctive arthropathy in some patients with the pseudogout syndrome. *AJR* 1970;109:587–605.
34. Weinberg S, Scott RA. Giant geode (subchondral cyst) in calcium pyrophosphate deposition disease of the wrist. *J Can Assoc Radiol* 1981;32:171–172.
35. Stern PJ, Weinberg S. Pathological fracture of the radius through a cyst caused by pyrophosphate arthropathy. *J Bone Joint Surg [Am]* 1981;63:1487–1488.
36. Leisen J. Calcium pyrophosphate dihydrate deposition disease: tumorous form. *AJR* 1982;138:962.
37. Ling D, Murphy WA, Kyriakos M. Tophaceous pseudogout. *AJR* 1982;138:162–165.
38. Yang B, Sartoris DJ, Djukic S, et al. Distribution of calcification in the triangular fibrocartilage region in 181 patients with calcium pyrophosphate deposition disease. *Radiology* 1995;196:547–550.

39. Smathers RL, Stelling CB, Keats TE. The destructive wrist arthropathy of pseudogout. *Skeletal Radiol* 1982;7:255–258.
40. Foldes K, Lenchik L, Jaovisidha S, et al. Association of gastrocnemius tendon calcification with chondrocalcinosis of the knee. *Skeletal Radiol* 1996;25:621–624.
41. Dirheimer Y, Bensimon C, Christmann D, et al. Syndesmoodontoid joint and calcium pyrophosphate dihydrate deposition disease (CPPD). *Neuroradiology* 1983;25:319–321.
42. Dirheimer Y, Wackenheim C, et al. Calcification of the transverse ligament in calcium dihydrate deposition disease (CPPD). *Neuroradiology* 1985;27:87.
43. El-Khoury GY, Tozzi JE, et al. Massive calcium pyrophosphate crystal deposition at the craniovertebral junction. *AJR* 1985;145:777–778.
44. Rivera-Sanfeliz G, Resnick D, Haghighi P, et al. Tophaceous pseudogout. *Skeletal Radiol* 1996;25:699–701.
45. Boutin RD, Kakitsubatay, Theodorou DJ, et al. CPPD crystal deposition in and around the atlantoaxial joint. Presented at the SSR meeting. Scottsdale AZ, March, 1999.
46. Ohira T, Ishikawa K. Hydroxyapatite deposition in articular cartilage by intra-articular injections of methylprednisolone. *J Bone Joint Surg* 1986;68:509–520.

Calcium Hydroxyapatite And Basic Calcium Phosphate Deposition Disease
47. McCarty DJ, Halverson PB. Basic calcium phosphate (apatite, octacalcium phosphate, tricalcium phosphate) crystal deposition diseases in arthritis and allied conditions, 12th ed. Philadelphia: Lea & Febiger, 1993:1857–1872.
48. Sarkar K, Uhthoff HK. Rotator cuff tendinopathies with calcification. In Rubin RP, Weiss G, Putney JW, eds. *Calcium in biological systems,* 11th ed. New York: Plenum, 1984.
49. Fam AG, Rubenstein J. Hydroxyapatite pseudopodagra. *Arthritis Rheum* 1989;32:741–747.
50. Halverson PB, McCarty DJ. Basic calcium phosphate (apatite, octacalcium phosphate, tricalcium phosphate) crystal deposition diseases. Rotator cuff tendinopathies with calcification. In Rubin RP, Weiss G, Putney JW, eds. *Calcium in biological systems*, 11th ed. New York: Plenum, 1984.
51. Caspi D, Rosenbach TO, Yaron M, et al. Periarthritis associated with basic calcium phospate crystal deposition and low levels of serum alkaline phosphatase. Report of three cases from one family. *J Rheumatol* 1988;15:823–828.
52. Nguyen VD. Rapid destructive arthritis of the shoulder. *Skeletal Radiol* 1996;25:107–112.
53. Dalinka MK, Stewart V, et al. Periarticular calcifications in association with intra-articular corticosteroid injections. *Radiology* 1984;153:615–618.

Hemochromatosis
54. Jensen PS. Hemochromatosis: a disease often silent but not invisible. *AJR* 1976;126:343–351.
55. Ross P, Wood B. Osteoarthropathy in idiopathic hemochromatosis. *AJR* 1970;109:575–580.
56. Twersky J. Joint changes in idiopathic hemochromatosis. *AJR* 1975;124:139–144.
57. Wardle EN, Patton JT. Bone and joint changes in haemochromatosis. *Ann Rheum Dis* 1969;28:15–23.
58. Sella EJ, Goodman AH. Arthropathy secondary to transfusion hemochromatosis. *J Bone Joint Surg [Am]* 1973;55:1077–1081.
59. Bywaters EGL, Hamilton EBD, Williams R. The spine in idiopathic haemochromatosis. *Ann Rheum Dis* 1971;30:453–465.

Ochronosis

60. Hollander JL, McCarty DJ. *Arthritis and allied conditions,* 8th ed. Philadelphia: Lea & Febiger, 1972.
61. Laskar FJ, Sargison KD. Ochronotic arthropathy: a review with 4 case reports. *J Bone Joint Surg [Br]* 1970;52:653–666.
62. Lagier R, Steiger U. Hip arthropathy in ochronosis: Anatomical and radiological study. *Skeletal Radiol* 1980;5:91–98.

Amyloid Arthropathy and Dialysis Arthritis; Arthropathies in Chronic Renal Failure

63. Resnick DL. Erosive arthritis of the hand and wrist in hyperparathyroidism. *Radiology* 1974;110:263–269.
64. Rubin LA, Fam AJ, Rubenstein J, et al. Erosive azotemic arthropathy. *Arthritis Rheum* 1984;27:1086–1094.
65. Huaux J, Noel H, Malghem J, et al. Erosive azotemic osteoarthropathy. Possible role of amyloidosis. *Arthritis Rheum* 1985;28:1975–1076.
66. Bardin T, Bardin T, Kunt D, Zingraff J, et al. Synovial amyloidosis in patients undergoing long-term hemodialysis. *Arthritis Rheum* 1985;28:1052–1058.
67. Kay J, Benson CB, Lester S, et al. Utility of high resolution ultrasound for the diagnosis of dialysis related amyloidosis. *Arthritis Rheum* 1992;35:926–932.
68. Chassagne P, Dhib M, Alt Said L, et al. Spinal cord compression revealing a destructive arthropathy of the atlanto-occipital joint associated with B2 microglobulin amyloidosis in a haemodialysed patient. *Br J Rheumatol* 1992;31:427–428.
69. Jadoul M, Malgheim J, Pirson Y, et al. Effect of renal transplantation on the radiological signs of dialysis amyloid osteoarthropathy. *Clin Nephrol* 1989;32:194–197.
70. Nelson SR, Sharpstone P, Kingswood JC. Does dialysis associated amyloidosis resolve after transplantation? *Nephrology, Dialysis, Transplantation* 1993;8:369–377.
71. Campistol JM, Munoz-Gomez J, Sole M, et al. Results of renal transplantation for dialysis arthropathy. *Transplant Proc* 1990; 22:1416.

72. Halverson PB, McCarty DJ. Basic calcium phosphate deposition diseases. *Arthritis and allied conditions.* 12th ed. Philadelphia: Lea & Febiger, 1993, 1857–1872.
73. Hoffman GS, Schumacher HR, Paul H, et al. Calcium oxalate microcrystalline-associated arthritis in end stage renal disease. *Ann Intern Med* 1982;97:36–42.
74. Netter P, DeLongea JL, Favre G, et al. Inflammatory effect of aluminum phosphate. *Ann Rheum Dis* 1983;42:114.
75. Netter P, Kessler M, Durnel D, et al. Aluminum in joint tissues of chronic renal failure patients treated with regular hemodialysis and aluminum compounds. *J Rheumatol* 1984; 11:66–70.

Radiologic Aspects

76. Goldman AB, Bansal M. Amyloidosis and silicone synovitis. *Radiol Clin North Am* 1996;34:375–394.
77. Cotton A, Flipo RM, Boutry N, et al. Natural course of erosive arthropathy of the hand in patients undergoing hemodialysis. *Skeletal Radiol* 1997;26:20–26.
78. Tigges S, Nance EP, Carpenter WP, et al. Renal osteodystrophy: imaging findings that mimic those of other diseases. *AJR* 1995;165:143–148.
79. Cameron EW, Resnik CS, Light PD, et al. Hemodialysis related amyloidosis of the sternoclavicular joint. *Skeletal Radiol* 1997;26:428–430.

Wilson's Disease

80. Aksoy M, Camli N, Dincol K, et al. Osseous changes in Wilson's disease: a radiologic study of 9 patients. *Radiology* 1972;102: 505–510.
81. Mindelzun R, Elkin M, Scheinberg IH, et al. Skeletal changes in Wilson's disease. *Radiology* 1970;94:127–132.

OSTEOARTHRITIS AND RELATED CONDITIONS

OSTEOARTHRITIS

Osteoarthritis (osteoarthrosis; OA) is the most common of the arthritides, affecting a majority of elderly persons. It can involve the peripheral joints as well as the central skeleton. It may be primary or secondary to a variety of conditions. It can lead to radiculopathy and neuropathy as well as low back pain. Several other conditions may show symptomatology that overlaps that of osteoarthritis. In the spine, these include spondylolysis, spondylolisthesis, and Kashin–Bek disease. Diffuse idiopathic skeletal hyperostosis (DISH) is also included in this chapter.

Low Back Pain

Frank B. Vasey

Low back pain is a major public health issue; 25% of adults experience it every year.[1] It is one of the top 10 reasons to visit a physician. Fortunately, serious disease is uncommon. Herniated discs, fractures, cancer, and infection combined represent less than 5% of back pain patients.[2]

Worrisome findings (red flags) have included age over 50, weight loss, fever, night pain, neuromuscular defects, severe writhing pain at rest (which suggests vascular catastrophe), and duration over 3 months with morning stiffness (which points toward one of the forms of inflammatory spondyloarthritis). The physical examination stresses localization of painful areas by palpation and spinal motion. Localized tenderness to a vertebral body may suggest fracture or infection. Loss of spinal mobility suggests muscle spasm or loss of structural integrity of the spine. Range of motion of the hip should detect patients with osteoarthritis and referral into the buttock from the hip. Straight leg raising suggests radicular involvement when restricted and painful. Careful neurological examination of muscle strength and reflexes in the lower extremity gives useful information on the seriousness of the problem and the likeli-

hood of orthopedic or neurosurgical referral as well as further radiographic evaluation with CT or MRI of the lumbar spine. Abdominal palpation is important to document an expanding abdominal aortic aneurysm, which can be demonstrated more precisely by abdominal ultrasound.

In one large outcome study of typical back pain without red flags, only 5% of patients had not reported functional recovery at 6 months, but 31% reported not being completely recovered.[3] The type of physician seen did not seem to impact the outcome.

In typical patients with low back pain with or without a radicular component initial bed rest, which may be as brief as 48 hours, is necessary. Patients need to recognize that pain is worsened by physical activities that increase pressure in the spine, including sitting, coughing, or straining. Use of narcotics or tricyclics could increase the likelihood of constipation at the same time, improving the patient's back pain. If helpful, acetaminophen or nonsteroidal antiinflammatory drugs (NSAIDs) should be used.

Medical management can be continued for 3 months without prejudicing surgical results.[4] In that case, an MRI may also be delayed. Prolonged delay in elective surgery is reasonable because spinal healing is slow and many patients gradually return to normal activities over several months. Classic large-scale studies of operative patients versus nonoperative with a randomized study design show that patients who undergo surgery improve more quickly, particularly regarding the radicular symptoms; however, by the end of the follow-up period of 5 to 10 years, there was no statistical difference between the groups (90% satisfactory result for operative treatment versus 85% satisfactory result with nonoperative treatment).

On the initial visit, spinal radiographs may be withheld in the absence of the red flags discussed in the preceding. If brief bed rest is ineffective, then lumbar spine films should be obtained after several weeks. Keep in mind 95% of 50-year-old patients will show evidence of disc space narrowing, calcification, and sclerosis known as degenerative changes or lumbar spondylosis. These changes increase with age and affect fewer than 5% of people under age 20.

Lumbar spine films are reassuring for the absence of evidence of metastatic tumor, osteomyelitis, osteoporotic fracture, or spinal instability. AP, lateral, and cone down views of L4-5 and L5-S1 with obliques can help identify anatomic defects in the pars interarticularis resulting in spondylolysis or spondylolisthesis as well as evidence of facet joint osteoarthritis.

Flexion and extension views are helpful in patients with an unstable spine. Ferguson and oblique views of the sacroiliac joints should be obtained in patients with persistent morning stiffness (over 3 months). An MRI should be considered in patients with persistent sharp pain, particularly radicular with positive straight leg raising accompanied by neurologic defects, usually in L4-5 or L5-S1. Findings include weakness of dorsiflexion of the hallux, and foot atrophy of anterior tibialis muscle without reflex changes. L5-S1 findings include weakness of plantar flexion with calf atrophy and loss of ankle jerks. Keep in mind that radicular symptoms may arise from causes other than degenerative disc disease. Some of these include spinothalamic tract lesions in the spinal cord and lumbosacral root lesions, including arachnoiditis and entrapment syndrome. The piriformis syndrome and tarsal tunnel syndrome may simulate disc disease.

The issue of timing of the MRI is difficult. The major consideration arguing in favor of obtaining the study is a serious consideration of surgery. In the setting of acute back pain, the surgical emergency is incontinence of bowel or bladder, with decreased sensation perianally. Urinary retention may also occur. An MRI may demonstrate a broad-based disc rupture with cord compression. Consultation with a spine surgeon should be promptly obtained.

The issue of various radiographic approaches is controversial and discussed in more detail elsewhere in this text. Myelography is most invasive and may provide some unique information. CT and MRI are both utilized and provide useful spinal images. MRI may have an advantage in detecting vertebral osteomyelitis and is the study of choice.

Clinical Aspects

Joanne Valeriano-Marcet

OA is a slowly progressive disorder affecting patients in their mid to later years. Clinically, patients present with pain, deformity, bony enlargement of the joints, and limitation of motion. The most frequently affected joints are the hips, knees, spine, and small joints of the hands and feet. In the absence of trauma or some form of congenital abnormality, the wrist (except the first carpometacarpal joint), elbow, shoulder, and ankle usually are spared.

Historically, most patients with OA state that symptoms have been present for some time and are very slowly pro-

gressive. The pain is almost always described as mild to moderate and dull and aching in character. It is almost always at least partially relieved by rest and exacerbated by movement, especially weight bearing.

The most frequent finding is limitation of motion. Crepitus can be felt as a crackling or crunching sensation with palpation of the joint in motion. In addition, joint enlargement occurs because of osteophytes or the presence of synovial effusion. Laboratory testing of patients with OA are used mainly to rule out other conditions. The CBC and ESR are usually normal. Tests for antinuclear antibodies, rheumatoid factor, and assessment of complement components are routinely normal. Synovial fluid in OA is noninflammatory (white blood cell [WBC] count < 2,000).

Radiography usually serves to confirm the clinical finding and assess the extent of joint degeneration in a patient who presents in the appropriate age range with a history and physical examination compatible with the diagnosis of osteoarthritis. When the initial clinical assessment cannot totally exclude the possibility of a mild inflammatory arthritis, radiologic findings of juxtaarticular osteopenia and erosions might help to further elucidate the diagnosis. The documentation of evidence of an inflammatory arthritis might significantly alter the management of the case. More sophisticated radiographic testing is needed in certain situations in evaluating the patient with osteoarthritis.

MRI or bone scan may detect OA in a patient with early disease who does not yet have abnormal radiographs. Patients with OA may present with an acute change in symptoms, such as increase in pain in a previously affected joint, pain in a previously uninvolved joint, or a new joint effusion. Bone scan or MRI can help diagnose avascular necrosis. MRI can help in the diagnosis of PVNS (pigmented villonodular synovitis) or other tumor, Baker's cyst, or internal derangement. Bone scan and MRI may be helpful in differentiating OA from Charcot's arthropathy in a patient with underlying diabetes mellitus or neuropathy. Techniques such as CT and MRI are useful in determining the extent of spinal OA as well as eliminating other diagnostic possibilities.

Radiologic Aspects

George B. Greenfield

Osteoarthritis is a progressive disorder of diarthrodial joints.[5-13] It is characterized by deterioration of articular cartilage, spur formation at the joint margins, subchondral sclerosis, and cysts. It is by far the most common arthritis. It may be primary or secondary. A rarer inflammatory form also exists.

Primary osteoarthritis occurs with initial intrinsic changes of articular cartilage. This painful form overwhelmingly affects women. Initial involvement of the hands is in the distal interphalangeal joints and the first carpometacarpal joints.

Osteoarthritis, particularly involving weight-bearing joints, may result from senescent changes in cartilage. Idiopathic osteoarthritis occurs in the shoulder in elderly persons.[12]

When a cause can be determined, the disease is called *secondary osteoarthritis*. Predisposing factors include obesity, excess activity and stress, deposition diseases, acromegaly, disordered proprioceptive sense, and inflammatory arthritides, as well as local structural abnormality, trauma, alkaptonuria, and hemorrhage. Osteoarthritis of the glenohumeral joint occurs secondary to the use of crutches and rotator cuff tears or atrophy. Joint space narrowing may also result from disuse atrophy of cartilage.

The nutrition of chondrocytes depends on diffusion of synovial fluid driven by the pressure of normal joint motion. Any long-term immobilization of the joint will result in cartilage atrophy.

Osteoarthritis is usually slowly progressive. The major clinical complaints are pain, stiffness after rest, aching in humid weather, crepitation, limitation of motion, and at times malalignment. The joints of major clinical concern are those of the hip, knee, and spine. Rarely, synovitis and joint effusion may be associated. In some cases, subchondral erosion in the center of the joint proceeds rapidly, with painful soft-tissue swelling. This condition is termed *inflammatory* or *erosive* osteoarthritis. Other causes of inflammation in osteoarthritis of the interphalangeal joints include CPPD and gout.[14]

Pathologic changes in osteoarthritis include fraying and fibrillation of cartilage, with depletion of chondrocytes and of protein-polysaccharides. The cartilage becomes yellow and opaque, with focal areas of malacia and roughening of the surface. The surface then frays and fibrillates, with deep cracks. Minute fragments of cartilage may induce an acute synovitis. In the final stages, the articular surface totally loses cartilage. Remodeling of subchondral bone is accompanied by eburnation. Bony spurs, at times very large, form at the joint margins and attachments of ligaments and tendons. Osteoporosis, paralysis, and local pressure inhibit this spur formation. The joint later may ankylose in very rare cases.

Radiologically, the changes of primary and secondary osteoarthritis are similar. The typical picture is nonuniform joint space narrowing with subchondral sclerosis and marginal osteophytes. Subchondral radiolucencies may either result from ingrowth of granulation tissue through defects in articular cartilage, or erosion from synovial fluid forced through these defects by intraarticular pressure. A subchondral cyst may collapse, resulting in flattening and irregularity of a segment of the articular surface. The cysts rarely may be large and expansile, termed geodes. Microfractures and focal areas of avascular necrosis may follow. Periosteal new bone formation is sparse. Loose bodies may become detached and fall free in the joint. There is a relative lack of osteoporosis in such cases. The end stage in certain areas may very rarely be bony ankylosis.

Primary osteoarthritis can be widespread and may involve small and large joints. Secondary osteoarthritis affects those joints subject to weight bearing and stress. The large joints most frequently involved with osteoarthritis are those of the hip and knee.

Peripheral Skeleton. In the *hands* in the primary form, there is an initial predilection of the distal interphalangeal joints (Fig. 5.1). The proximal interphalangeal joints may be involved later (Fig. 5.2), and less frequently the metacarpophalangeal joints.[15] Rarely, the proximal interphalangeal joints can be involved alone. The basic changes are joint space narrowing, subchondral sclerosis, and marginal spur formation. Bony protuberances at the dorsal margins of the distal interphalangeal joints later commonly develop, and are referred to as Heberden's nodes (Fig. 5.3). Lateral deviation (Fig. 5.4) and flexion of the distal phalanges may occur. The index and middle fingers are most severely involved. Less frequently, similar nodes, referred to as Bouchard's nodes (Fig. 5.5), are seen in the proximal interphalangeal joints. Marginal erosions are not seen. Rarely, bony ankylosis of the interphalangeal joints can be seen.[16]

One or more of the metacarpophalangeal joints uncommonly shows uniform narrowing. The uniform narrowing may be on the basis of disuse atrophy of cartilage. Osteophytes may be present, as well as small, discrete subchondral radiolucencies, usually 1 to 3 mm in diameter. Occasionally, "hooklike" osteophytes such as those seen in CPPD and hemochromatosis may be present (Figs. 5.6 and 5.7). Marginal erosions are not present, nor are flexion deformities, volar subluxations, nor ulnar deviation.

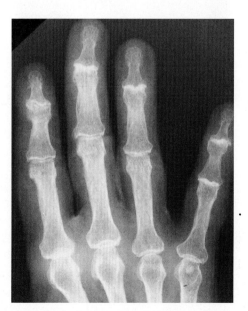

FIGURE 5.1. Osteoarthritis. Hand. There is narrowing of the distal interphalangeal joints with central erosions.

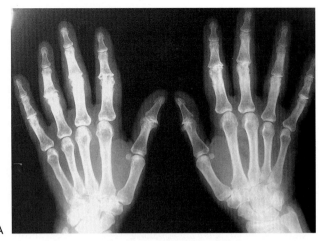
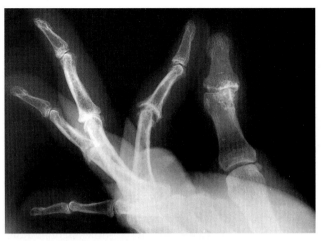

A

B

FIGURE 5.2. Osteoarthritis. **A:** Osteoarthritic changes with minimal erosions are seen involving the proximal interphalangeal joints bilaterally. The interphalangeal joints and the metacarpophalangeal joints show no changes. The interphalangeal joints of the thumbs also show osteoarthritis. **B:** Lateral view showing details of spur formation at the proximal interphalangeal joints.

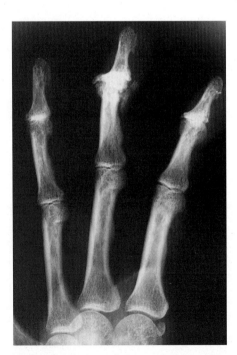

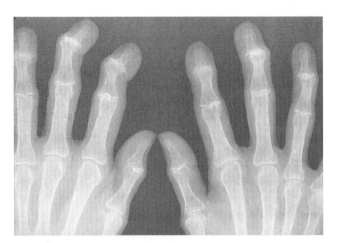

FIGURE 5.3. Osteoarthritis. Hand. Involvement of the distal interphalangeal joints is noted and there is marked spur formation at the middle finger. This is a Heberden's node.

FIGURE 5.4. Osteoarthritis. Hands. Involvement of multiple distal interphalangeal joints with lateral deviation and flexion of the distal phalanges is seen. The proximal interphalangeal joints of both index fingers are also involved.

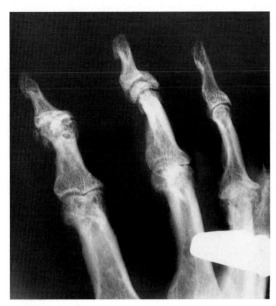

FIGURE 5.5. Osteoarthritis. Hand. Bony spurs at the proximal interphalangeal joints are seen, most marked in the ring finger. These are Bouchard's node. Heberden's nodes are seen in the distal interphalangeal joints of the index and middle fingers.

Unusual appearances that may mimic rheumatoid arthritis include ulnar deviation of the fingers (Figs. 5.8 and 5.9), and boutonierre deformity (Figs. 5.10 and 5.11). Osteoarthritis in the hand and wrist with osteophyte formation and with joint space widening rather than narrowing is typical of acromegaly (Fig. 5.12).

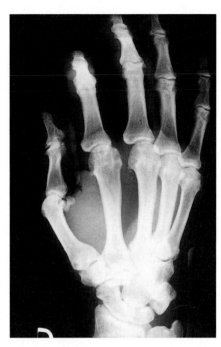

FIGURE 5.7. Osteoarthritis. Hand. "Hooklike" osteophytes are seen at the second and third metacarpal heads. Subchondral cysts are also noted at these sites as well as in the first metacarpal.

Erosive osteoarthritis is an inflammatory form of primary osteoarthritis generally limited to the hands and predominantly affecting postmenopausal women.[17,18] The interphalangeal joints, both proximal and distal, and the trapeziometacarpal joint are chiefly involved. Clinically,

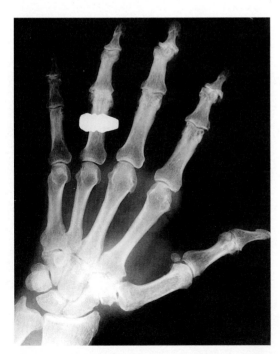

FIGURE 5.6. Osteoarthritis. Hand. A "hooklike" osteophyte at the third metacarpal head is present. Typical osteoarthritic changes at the distal and proximal interphalangeal joints are also seen.

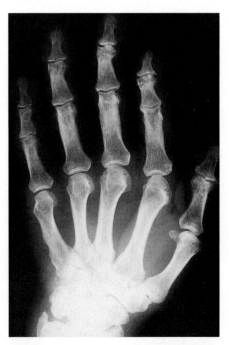

FIGURE 5.8. Osteoarthritis. Hand. Involvement of the distal interphalangeal joints of the index and middle fingers are seen, as well as the interphalangeal joint of the thumb. There is ulnar deviation of the fingers.

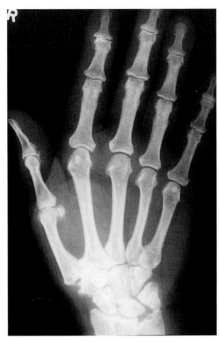

FIGURE 5.9. Osteoarthritis. Hand. Ulnar deviation of the fingers is seen. Involvement of the distal interphalangeal joints of the index and middle fingers with osteoarthritis is seen.

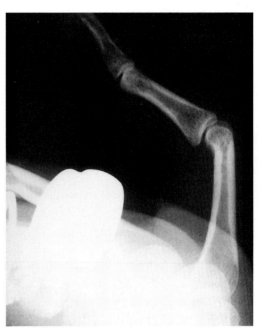

FIGURE 5.11. Osteoarthritis. There is a boutonniere deformity of the little finger.

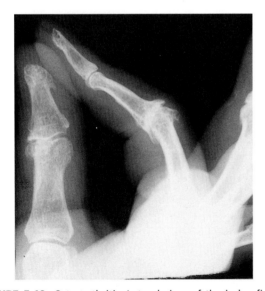

FIGURE 5.10. Osteoarthritis. Lateral view of the index finger. Osteoarthritis in the proximal interphalangeal joint is seen. A boutonierre deformity is present.

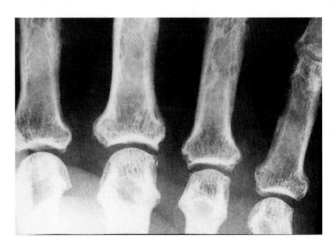

FIGURE 5.12. Acromegaly. Metacarpophalangeal joints. Hypertrophic marginal spurs are seen with joint space widening.

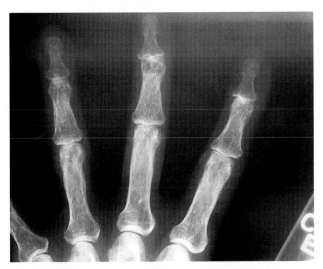

FIGURE 5.13. Erosive osteoarthritis. Osteoarthritis with joint space narrowing and marginal spur formation is seen at the distal interphalangeal joints. Radiolucencies indicating erosion are noted at the distal aspects of the middle phalanges of the index and middle fingers, as well as an erosion at the radial aspect of the proximal interphalangeal joint of the index finger.

symmetrically distributed synovitis of the interphalangeal joints of the hand, wrist, and knees occurs.[19] The erosive changes seen are not symmetrical (Fig. 5.13). Joint space narrowing occurs. Irregular destruction of the subchondral cortex may be associated with soft-tissue swelling (Fig. 5.14). Bone erosion, which may involve the entire width,

may develop over time (Figs. 5.15 and 5.16). Osteophyte formation and sclerosis follow.

There is contact erosion resulting in a "gull wing" appearance (Fig. 5.17), principally in the distal interphalangeal joints. Local osteoporosis may result (Fig. 5.18).

Erosive osteoarthritis can be differentiated from psoriatic arthritis by central erosion and osteophyte formation, in

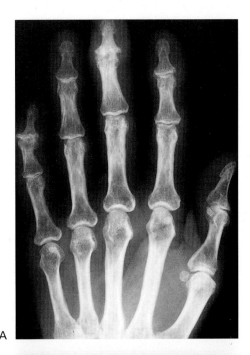

A

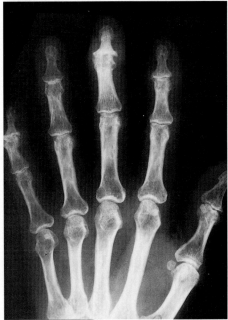

B

FIGURE 5.15. Erosive osteoarthritis. Distal interphalangeal joints of the middle and little fingers. **A:** Film taken in November 1992 shows erosions of the distal aspects of the middle phalanges with erosion of the articular cortex at those sites. **B:** Film taken in March 1993 shows progress of erosions.

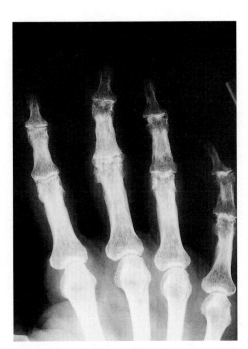

FIGURE 5.14. Erosive osteoarthritis. Hand. Bone erosions at the proximal and distal interphalangeal joints are seen varying in size.

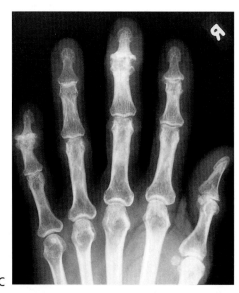

C

FIGURE 5.15. *(continued)* **C:** Film taken in December 1993 shows further progress of erosions with destruction of the articular cortex. Osteophytes at the bases of the distal phalanges are also seen.

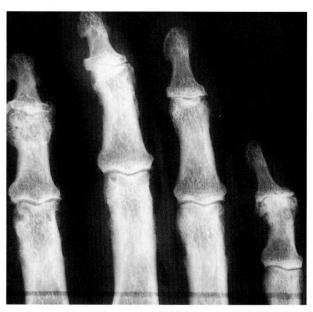

FIGURE 5.17. Erosive osteoarthritis. Hand. There is involvement of the distal interphalangeal joints of the index and little fingers with contact erosion resulting in a "gull wing" appearance.

contrast to marginal erosion and no true osteophytes in psoriasis, but bony proliferation.

In the wrist, erosions at the first carpometacarpal joint may occur, which can progress to subluxation.

Erosive osteoarthritis with destructive changes in the large joints, including the shoulders, hips, spine, and knees,

has been reported.[20] Silicone-induced erosive arthritis as a complication of silicone polymer implants has been reported as a rare complication of that procedure. Radiologic changes include well-defined marginal erosions and subchondral cysts, deformity, dislocation, or decrease of implant size. Removal of the prosthesis stops the process.[21]

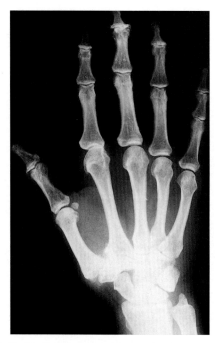

FIGURE 5.16. Erosive osteoarthritis. Hand. A large erosion at the distal interphalangeal joint of the middle finger is seen with osteophyte formation at the base of the distal phalanx. A smaller erosion at the distal interphalangeal joint of the index finger is also seen.

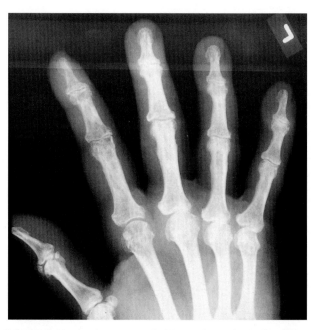

FIGURE 5.18. Erosive osteoarthritis involving the index finger. Erosions around the proximal and distal interphalangeal joints are seen that have resulted in local osteoporosis of the index finger.

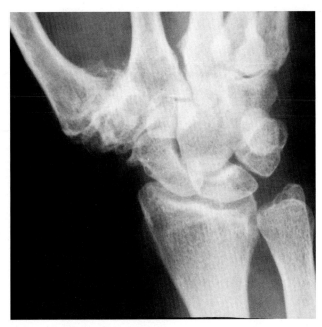

FIGURE 5.19. Erosive osteoarthritis. Erosions at the trapezium and the outer aspect of the scaphoid are seen.

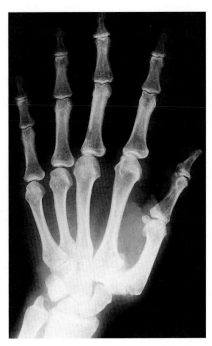

FIGURE 5.21. Erosive osteoarthritis. Wrist. Erosions at the first carpometacarpal joint are seen that have resulted in subluxation.

Osteoarthritis may involve the *wrist* at its radial aspect at the first carpometacarpal joint with osteophytes, erosion (Figs. 5.19 and 5.20), subluxation (Fig. 5.21), fragmentation (Fig. 5.22), and sclerosis (Fig. 5.23). The trapezio scaphoid joint (Fig. 5.24) may also be involved. Diffuse involvement of the intracarpal joints, and radiocarpal and distal radioulnar joint involvement are not seen in primary osteoarthritis, but may be secondary. Rarely, a "reverse 3"

erosion at the radial articular surface is seen (Fig. 5.25), which mimics CPPD.

Vibration syndrome occurs in jackhammer workers and involves the wrist.[22] It comprises clinical Raynaud's phenomenon with or without bony changes. It progresses to se-

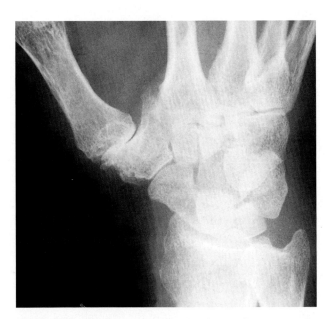

FIGURE 5.20. Osteoarthritis. Wrist. Erosion at the outer aspect of the trapezium is noted.

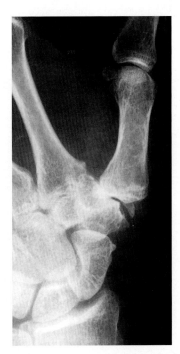

FIGURE 5.22. Osteoarthritis. Wrist. A single bone fragment at the first carpometacarpal joint is noted.

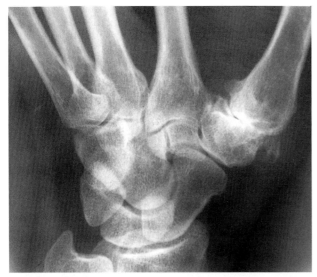

FIGURE 5.23. Osteoarthritis. Wrist. Involvement of the first car-pometacarpal joint is seen with spur formation and small cysts.

vere osteoarthritis of the wrist with avascular necrosis of the carpal bones and marked subchondral cyst formation. It is caused by chronic repeated trauma (Fig. 5.26).

Involvement of the *shoulder* is much less common (Figs 5.27 and 5.28), except for the acromioclavicular joint (Fig. 5.29). Spur formation at that site can compromise the rotator cuff tendon, causing shoulder impingement syndrome. Osteoarthritis of the shoulder is more often seen in people who use crutches (Figs. 5.30 and 5.31). Spur formation at the medial aspect of the margin of the humeral head is seen. Changes can also be secondary to trauma (Fig. 5.32).

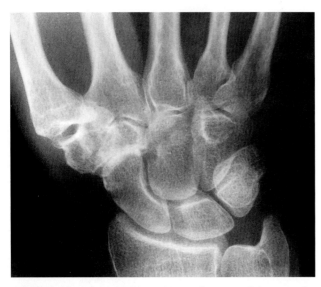

FIGURE 5.24. Osteoarthritis. Wrist. Involvement of the trapezio-scaphoid joint with narrowing and sclerosis is seen.

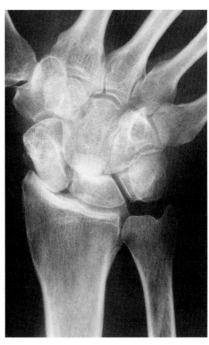

FIGURE 5.25. Osteoarthritis. Wrist. There is erosion of the articular surface of the radius in a "reverse 3" pattern. Erosion of the scaphoid is also noted. This picture is similar to that seen in CPPD.

Shoulder impingement syndrome is a common cause of shoulder pain, which can lead to secondary rotator cuff tendon tears.[22,23] It occurs when there is compression of the supraspinatus tendon and long head of the biceps tendon between the acromion process and humeral head (Fig. 5.33). Hypertrophic changes at the acromioclavicular joint and soft-tissue structures of the superior aspect of the shoulder encroach on the coracoacromial ligamentous arch when the arm is abducted. Subacromial bursitis, bicipital tendinitis, and rotator cuff disruptions are common sequelae.

Bony spurs arising from the anteroinferior aspect of the acromion and flattening and sclerosis of the greater tuberosity of the humerus are conventional radiographic signs. MRI can show structural details.[24,25]

In the *hips,* the etiology may be primary or secondary to a wide variety of disturbances, some of which are summarized in Table 5.1.[26–28] Involvement is often unilateral. Seventy percent of cases of osteoarthritis of the hip are primary.[29] Severe osteoarthritis in old age occurs at times, particularly after vigorous athletic stress in early life.

Nonuniform narrowing of the joint space is seen, with the greatest narrowing at the superior, weight-bearing surface.[30] There is usually no very pronounced medial migration of the femoral head, as is seen in rheumatoid arthritis (Fig. 5.34).

A measurement of the resultant drift of the femoral head is the center-edge angle (C–E angle).[31] A vertical line is drawn from the central point of the femoral head, and another line is drawn from the central point to the acetabular

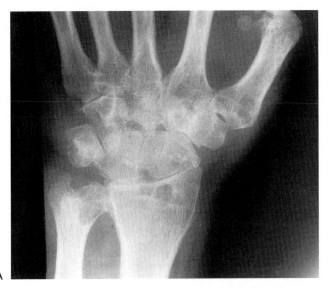
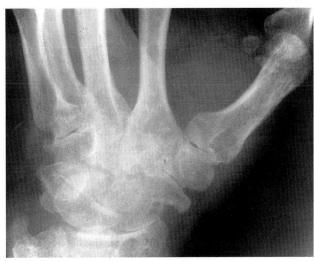

A

B

FIGURE 5.26. Vibration syndrome. **A:** AP view of the wrist shows osteoporosis and multiple cysts and erosions. Scaphoid lunate separation has occurred. **B:** Oblique view shows further details of cysts and erosions in the carpus. Cysts in the distal radius and ulna, as well as in the proximal first metacarpal are seen.

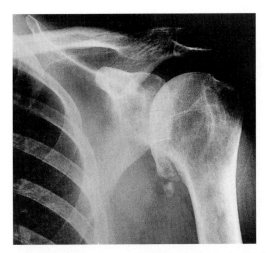
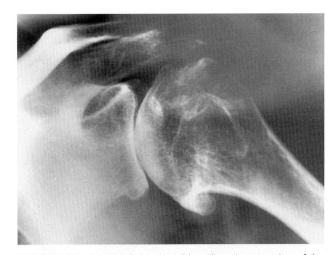

FIGURE 5.27. Osteoarthritis. Shoulder. Flattening of the humeral head, a large spur at the inferior aspect of the humeral head with a smaller detached fragment, and sclerosis at the glenoid fossa are seen.

FIGURE 5.28. Osteoarthritis. Shoulder. There is narrowing of the glenohumeral joint, with subchondral sclerosis. A large spur at the inferior aspect of the margin of the humeral head is noted as well as an erosion at the greater tuberosity.

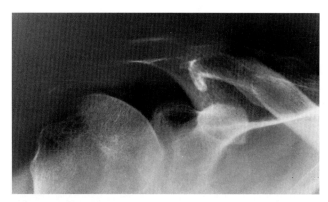

FIGURE 5.29. Osteoarthritis. Shoulder. A hypertrophic spur at the acromioclavicular joint protruding downward into the rotator cuff tendon region is noted.

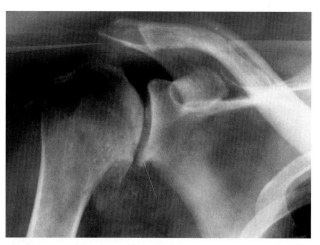

FIGURE 5.31. Osteoarthritis of the shoulder in a crutch user. There is marked inferior spur formation at the margin of the humeral head, as well as at the glenoid margin. Soft-tissue calcific debris is noted at the inferior and superior aspects of the shoulder joint.

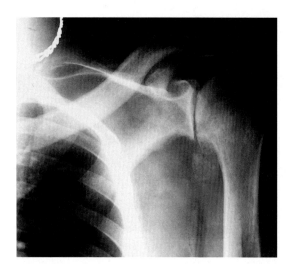

FIGURE 5.30. Osteoarthritis of the shoulder in a crutch user. There is narrowing of the glenohumeral joint and a large spur at the inferior aspect of the humeral head. There is flattening of the humeral head and a detached bony fragment inferior to the spur.

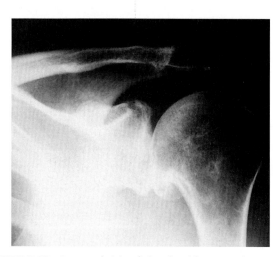

FIGURE 5.32. Osteoarthritis of the shoulder secondary to old trauma. Old fracture deformities of the glenoid are seen as well as large spurs at the inferior aspect of the glenoid fossa and humeral head.

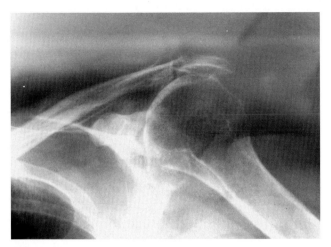

FIGURE 5.33. Osteoarthritis with shoulder impingement syndrome. There is elevation of the humeral head with little room for the rotator cuff tendon. Osteoarthritic changes at the acromioclavicular joint are also seen.

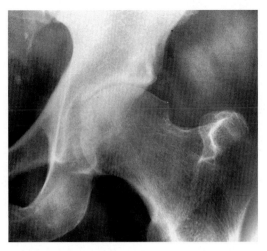

FIGURE 5.34. Osteoarthritis. Hip. AP view of the left hip shows narrowing of the superior aspect of the hip joint space without narrowing of the medial aspect. There is sclerosis of the acetabular margin and a small marginal osteophyte. Osteophytes at the superior and inferior aspects of the femoral head are also seen.

edge. The normal range of this angle is between 20 and 40 degrees, with an average of 36 degrees.[32] The distribution curves in Black and white populations are similar.[33]

In a small number of patients, the medial aspect of the joint may show greatest narrowing. Anterior–superior or posterior–medial migration patterns may occur.[34] The femoral head migrates in the acetabulum, usually superiorly or laterally, and rarely medially.[35] Subchondral sclerosis and well-marginated cystlike radiolucencies are present (Fig. 5.35). A large cyst may be connected to the joint cavity by a narrow "bottleneck" opening. Cysts may be present before marked joint space narrowing. A massive subarticular cyst in the supraacetabular ilium may be seen.[36] These large cystlike lesions are called *geodes*. They may be seen in os-

teoarthritis, RA, CPPD, and gout.[37] They are caused by intraosseous hemorrhages in hemophilia.

Collapse of a cyst results in deformity of the articular surface (Fig. 5.36). Further deformities may develop, including flattening of the femoral head, varus angulation, and "flat exostosis" formation at the superior margin of the junction between the femoral head and neck, a projected double contour of the medial aspect of the femoral head, medial spur formation, and buttressing of the medial femoral neck. Osteophytes at the acetabular margins are also frequent. Erosion of the femoral head with marked diminution in size

TABLE 5.1. ETIOLOGY OF SECONDARY OSTEOARTHRITIS OF THE HIP

Acetabular dysplasia
Acromegaly[26]
Athletic activity in adolescence[27,28]
Congenital dislocation of the hip
Disturbances of stress forces
Endocrine disturbances
Fracture or trauma
Idiopathic coxa vara
Ischemic necrosis of the femoral head
Legg-Perthes disease
Multiple epiphyseal dysplasia
Obesity
Ochronosis
Previous rheumatoid arthritis
Previous septic arthritis
Slipped capital femoral epiphysis

From Greenfield GB. Radiology of bone diseases, 5th ed. Philadelphia: JB Lippincott, 1990, with permission.

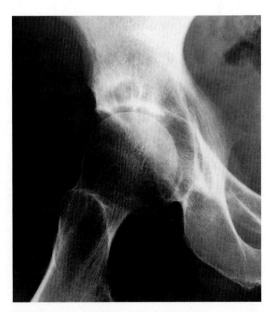

FIGURE 5.35. Osteoarthritis. Hip. There is narrowing of the superior aspect of the hip joint space. Sclerosis of the superior articular surface of the acetabulum is seen with well-defined subchondral cysts.

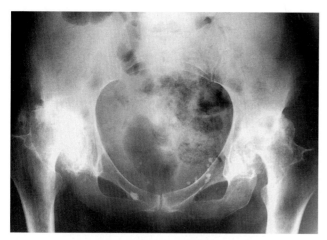

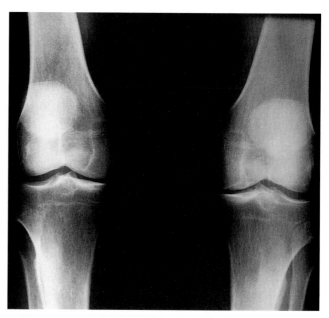

FIGURE 5.36. Severe osteoarthritis of the hips in a former ballet dancer. There is loss of joint space in the superior aspect on both sides, with erosions of both the acetabular grooves and the femoral heads and resultant flattening. This appears as upward subluxation of both femoral heads. A large cyst in the femoral head on the left side is seen as well as several cysts in the supraacetabular region on the right side. Soft-tissue calcification above the right greater trochanter is also seen.

FIGURE 5.37. Osteoarthritis. Knees. Narrowing of the medial compartments of both knee joints is noted.

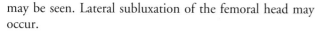

may be seen. Lateral subluxation of the femoral head may occur.

Bursal extension into the pelvis, presenting as an intrapelvic mass, has been described in osteoarthritis as well as in rheumatoid arthritis.[38]

Narrowing of the hip joint space may rarely occur after hip pinning for slipped femoral capital epiphysis, and may progress rapidly with acute symptoms. It is then known as *acute chondrolysis.* Joint space narrowing also

may occur with slipped capital femoral epiphysis without treatment.

Stress or insufficiency fractures may simulate the clinical symptoms of osteoarthritis of the hip. These may also be in the adjacent ischium or pubis. Persistent "hip" pain may be present in an osteopenic patient, with no fracture visible in the hip joint on conventional radiographs. After an interval, the fractures become evident with callus formation. However, MRI can detect these fractures immediately.

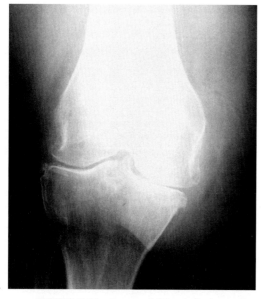

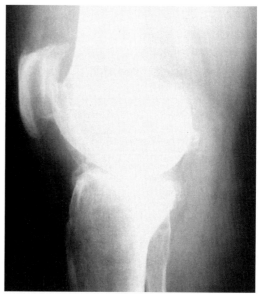

A

B

FIGURE 5.38. Osteoarthritis of the knee. **A:** AP view of the knee. **B:** Lateral view of the knee. Narrowing of the medial and lateral compartments of the knee joint space and osteophyte formation medially and at the patellar articular surface are seen.

The *knee* has three compartments: the lateral and medial femorotibial, and the patellofemoral. Narrowing of the knee joint space in osteoarthritis does not involve all three uniformly. The weight-bearing portion with greatest stress, usually the medial compartment, shows initial and greatest narrowing (Fig. 5.37). Weight-bearing radiographs show this best. Varus deformity may develop, with later subluxation. Occasionally, the lateral compartment may initially be narrowed, and in late stages, both medial and lateral compartments may develop narrowing (Fig. 5.38).

Marked spur formation at the joint margins and intercondyloid eminences may ensue, as well as at the margins of the patella. Subchondral sclerosis and cyst formation also are characteristic (Fig. 5.39), and erosions may occur (Fig. 5.40). A Baker's cyst and superior distension of the joint capsule may be present.

Chondrocalcinosis is frequently associated with advanced disease, involving the articular cartilage and the menisci. Erosion of the anterior aspect of the lower femur superior to the patella occurs associated with patellofemoral osteoarthritis.[39] Osteophyte formation at the patellar insertion of the quadriceps tendon can result in severe vertical ridging at the anterior superior surface of the patella.[40] Ossification of the medial collateral ligament, or Pellegrini–Stieda disease may be associated (Fig. 5.41). Stress fractures of the tibia have been reported to be associated with osteoarthritis of the knee, some following intraarticular steroid injections.[41] They may also occur at the dis-

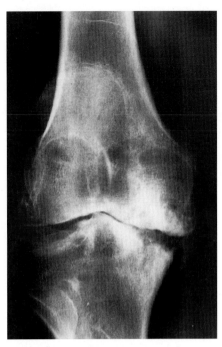

FIGURE 5.40. Osteoarthritis. Knee. Advanced. There is marked narrowing of the knee joint space with erosions at the margins. Subchondral cyst formation on both sides of the joint is seen as well as marginal spurs. There is a ridge at the superior aspect of the patella.

tal tibia, showing periosteal new bone formation. There may be rupture of the joint capsule, and arthrogram may show extravasated contrast material (Fig. 5.42).

Chondromalacia patellae is a related condition that occurs in younger patients.[42] "Softening" of cartilage at the articular surface of the patella occurs. Hypertrophic spurs at the patellar margins in a young person should raise suspicion of this possibility. Irregularity or loss of the patellar articular margin may also be seen. This condition is thought to be related to trauma. MRI can show details of the articular cartilage, articular cortex, and joint effusion, if present. Cartilage irregularities can be readily detected. These may range from a minimal articular cartilage brush-like surface to irregularity and loss of cartilage substance (Fig. 5.43).

In the *foot* and *ankle,* the most common site of involvement is the first metatarsophalangeal joint, usually associated with hallux valgus (Fig. 5.44). The first tarsometatarsal and talonavicular joints are commonly involved (Fig. 5.45). The tarsus may be involved secondary to congenital anomalies (Fig. 5.46). Spur formation at the dorsum of the talonavicular joint is seen in tarsal coalition, and may indicate that condition (Fig. 5.47). This is called the "talar beak" and is caused by overriding of the navicular on the talus. Pain at the first metatarsophalangeal joint may also be caused by reactive osteitis of the sesamoid bone (Fig. 5.48).

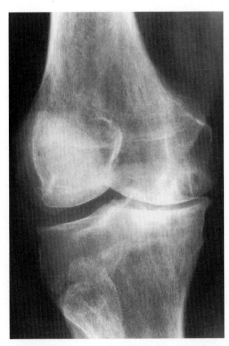

FIGURE 5.39. Osteoarthritis. Knee. There is narrowing of the medial compartment of the joint space with a large cyst at the articular surface of the distal femur and a small amount of spur formation.

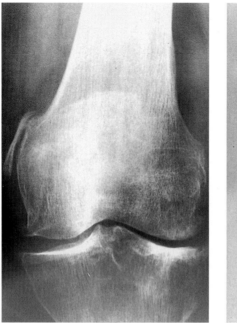
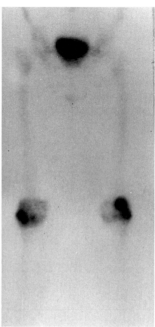

A   B

FIGURE 5.41. Osteoarthritis with associated Pellegrini–Stieda disease. **A:** Joint space narrowing most marked in the lateral compartment is noted as well as medial marginal spur formation. There is ossification of the medial collateral ligament. **B:** Radionuclide bone scan showing increased activity in both knees at their lateral aspects.

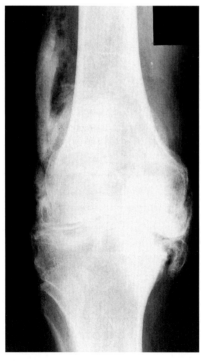

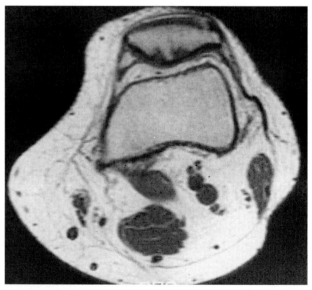

FIGURE 5.42. Osteoarthritis. Knee. Arthrogram. Marked joint space narrowing and spur formation are noted medially. Extravasated contrast material and air are seen extending superiorly along the lateral side.

FIGURE 5.43. Chondromalacia patellae. MRI. T1-weighted image. Irregularity of the articular surface of the patella with two central low-signal intensity defects is seen.

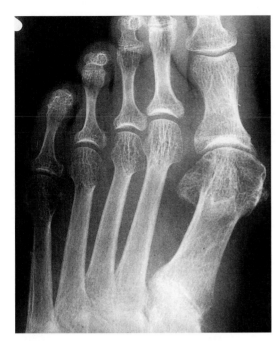

FIGURE 5.44. Osteoarthritis and hallux valgus of the first metatarsophalangeal joint are noted.

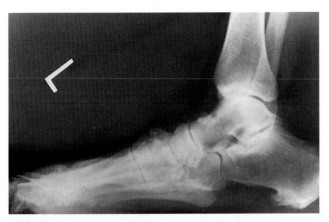

FIGURE 5.45. Osteoarthritis. Foot. Spur formation is seen in the tarsometatarsal area as well as plantar and dorsal calcaneal spurs.

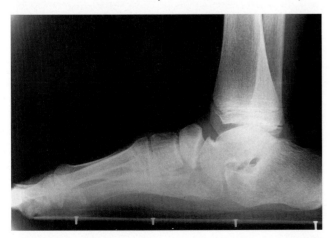

FIGURE 5.46. Foot. Lateral view shows a dorsal spur at the distal calcaneus with dorsal subluxation of the navicular bone in this patient with pes planovalgus.

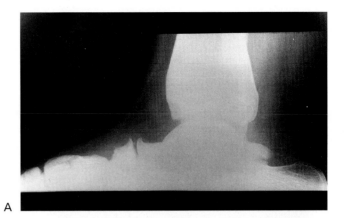

A

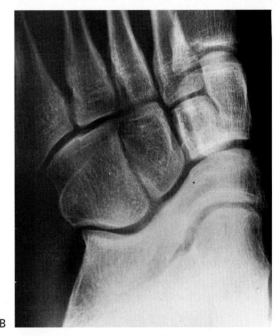

B

FIGURE 5.47. Calcaneonavicular coalition or bar. **A:** Lateral view shows spur formation at the dorsum. **B:** Oblique view. A calcaneonavicular coalition is noted.

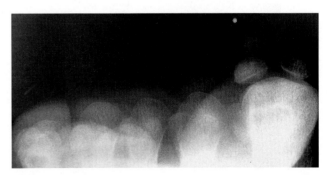

FIGURE 5.48. Reactive osteitis of the lateral sesamoid bone. Sesamoid axial view showing osteosclerosis at that site. A marker at the point of pain is present.

The *temporomandibular joint* may be involved with osteoarthritis (Fig. 5.49). Open-mouth and closed-mouth conventional views can demonstrate joint contours and range of motion. CT can yield better bony detail. MRI can show internal structural detail, including the fibrocartilaginous disc, lateral pterygoid muscle, capsule, bony contours, and range of motion. Visualization of the disc is of prime importance in evaluating internal derangements. It is composed of thicker anterior and posterior bands joined by a thin zone. The posterior band lies directly above the mandibular condyle in the closed-mouth position.

Central Skeleton. In the *spine,* there are two distinct articular systems: the apophyseal joints, which are diarthrodial, and the intervertebral discs. Thus, there are two distinct processes; facet joint osteoarthritis, and spondylosis, which involves the vertebral margins.

The spinal canal is formed anteriorly by the vertebral bodies and the posterior longitudinal ligament. The neural arch surrounds the canal laterally and posteriorly. This consists of the pedicles, the facet joint complex, and the lamina. The facet joint complex comprises the superior articular facets, pars interarticulars, and inferior articular facets. The ligamentum flavum lies on the inner aspect of the lamina on each side.

The facet joints are true synovial joints, surrounded by a capsular ligament. Osteoarthritic changes are similar to those in peripheral joints.

The intervertebral disc is composed of a central nucleus pulposus surrounded by the annulus fibrosus. The annulus

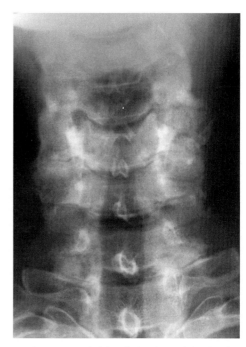

FIGURE 5.50. Osteoarthritis of the facet joint in the cervical spine. Osteosclerosis and lateral spur formation on the left side in the mid cervical spine are noted.

fibrosus comprises collagenous and fibrocartilaginous fibers. These are thinnest posteriorly, and are reinforced by the posterior longitudinal ligament. The cartilaginous end plates form the superior and inferior boundaries.

The lateral recess of the spinal canal is formed anteriorly by the posterior aspect of the vertebral body, and at the disc by the annulus fibrosus. The posterolateral borders include the pedicle and the facet joint.

The spinal nerve roots travel inferiorly within the lateral recesses and exit through the intervertebral foramina. These foramina are formed by the inferior aspect of the vertebral

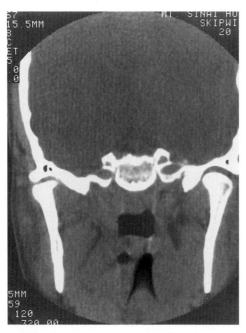

FIGURE 5.49. Osteoarthritis of the right temporomandibular joint. CT. Flattening and medial spur formation of the right mandibular head are seen.

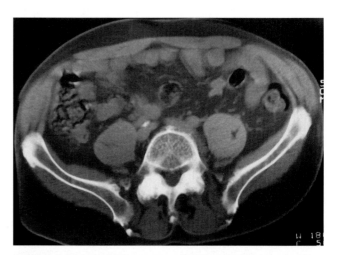

FIGURE 5.51. Facet joint osteoarthritis. CT axial image shows facet joint arthritis bilaterally with joint space narrowing, hypertrophy, and sclerosis. A vacuum sign is seen on the left side.

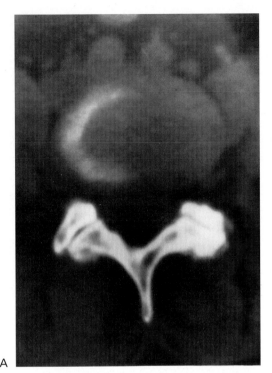
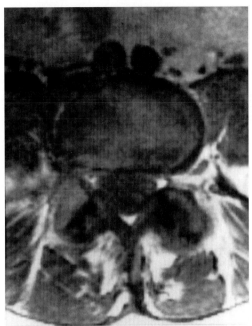

A   B

FIGURE 5.52. Facet joint osteoarthritis. **A:** CT axial image shows facet joint arthritis on the left side with joint space narrowing, hypertrophy, and sclerosis. **B:** MRI. Proton density-weighted image. Enlargement of the facet joint with irregularity is seen.

body and intervertebral disc anteriorly, the respective pedicles superiorly and inferiorly, and the facet joint posteriorly.

Conventional radiographs in the anteroposterior, lateral, and oblique projections demonstrate the bony structures. Malalignment, neural arch defects, spondylosis, facet joint arthritis, disc space narrowing, as well as vertebral body changes can be well shown.

CT and MRI can directly relate bony changes to spinal canal and foramen involvement.

Spinal osteoarthritis of the facet joints is similar to osteoarthritis in peripheral joints. Conventional radiography can show joint space narrowing, sclerosis, cysts, and osteophytes (Fig. 5.50). CT and MRI can better demonstrate the changes, as well as a vacuum sign (Figs. 5.51 and 5.52), hypertrophy, or a synovial cyst.[43] The latter two conditions may impinge on the lateral recess and cause lateral recess stenosis of the spinal canal. This causes symptoms of nerve root compression.

RELATED CONDITIONS

Spinal Stenosis

Clinical Aspects

Frank B. Vasey

Low back pain worsened by walking with improvement at rest initially suggests vascular compromise to the exercising muscle. It has been increasingly recognized since the 1950s

that spinal cord and nerve root compression can produce similar symptoms. Clinical clues suggesting neurogenic claudication include less predictability as to onset of pain in relation to distance walked. Postural relief in a flexed position increases the likelihood of spinal stenosis (SS). Patients with neurogenic claudication function better at the grocery store when they lean on the cart while walking.

Multiple factors contribute to spinal canal insufficiency. These include: congenital factors such as short pedicles, a triangular (trefoil) shape, to a completely narrow canal. Acquired problems include bulging discs, hypertrophic facet joints and spinal ligaments, and spinal instability in the form of spondylolysis and spondylolisthesis. It remains unclear if symptoms are caused by direct compression of neural elements or indirect vascular compromise.

Plain radiographs suggest the possibility of spinal stenosis by demonstrating disc space narrowing and hypertrophy of facet joints. More definitive information can be obtained by CT and MRI.

Surgical decompression is the ultimate treatment. Patients need to recognize that it will not resolve their pain completely because of persisting facet joint osteoarthritis.

Radiologic Aspects

George B. Greenfield

Spinal stenosis, or narrowing of the spinal canal is clinically important in the cervical and lumbar areas.[44,45] Congenital or developmental spinal stenosis may occur in conditions such as achondroplasia with developmentally short pedicles; however, most cases are acquired. The stenosis may be localized, and in the lumbar spine it is more likely to occur in the lowermost two segments.

The anatomic regions of interest in spinal stenosis are the sagittal diameter or central canal, the lateral recesses, and the intervertebral foramina. Degenerative lesions leading to stenosis have been described as a function of the three-joint complex (intervertebral disc and the two apophyseal facet joints).[45]

Central canal stenosis may result from posterior hypertrophic spur formation of the vertebral body, spondylolisthesis, intervertebral disc protrusion or herniation, ligamentum flavum hypertrophy, or other diseases, such as Paget's disease. An anteroposterior diameter of 11.5 mm is considered absolute stenosis, whereas a diameter 13 to 14 mm is considered to be relative stenosis. Lateral recess stenosis usually results from hypertrophic changes of the inferior articular facets. A synovial cyst of the facet joint may also result in this condition. A lateral recess of less than 3 mm is considered stenotic.[46] A trefoil contour of the spinal canal is seen on axial CT images. Intervertebral foramen stenosis or impingement may develop from hypertrophic spur formation, particularly in the cervical spine. Lateral disc herniation, or narrowing of the intervertebral space with subsequent diminution of height of the lateral canal can also be causative.

Spondylosis results from the avulsion of fibers of the annulus fibrosus from the marginal ridge of the vertebral body.[47] It is usually located in the lower cervical, lower thoracic, and lower lumbar and lumbosacral segments. Protuberances from the vertebral margins, termed *osteophytes*, are seen. They blend with the vertebral bodies, with a continuous cortex. Their departure is horizontal, although later they curve and may fuse with one another (Figs. 5.53, 5.54, and 5.55).

Osteophytes are to be differentiated from *syndesmophytes*, which have a vertical direction and occur in inflammatory disease of the spine. Another type of osteophyte is called the *traction spur*.[48] These are also initially horizontally directed, but arise approximately 2 mm away from the vertebral margin at the site of attachment of the outermost fibers of the anulus fibrosus. They signify segmental instability. Both types of osteophytes may coexist, and they represent different stages of the same process.[49]

Spondylosis of the *cervical spine* is most likely to cause severe symptoms because of the relatively narrow cervical neural canal and intervertebral foramina.

Posterior osteophytes may form a ridge (Fig. 5.56) that causes narrowing, and may compress the cervical cord. Spurs on the lateral lips of the uncovertebral "joints" of Luschka may narrow or encroach on the intervertebral foramina, resulting in neurological symptoms (Figs. 5.57 and 5.58). These spurs have a radiolucent cartilage cap; therefore, their true size is not indicated on conventional radiographs. Subluxations may also occur.

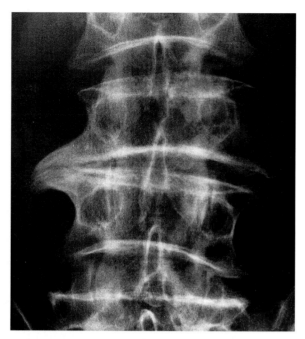

FIGURE 5.53. Lumbar spine. Osteophytes. A large osteophyte with a horizontal takeoff is seen on the right side at L3-4. Smaller osteophytes on the left side are also noted. These are seen at the margins of the vertebral bodies. On the left side at L-1 a small traction spur is noted approximately 2 mm proximal to the vertebral margin.

Osteophytosis surrounding the odontoid process and the superior margin of the anterior arch of the atlas may be seen.[50]

Disc degeneration may be evident as narrowing of the intervertebral space, or as a radiolucency in the disc, termed

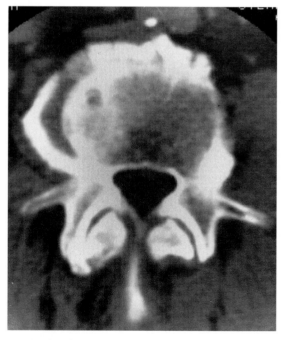

FIGURE 5.54. Lumbar spine. CT. A large lateral osteophyte is seen removed from the vertebral body at this level as well as large anterior osteophytes.

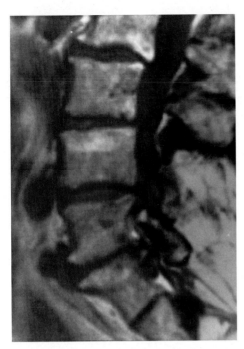

FIGURE 5.55. Lumbar spine. MRI. Sagittal T1-weighted image. Narrowing of the intervertebral space between L-5 and the sacrum is seen as well as anterior osteophytes at that level. The osteophytes contain normal marrow signal within them.

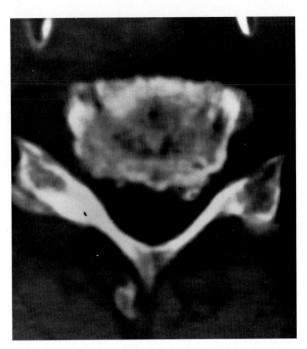

FIGURE 5.56. Cervical spine. CT. Posterior osteophytes have formed a ridge compressing the lateral recess and the neural canal.

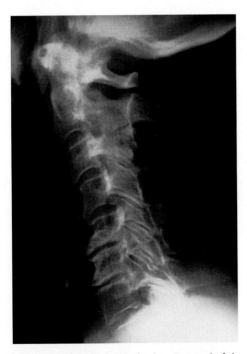

FIGURE 5.57. Spondylosis. Cervical spine. Reversal of the cervical lordotic curvature, narrowing of the intervertebral discs at C5-6 and C6-7 is noted, as well as hypertrophic spur formation at these levels.

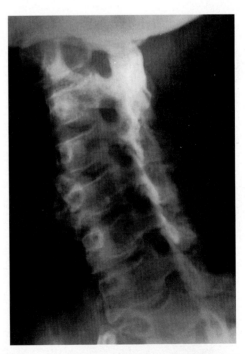

FIGURE 5.58. Cervical spine. Oblique view. Posterior osteophytes are seen encroaching into the intervertebral foramen at C4-5 from its anterior aspect. There is also facet joint osteoarthritis posteriorly with encroachment into the intervertebral foramen at C4-5 and to a greater extent at C5-6, from the posterior aspects.

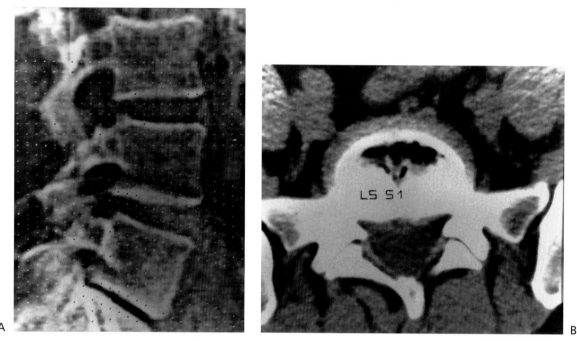

FIGURE 5.59. Vacuum sign. Lumbar spine. CT. **A:** Scout view. A vacuum sign is seen between L-5 and the sacrum as a low density line. **B:** Axial section shows air density in the anterior part of the intervertebral disc.

the *vacuum sign* (Fig. 5.59). Gas, principally nitrogen, accumulates within disc fissures, particularly under conditions of reduced pressure.

Herniation of the intervertebral disc through the end plates results in Schmorl's nodes (Fig. 5.60). If the herniation occurs at the anterior aspect of the vertebral body, an

appearance of a detached corner is seen (Fig. 5.61). Such a configuration is called a "limbus vertebra."

Calcification of the intervertebral disc may result from a variety of conditions, such as ochronosis, ankylosing spondylitis, trauma, and chronic stress.[51]

A transitional lumbosacral vertebra may form a pseu-

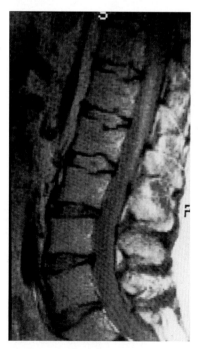

FIGURE 5.60. Lumbar spine. MRI. T1-weighted image. Multiple herniations of the nucleus pulposus into the vertebral bodies are seen representing Schmorl's nodes.

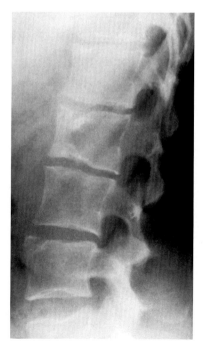

FIGURE 5.61. Lateral view of the lumbar spine. Schmorl's nodes are seen at L-1 and L-2. An anterior Schmorl's node at L-4 has resulted in a "limbus vertebra" configuration.

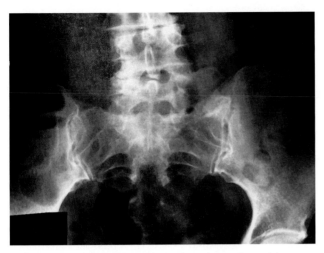

FIGURE 5.62. A transitional lumbosacral vertebra with an enlarged left transverse process forms a pseudarthrosis with the sacral wing.

darthrosis between its large transverse process and the sacral wing, and develop symptomatic osteoarthritis at that site (Fig. 5.62). A neural arch defect may result in reactive sclerosis, usually on the contralateral side, but occasionally on the ipsilateral side (Fig. 5.63).

The *sacroiliac joints* may be involved with osteoarthritis. Joint space narrowing, subchondral sclerosis, and osteophyte formation at the inferior margins are seen (Fig. 5.64). The osteophytes may be bridging. Plain films may show these bridging osteophytes as simulating joint fusion (Fig. 5.65), but CT can show the true anatomical changes (Fig. 5.66).

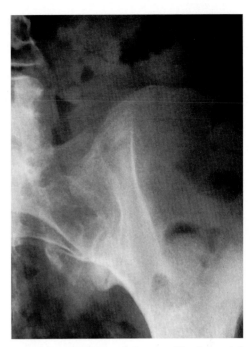

FIGURE 5.64. Osteoarthritis of the sacroiliac joint. A large osteophyte at the inferior aspect of the sacroiliac is seen.

Osteitis condensans ilii represents reactive sclerosis to stress of the SI joint. It occurs on the iliac side of the joint because of the thinner cartilage in that location. On AP view, it can be projected over the sacral wing. The SI joint itself can be seen to be normal (Fig. 5.67).

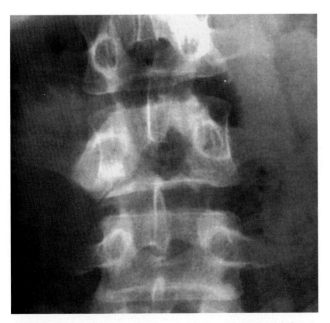

FIGURE 5.63. AP view of the lumbar spine. There is a defect in the right pars interarticularis of L3 on the right side with reactive sclerosis present.

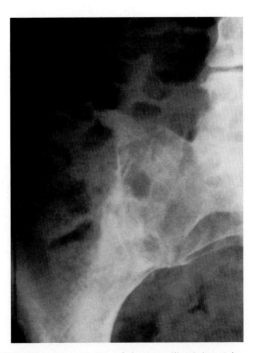

FIGURE 5.65. Osteoarthritis of the sacroiliac joint. A bony mass is seen across the sacroiliac joint that represents a bridging osteophyte of the joint. The contours of the joint can be seen through the bony density.

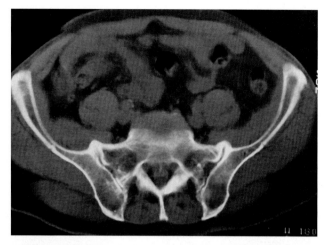

FIGURE 5.66. Osteoarthritis. Sacroiliac joints. CT. Osteophytes bilaterally at the anterior aspects of the sacroiliac joints with bony bridging are seen.

Case Reports

Joanne Valeriano-Marcet

Case 1. A 65-year-old woman with generalized OA involving the hands, hips, cervical and lumbar spine, who was status post lumbar laminectomy and fusion, presented with increasing neck pain radiating into both upper extremities. She experienced intermittent numbness in the lateral aspect of both arms.

Physical Examination. Physical examination revealed marked decrease in lateral flexion of the cervical spine with cervical paraspinal muscle spasm.

Radiograph. Cervical spine radiograph revealed severe hyperostosis of the cervical spine from C3-7 with severe disc space narrowing at C5-6 and C6-7. Significant posterior hyperostosis with impingement on the neural foramina was present at C5-6 and C6-7. There was bony sclerosis at C-5 and C-6.

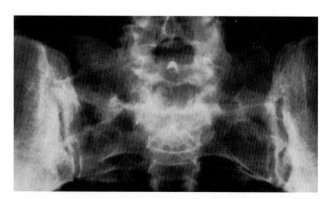

FIGURE 5.67. Osteitis condensans ilii. AP view of the pelvis. Sclerosis at the iliac side of the sacroiliac joints bilaterally is noted. The sacroiliac joints are normal. Sclerosis and spur formation at the symphysis pubis are also seen.

MRI. Cervical MRI revealed spondylosis at the C5-6 level, which indented the ventral margin of the cervical spinal cord and resulted in canal and bilateral foramina stenosis at this level. Less prominent foramina encroachment was also identified on the right at the C6-7 and on the left at C3-4 (Fig. 5.68).

The patient had continued neck pain radiating into the upper extremities as well as upper extremity weakness despite 8 weeks of treatment with NSAIDs, Tylenol, a muscle relaxant, physical therapy, and use of a cervical pillow. The patient was referred to neurosurgery for further evaluation.

Case 2. A 67-year-old woman with a history of OA involving the hands and cervical and lumbar spine presented with progressive increase in low back pain radiating into the buttocks. The pain was exacerbated by walking and relieved with rest. The patient denied bowel or bladder incontinence. There was no numbness or tingling or weakness of the lower extremities. She denied calf claudication.

Physical Examination. Physical examination revealed tenderness of the lumbar paraspinal muscles, good ROM of the hips, (exacerbation of back pain with lumbar extension) back pain with negative straight leg raising, and lower lumbar dextroscoliosis.

MRI Reading. Lumbar intervertebral disc herniations were demonstrated by MRI (Fig. 5.69).

Diffuse Idiopathic Skeletal Hyperostosis
Clinical Aspects

Frank B. Vasey

Diffuse idiopathic skeletal hyperostosis (DISH) is a common finding in elderly patients. It was originally described in 1950 by a French clinician, Forestier. The current radiographic understanding and terminology for the condition were described by Resnick in 1975 and 1976. This important work, however, did not emphasize the fact that the patient may be symptomatic. Chronic thoracic spine pain is unusual in comparison to lumbar or cervical pain, likely related to better spine support from the ribs. In Resnick's study, T-7 to T-12 was the most frequently involved area. These typically elderly patients have chronic mild pain and stiffness, which may take an inflammatory pattern by improving during the day but worsening with inactivity. Conversely, the pain may be aggravated by strenuous overactivity. Eventual loss of motion in the spine occurs, but not usually to the extent of complete spinal fusion, as seen in ankylosing spondylitis.

The process in the cervical spine may be rarely so exuberant as to cause dysphagia. Extraspinal involvement occurs in the form of enthesopathy (tendinous insertion into bone). Heel spurs, elbow spurs, and a ragged appearance to

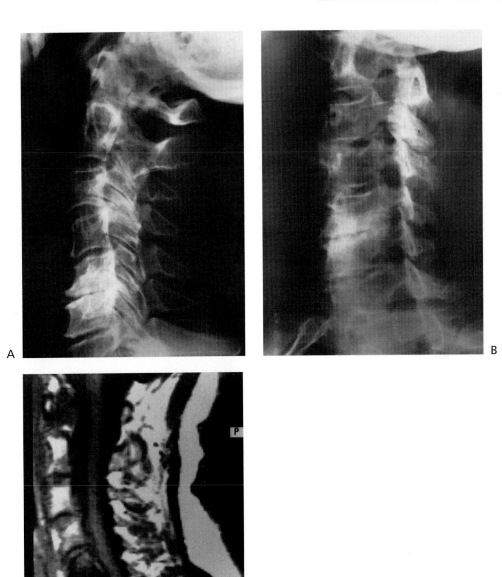

FIGURE 5.68. A: Cervical spine. Lateral view. Severe hyperostosis of the cervical spine from C3-7 with disc space narrowing at C5-6 and C6-7 is seen. **B:** Oblique view. Posterior hyperostosis with impingement on the neural foramina is present at C5-6 and C6-7. There is bony sclerosis at C-5 and C-6. **C:** MRI. Spondylosis at the C5-6 level indents the ventral margin of the cervical spinal cord. Less prominent encroachment is also identified at C3-4.

the pelvis all may reflect this condition. The diagnosis is made by plain spinal radiographs. Resnick's criteria include flowing calcification along four contiguous vertebral bodies, preservation of intervertebral disc height (as opposed to degenerative disc disease) and absence of apophyseal or sacroiliac joint fusion in the synovial compartment (as opposed to ankylosing spondylitis). The calcification of the spine occurs in the anterior spinal ligament, which provides an important radiographic clue, namely a zone of lucency where the ligament rolls away from the vertebral body and disc. Again, this is distinct from ankylosing spondylitis where the calci-

fication occurs in the annulus fibrosus tightly adherent to the disc.

Radiologic Aspects

George B. Greenfield

DISH, originally termed ankylosing hyperostosis or Forestier's disease, represents ossification of the anterior longitudinal ligament of the spine, other ligaments, and enthesitis.[52–54] It commonly affects older patients. The basic process is ligamentous ossification. This can occur at enthesis,

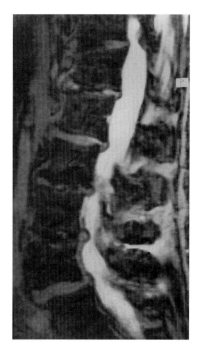

FIGURE 5.69. Lumbar spine. MRI. Sagittal T2-weighted image. Disc herniations at L2-3 and L3-4 are seen. Spinal stenosis has resulted at the lower level.

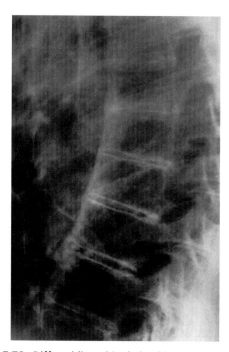

FIGURE 5.70. Diffuse idiopathic skeletal hyperostosis. Thoracic spine. Calcification of the anterior longitudinal ligament is seen. There is a radiolucent line separating the anterior vertebral bodies from the calcified anterior longitudinal ligament.

or ligamentous attachments, as well as tendons and ligaments in the pelvis, superior third of the sacroiliac joints, symphysis pubis, calcaneus, tarsals, patella, olecranon, humerus, and hands.

It is a reaction to stress; it is not an arthritis. It commonly affects older patients. It is present in 25% to 35% of elderly white men. It is less frequent in women and Blacks.[55] It is considered by many to be asymptomatic; however, some patients with thoracic spine pain do have DISH.

Central Skeleton. In the *spine,* classic criteria include involvement over four contiguous vertebral bodies, relative intervertebral disc preservation, and no relation to arthritis, which may be coincidentally present. The thoracic spine is most often involved, either with large pointed and fused spurs or smooth anterior longitudinal ligament ossification. This may vary in thickness from a few millimeters up to 2 cm. The ossified anterior longitudinal ligament is separated from the vertebral margin by a thin radiolucent line (Figs. 5.70 and 5.71). All segments of the spine may be involved. When the cervical spine is involved, dysphagia owing to anterior infringement on the esophagus may result, particularly if only one segment remains mobile and large osteophytes develop at that site (Figs. 5.72 and 5.73).[54] The apophyseal joints are not fused, and the intervertebral spaces are not narrowed. CT can demonstrate the ossification to good advantage (Fig. 5.74).

Ossification of the posterior longitudinal ligament also may occur (Figs. 5.75 and 5.76). This ossification may be extensive and result in spinal stenosis (Fig. 5.77). It may be associated with DISH or it may be isolated. This is more

commonly seen in Japan. CT can show anatomic details of the narrowed spinal canal. MRI can provide information about the severity of spinal cord compression by the abnormal signal intensity of the spinal cord.[56]

The ossified ligament may be involved with metastases (Fig. 5.78).

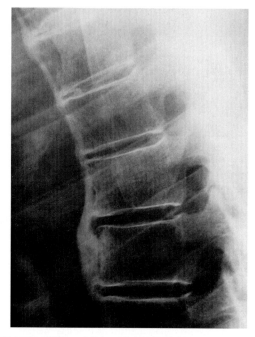

FIGURE 5.71. Diffuse idiopathic skeletal hyperostosis. Thoracic spine. Ossification of the anterior longitudinal ligament is seen with a clear zone of separation from the anterior margin of the vertebral body. The ossification is thicker at its inferior aspect.

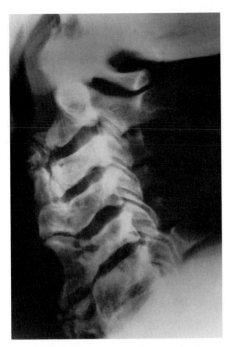

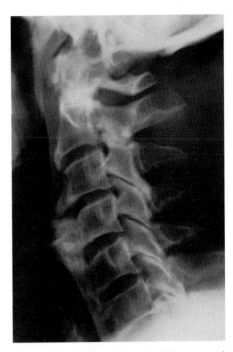

FIGURE 5.72. Diffuse idiopathic skeletal hyperostosis. Cervical spine. Large exuberant bone formation is noted at the anterior aspect of the cervical spine with several pseudoarthroses. The patient complained of dysphagia.

FIGURE 5.73. Diffuse idiopathic skeletal hyperostosis. Cervical spine. Lateral view shows dense ossification of the anterior longitudinal ligament from C-4 downward. Motility is maintained at C3-4 where a large spur has developed resulting in dysphagia. The intervertebral spaces are preserved, as is the bone density.

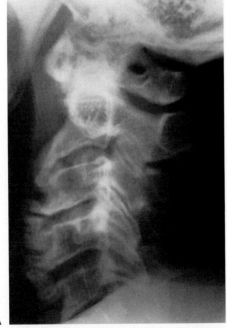

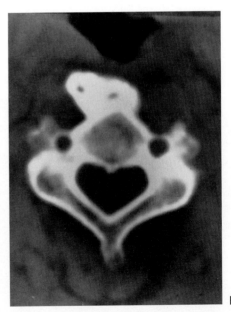

A   B

FIGURE 5.74. Diffuse idiopathic skeletal hyperostosis. Cervical spine. **A:** Lateral view showing exuberant ossification of the anterior longitudinal ligament over four vertebral bodies. There is no osteoporosis, and the intervertebral spaces are intact. **B:** CT of the same patient is showing dense ossification of the anterior longitudinal ligament.

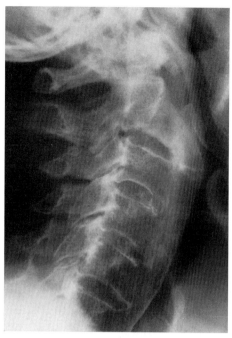

FIGURE 5.75. Diffuse idiopathic skeletal hyperostosis in an 82-year-old woman. Ossification of the posterior longitudinal ligament is seen as well as dense ossification of the entire anterior longitudinal ligament. Osteoporosis of the cervical spine is also seen.

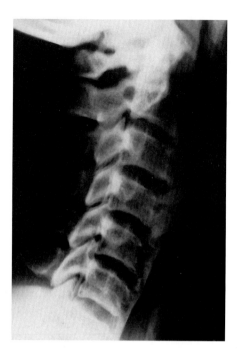

FIGURE 5.76. Diffuse idiopathic skeletal hyperostosis. Ossification of the posterior longitudinal ligament (OPL) is seen as well as ossification of the anterior longitudinal ligament and a large spur in the ossified mass at C3-4. The intervertebral discs are preserved.

Retinoid intake may also result in ossification of this ligament.[57]

The *pelvis* is not uncommonly involved with a whiskered appearance of the iliac and ischiac bones (Fig. 5.79), as well as the trochanters of the femur. The symph-ysis pubis may be bridged. Ossification of the ligaments at the superior third of the *sacroiliac joints* with fusion may be seen in DISH, in contrast to involvement of the lower two-thirds, as in the inflammatory arthritides (Figs. 5.80 and 5.81).

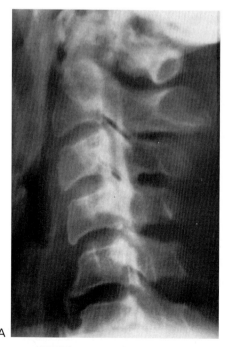

A

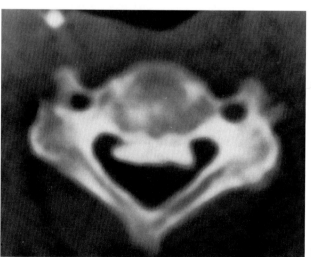

B

FIGURE 5.77. Diffuse idiopathic skeletal hyperostosis. **A:** Lateral view of the cervical spine shows ossification of the posterior longitudinal ligament. **B:** CT shows ossification of the posterior longitudinal ligament causing spinal stenosis.

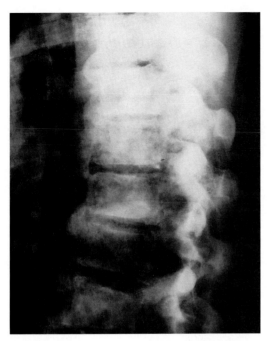

FIGURE 5.78. Patient with prostate carcinoma with blastic metastases to the spine. Diffuse idiopathic skeletal hyperostosis in the spine is also involved.

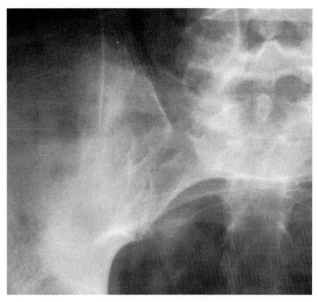

FIGURE 5.80. Diffuse idiopathic skeletal hyperostosis. Sacroiliac joint. Ossification at the superior aspect of sacroiliac joint is noted, whereas the inferior aspect remains intact.

Peripheral Skeleton. The *hands* may be involved, with broadening of the terminal tufts, increased cortical width, enlarged sesamoid bones, exostoses, and capsular new bone formation (Fig. 5.82).[58]

In the *shoulder,* enthesitis may be seen, particularly as calcifications at the inferior aspect of the glenoid margin (Fig. 5.83). Enthesitis at the acromioclavicular joint and calcification of the rotator cuff tendon may also occur.

In the *elbow,* extensive ossific spur formation may occur, particularly about the olecranon.

Hyperostosis of the attachments of the interosseous membranes of the forearm and leg also occurs.

In the *foot* and *ankle,* bony spurs at the attachments of the Achilles tendon and the plantar aponeurosis to the calcaneus are seen. In the forefoot, spurring of the terminal tufts of the toes occurs without marked subchondral sclerosis.[59] Spurs at the dorsal margins of the tarsal bones and at the tibiotalar joint may be seen.

In the *knee,* bony spurs at the attachments of the quadriceps tendon and the patellar ligament may be seen, also at the tibial tubercle. There may be ossification of the medial collateral ligament, and at the tibial tuberosity.

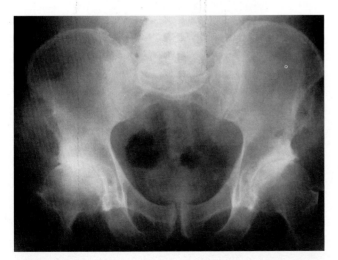

FIGURE 5.79. Diffuse idiopathic skeletal hyperostosis. Pelvis. Whiskering at the lateral margins of both iliac bones are noted. Osteoarthritis of both hips with marginal spur formation, and enthesitis at the acetabular margins are also seen.

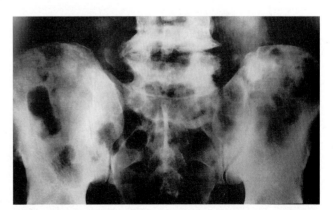

FIGURE 5.81. Diffuse idiopathic skeletal hyperostosis. Sacroiliac joints. There is fusion of the superior third of the sacroiliac joints, whereas the lower two-thirds, which are synovial joints, are not involved. Spondylosis at L4-5 is also noted.

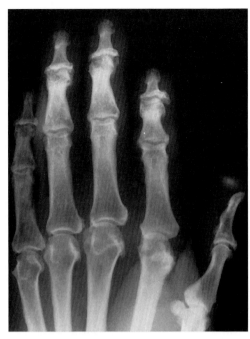

FIGURE 5.82. Diffuse idiopathic skeletal hyperostosis. Hand. Osteoarthritis at the distal interphalangeal joints and at the metacarpal phalangeal joints are noted. Ossifications at the radial aspect of the distal interphalangeal joints of the middle and ring fingers are seen as well as a very exuberant osteophyte at the distal interphalangeal joint of the index finger. A triangular protrusion at the distal fifth metacarpal is also seen. Paraarticular calcification at the base of the proximal phalanx of the middle finger is present.

Spondylolysis and Spondylolisthesis

George B. Greenfield

Spondylolysis refers to a defect in the pars interarticularis.[60] This is now considered to be secondary to a stress fracture. This is a common condition, affecting an estimated 14 mil-

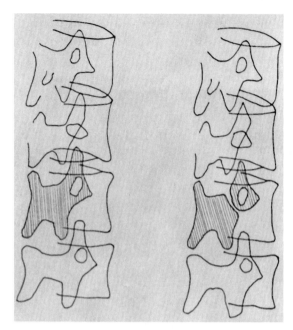

FIGURE 5.84. Diagram of normal scotty dog sign and spondylolysis. (Photo, courtesy of Dr. Pakorn Sirijintakarn.)

lion people in the United States. Up to one-fourth of people involved experience low back pain at some time in their lives.[61] The defect is usually at the L5 level. It is best demonstrated by oblique radiographs, showing the "scotty dog" sign with a defect at its neck (Figs. 5.84 and 5.85).

Spondylolisthesis is forward displacement of a vertebral body with respect to the one below.[60] True spondylolisthe-

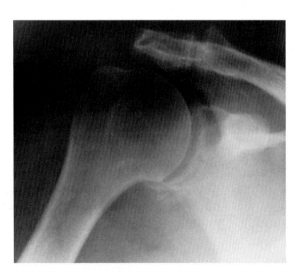

FIGURE 5.83. Diffuse idiopathic skeletal hyperostosis. Shoulder. Calcifications at the inferior margin of the glenoid fossa are noted representing enthesitis. Acromioclavicular arthritis and enthesitis is also present.

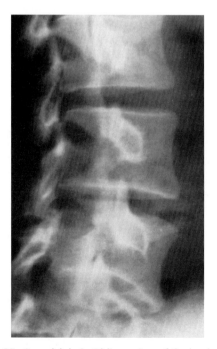

FIGURE 5.85. Spondylolysis. Oblique view of the lumbar spine. A pars interarticularis defect at L-5 is seen. This is the neck of the "scotty dog" sign.

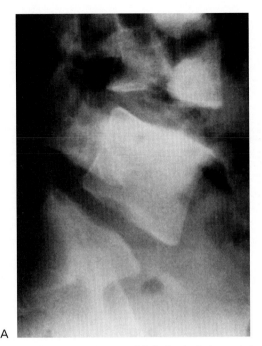

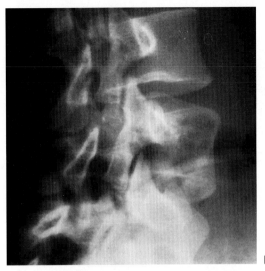

FIGURE 5.86. Spondylolisthesis. **A:** Lateral view of the lumbosacral region shows grade I spondylolisthesis with forward slippage of L-5 on the sacrum of less than 25%. **B:** Oblique view of the facet joints shows a defect in the pars interarticularis of L-5.

sis is usually at the L5-S1 level, and may be seen in a younger age group.

Degenerative spondylolisthesis or *pseudospondylolisthesis* results from degeneration of the intervertebral disc and loosened connecting ligaments.[62] This form is usually seen in patients older than 45 years of age. Osteoarthritis of the facet joints and thickening of the ligamentum flavum are seen. The amount of displacement is usually not great. The classic appearance of spondylolisthesis on conventional radiography is forward displacement of the superior body on the one inferior, seen on lateral view, with a defect in the pars interarticularis seen on oblique view (Fig. 5.86). The

"Napoleon hat sign" is seen in the anteroposterior view of the lumbosacral region. A bell-shaped curved contour of the overlap is noted (Fig. 5.87). On CT, a double contour of the vertebral bodies is seen, as well as the pars interarticularis defect (Fig. 5.88). The spinal canal may be stenosed.

The displacement can be graded on a scale of 1 to 4. Grade 1 is up to 25%, grade 2 is 50%, and so on.

Reverse spondylolisthesis or *retrolisthesis* is a result of degenerative changes in the disc.[60] A steplike interruption of the posterior vertebral contour is seen owing to posterior vertebral displacement. This results in narrowing of the intervertebral foramina, with an hourglass shape.

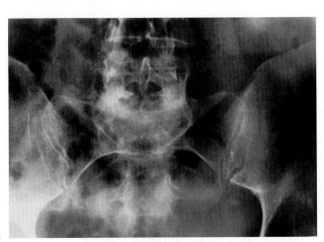

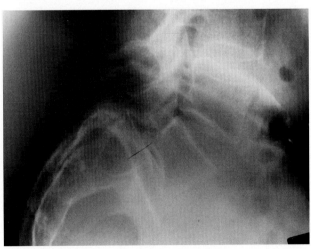

FIGURE 5.87. Spondylolisthesis of L-5 on S-1. **A:** AP view. **B:** Lateral view. Note the triangular configuration projected over the sacral promontory. This is the inverted "Napoleon hat sign".

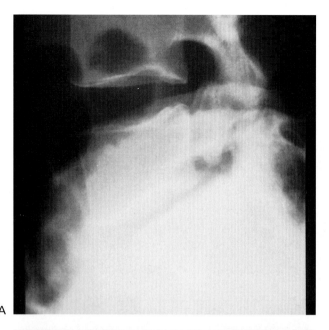

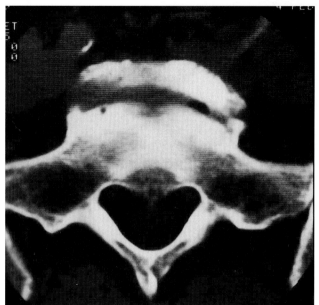

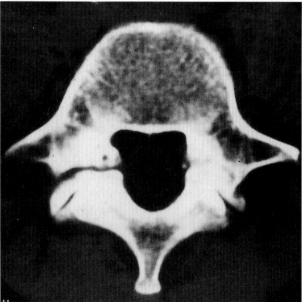

FIGURE 5.88. Spondylolisthesis of L-5 on S-1. **A:** Lateral view of the lumbosacral spine reveals grade I spondylolisthesis of L-5 on the sacrum. **B:** CT shows a double contour of L-5 and S-1 with the intervertebral space containing a small amount of gas between them. **C:** CT shows the pars interarticularis defect on the right side.

All of the preceding displacements may cause symptoms owing to compression of the contents of the spinal canal and nerve roots.

Kashin–Bek Disease

George B. Greenfield

Kashin–Bek disease is caused by excessive iron intake in the drinking water.[63] It results in necrosis and degeneration of cartilage in the joints of the spine and extremities. It almost always occurs in children. It is slowly progressive and results in metaphyseal and epiphyseal deformities, with shortening of the extremities and reduction of height. The hands and wrists are also often involved. It is endemic in parts of Asia, including China, Siberia, and North Korea.

REFERENCES

Osteoarthritis

1. Suarez-Almazor ME, Belseck E, Russell AS, et al. Use of lumbar radiographs for the early diagnosis of low back pain. *JAMA* 1997; 277:1782–1786.
2. Frazier LM, Carey TS, Lyles MF, et al. Selective criteria may increase lumbo sacral spine: roentgenogram use in acute low back pain. *Arch Int Med* 1989;149:47–50.
3. Carey TS, Garrett J, Jackman A, et al. The outcomes and costs of

care for acute low back pain among patients seen by primary care practitioners, chiropractors, and orthopedic surgeons. *NEJM* 1995;333:913–917.

4. Van Tulder MW, Assendelft WJ, Koeo BW, et al. Spinal radiographic findings and non-specific low back pain. *Spine* 1997; 22:427–434.

Hypertrophic Arthritis

5. Forrester DM, Brown JC, Nesson JW. *The radiology of joint disease,* 2nd ed. Philadelphia: WB Saunders, 1978.
6. Greenspan A, Norman A, Tchans FK. Tooth sign in patellar degenerative disease. *J Bone Joint Surg [Am]* 1977;59: 483–485.
7. Jaffe HL. *Metabolic, degenerative, and inflammatory diseases of bones and joints.* Philadelphia: Lea & Febiger, 1972.
8. Resnick D. Patterns of migration of the femoral head in osteoarthritis of the hip: roentgenographic–pathologic correlation and comparison with rheumatoid arthritis. *AJR* 1975;124: 62–74.
9. Resnick D, Niwayama G, Goergen TG. Comparison of radiographic abnormalities of the sacroiliac joint in degenerative disease and ankylosing spondylitis. *AJR* 1977;128:189–196.
10. Thomas RH, Resnick D, Alazraki NP, et al. Compartmental evaluation of osteoarthritis of the knee: a comparative study of available diagnostic modalities. *Radiology* 1975;116:585–594.
11. Udoff EJ, Genant HK, Kozin F, et al. Mixed connective tissue disease: the spectrum of radiographic manifestations. *Radiology* 1977;124:613–618.
12. Kerr R, Resnick D, Pineda C, et al. Osteoarthritis of the glenohumeral joint: a radiologic–pathologic study. *AJR* 1985;144: 967–972.
13. Palmer PES, Stadalnick R, Arnon S. The genetic factor in cervical spondylosis. *Skeletal Radiol* 1984;11:178–182.
14. Foldes K, Petersilge CA, Weisman MH, et al. Nodal osteoarthritis and gout: a report of four new cases. *Skeletal Radiol* 1996; 25:421–424.
15. Martel W, Snarr JW, Horn JR. The metacarpophalangeal joints in interphalangeal osteoarthritis. *Radiology* 1973;108:1–7.
16. Smukler NM, Edeiken J, Guiliano VJ. Ankylosis in osteoarthritis of the finger joints. *Radiology* 1971;100:525–530.

Erosive Osteoarthritis

17. Kidd KL, Peter JB. Erosive osteoarthritis. *Radiology* 1966; 86:640–674.
18. Swezey RL, Alexander SJ. Erosive osteoarthritis and the main-en-lorgnette deformity (opera glass hand). *Arch Intern Med* 1971; 128:269–272.
19. Utsinger PD, et al. Roentgenologic, immunologic, and therapeutic study of erosive (inflammatory) osteoarthritis. *Arch Intern Med* 1978;138:693–997.
20. Keats TE, Johnstone WH, O'Brien WM. Large joint destruction in erosive osteoarthritis. *Skeletal Radiol* 1981;6:276–269.
21. Schneider HJ, Weiss MA, Stern PJ, et al. Silicone-induced erosive arthritis: radiologic features in seven cases. *AJR* 1987;148: 923–925.
22. Rifkin MD, Levine RB. Driller wrist (vibratory arthropathy). *Skeletal Radiol* 1985;13:59–61.
23. Cone RO, Resnick D, Danzig L. Shoulder impingement syndrome: radiographic evaluation. *Radiology* 1984;150:29–33.
24. Kieft GJ, Bloem JL, et al. Rotator cuff impingement syndrome: MR imaging. *Radiology* 1988;166:211–214.
25. Seeger LL, Gold RH, Bassett LW, et al. Shoulder impingement syndrome: MR findings in 53 shoulders. *AJR* 1988;150: 343–347.
26. Jeffery AK. Osteogenesis in the osteoarthritic femoral head. *J*

Bone Joint Surg [Br] 1973;55:262–272.
27. Meachim G, Hardinge K, Williams DR. Methods for correlating pathological and radiological findings in osteoarthrosis of the hip. *Br J Radiol* 1972;45:670–676.
28. Murray RO. The aetiology of primary osteoarthritis of the hip. *Br J Radiol* 1965;38:810–824.
29. Meachim G, Whitehouse GH, Pedley RB, et al. An investigation of radiological, clinical and pathological correlations in osteoarthrosis of the hip. *Clin Radiol* 1980;31:565–574.
30. Hermodsson I. Roentgen appearances of arthritis of the hip. *Acta Radiol [Diagn]* 1972;12:865–881.
31. Armbuster TG, et al. The adult hip: an anatomic study. I. The bony landmarks. *Radiology* 1978;128:1–10.
32. Guerra J, et al. The adult hip: an anatomic study. II. The soft-tissue landmarks. *Radiology* 1978;128:11–20.
33. Skirving AP. The centre-edge angle of Wiberg in adult Africans and Caucasians. *J Bone Joint Surg [Br]* 1981;63:567–568.
34. Hayward I, Bjorkengren AG, Pathria MN, et al. Patterns of femoral head migration in osteoarthritis of the hip: a reappraisal with CT and pathologic correlation. *Radiology* 1988;166: 857–860.
35. Resnick D. Patterns of migration of the femoral head in osteoarthritis of the hip: roentgenographic–pathologic correlation and comparison with rheumatoid arthritis. *AJR* 1975;124: 62–74.
36. Stark DD, Genant HK, Spring DB. Primary cystic arthrosis of the hip. *Skeletal Radiol* 1984;11:124–127.
37. Bullough RG, Bansal M. The differential diagnosis of geodes. *Radiol Clin North Am* 1988;26:1165–1184.
38. Armstrong P, Saxton H. Iliopsoas bursa. *Br J Radiol* 1972;45: 493–495.
39. Rose CP, Cockshott WP. Anterior femoral erosion and patellofemoral osteoarthritis. *J Can Assoc Radiol* 1982;33:32–34.
40. Greenspan A, Norman A, Tchans FK. Tooth sign in patellar degenerative disease. *J Bone Joint Surg [Am]* 1977;59:483–485.
41. Satku K, Kumar VP, et al. Stress fractures of the tibia in osteoarthritis of the knee. *J Bone Joint Surg* 1987;69:309–311.
42. Outerbridge RE. The etiology of chondromalacia patellae. *J Bone Joint Surg [Br]* 1961;43:752–757.
43. Vallee C, Chevrot A, et al. Aspects tomodensitometriques des kystes synoviaux articulaires lombaires a developpement intrarachidien. *J Radiol* 1987;68:519–526.
44. Epstein BS, Epstein JA, Jones MD. Lumbar spinal stenosis. *Radiol Clin North Am* 1977;15:227–239.
45. Kirkaldy-Willis WH. Lecture series. University Hospital, Saskatchewan, Canada.
46. Dorwart RH, Genant HK. Anatomy of the lumbar spine. *Radiol Clin North Am* 1983;21:201–220.
47. Jaffe HL. *Metabolic, degenerative, and inflammatory diseases of bones and joints.* Philadelphia: Lea & Febiger, 1972.
48. Macnab I. The traction spur: an indicator of segmental instability. *J Bone Joint Surg [Am]* 1971;53:663–670.
49. Pate D, Goobar J, Resnick D, et al. Traction osteophytes of the lumbar spine: radiographic–pathologic correlation. *Radiology* 1988;166: 843–846.
50. Skaane VP, Klott KJ. Die peridental aureole (crowned odontoid process) bei der vorderen atlantodentalarthrose. *Fortschritte Gebeit Röntgenstrahlen* 1981;134:62–68.
51. Kerns S, Pope TL Jr, et al. Annulus fibrosus calcification in the cervical spine: radiologic–pathologic correlation. *Skeletal Radiol* 1986;15:605–609.

Diffuse Idiopathic Skeletal Hyperostosis

52. Resnick D, Shaul SR, Robins JM. Diffuse idiopathic skeletal hyperostosis (DISH): Forestier's disease with extraspinal manifesta-

tions. *Radiology* 1975;115:513–524.

53. Tsukamoto Y, Onitsuka H, Lee K. Radiologic aspects of diffuse idiopathic skeletal hyperostosis in the spine. *AJR* 1977;129:913–918.

54. Meeks LW, Renshaw TS. Vertebral osteophytosis and dysphagia: two case reports of the syndrome recently termed ankylosing hyperostosis. *J Bone Joint Surg [Am]* 1973;55:197–201.

55. Weinfeld RM, Olson PM, Maki DD, et al. The prevalence of diffuse idiopathic skeletal hyperostosis (DISH) in two large American midwest metropolitan hospital populations. *Skeletal Radiol* 1997;26:222–225.

56. Hirai T, Korogi Y, Yamashita Y, et al. Ossification of the posterior longitudinal ligaments: evaluation with MRI. *JMRI* 1998; 8:398–405.

57. Pennes DR, Martel W, et al. Retinoid-induced ossification of the posterior longitudinal ligament. *Skeletal Radiol* 1985;14:

191–192.

58. Littlejohn GO, Urowitz MB, Symthe HA, et al. Radiographic features of the hand in diffuse idiopathic skeletal hyperostosis (DISH). *Radiology* 1981;140:623–629.

59. Fischer VE. Manifestation der diffusen idiopathischen skeletthyperostose am vorfub. *Fortschritte Gebeit Röntgenstrahlen* 1987; 147:532–536.

Spondylolysis and Spondylolisthesis

60. Koehler A, Zimmer EA. *Borderlands of the normal and early pathologic in skeletal roentgenology.* New York: Grune & Stratton, 1958.

61. Ulmer JL, Matthews VP, Elster AD, et al. MR imaging of lumbar spondylosis. *AJR* 1997;169:233–239.

62. Epstein BS, Epstein JA, Jones MD. Degenerative spondylolisthesis with an intact neural arch. *Radiol Clin North Am* 1977; 15:275–287.

63. Sella EJ, Goodman AH. Arthropathy secondary to transfusion hemochromatosis. *J Bone Joint Surg [Am]* 1973;55:1077–1081.

6

NEUROPATHIC ARTHROPATHY (CHARCOT'S JOINT)

Clinical Aspects

Joanne Valeriano-Marcet

Neuroarthropathy refers to destructive and productive articular abnormalities occurring in association with loss of pain, proprioception, or both.[1-8] Contributing factors to the pathogenesis include the cumulative effect of trauma and joint laxity. The articular distribution depends on the underlying condition (Table 6.1). Other causes of neuropathic skeletal alterations include amyloid, peripheral nerve injury, myelopathy of pernicious anemia, Charcot-Marie-Tooth disease, arachnoiditis, paraplegia, familial interstitial hypertrophic polyneuropathy of Dejerine and Sottas, leprosy, and Yaws. An idiopathic variety of neuroarthropathy of the elbow has been identified.[9] Intraarticular steroid injections may result in neuropathiclike changes.[10]

Radiographic changes of bony eburnation, fracture, subluxation, and joint disorganization are virtually pathognomonic in the patient with advanced neuroarthropathy. The mild and moderate stages of disease are more difficult to differentiate from other processes, including Osteoarthritis (OA) and calcium pyrophosphate in cartilage (CPPD) crystal deposition disease. Differentiating a Charcot's foot from an underlying infectious process such as septic arthritis or osteomyelitis is a special concern in a diabetic patient.

Neuropathic arthropathy can present in two forms, depending on the pathogenesis. Acute neuroarthropathy (atrophic and resorptive form) presents rapidly in a period of a few weeks. The joint may be painful, swollen, warm, and erythematous. This form usually involves non–weight-bearing joints and must be distinguished from infection or tumor. Chronic neuroarthropathy (hypertrophic form) usually develops over a longer period of time and involves weight-bearing joints. Initially, the joint may mimic osteoarthritis; however, subsequently the joint develops effusion and/or hypertrophic osteophytes. Progression of the disease is variable. Sudden collapse of the joint may result from intraarticular or juxtaarticular fractures. Others may progress more slowly. Common complications include fractures, dislocation, and infection.

Laboratory tests are useful only to determine underlying etiology, such as diabetes. Elevated white blood cells

(WBC) might raise the suspicion of an infectious process in the acute form. Noninflammatory fluids and serosanguinous or hemorrhagic effusion are most frequently seen. Bone and cartilage fragments as well as CPPD crystals can be identified in synovial fluid.[11] Again, synovial fluid aspiration is an important means of ruling out an infectious process.

Radiologic Aspects

George B. Greenfield

Radiologically, the joint predilection depends on the etiology.[12-16] The more common neurotrophic arthropathies are summarized in Table 6.1.

Intraarticular steroid injection may result in changes that resemble neurotrophic joint. The neurotrophic joint may, paradoxically, be painful because of capsular distension and soft-tissue trauma.

There are two forms: *atrophic* and *hypertrophic* arthropathy, although combinations may occur. Atrophic arthropathy is encountered early, is more acute, and is seen more often in the upper extremities, although it can also be seen in the foot in patients with diabetes, in the hip in patients with paraplegia, and in lepers. Hypertrophic arthropathy is seen more often in the lower extremities. The spine shows only hypertrophic changes. The underlying disease does not determine which form predominates.

Atrophic arthropathy is seen as resorption of the ends of bone. This may have a sharp margin or a pointed end. Joint effusion usually precedes destructive changes. Destruction proceeds to dislocation. No osteophytes, sclerosis, fragmentation, or soft-tissue debris are present in the pure atrophic form. This may proceed to a bone-forming stage. Tapering of the distal aspect of the bone is seen in a "mortar-and-pestle" or "pencil-in-cup" deformity. There is a pointing of the convex member and a hollowing or broadening of the concave member of a small joint. Resorption of large portions of bone also may occur.

Hypertrophic arthropathy begins with effusion. The progress is usually slow but may rarely be rapid. The joint space becomes widened then narrowed. Subluxation may occur. Marked bony sclerosis occurs. Osteoporosis does not

TABLE 6.1. ARTICULAR DISTRIBUTION OF NEUROARTHROPATHY

Disease	Patients with Neuroarthropathy	Joints Most Commonly Affected
Neurosyphilis	(5–10%)[1–3]	Knee, hip
Syringomyelia	(20–50%)[4]	Glenohumeral joint, elbow, wrist, and cervical spine
Diabetes mellitus	(1%)[5–7]	Midfoot/forefoot
Alcohol-related	(Rare)[8]	Foot
Congenital insensitivity to pain	100%	Ankle, tarsal, knee, and hip

occur, even with advanced changes. Pathological fractures and fragmentation of the articular surfaces follow. A large amount of bony soft-tissue debris forms, which later fuses into a large, dense, well-organized bony mass with an integral cortex. This mass may fuse with the bone. The bone fragments may break out of the periarticular space and dissect along muscle planes.[17] Some may be resorbed. Periosteal new bone formation may occur. Subluxation and dislocation proceed to destruction, and finally to total disorganization of the joint.

Peripheral Skeleton. In the shoulder, the humeral head may be resorbed (Fig. 6.1) in the atrophic type of neurotrophic arthropathy, particularly in syringomyelia. Repair (Fig. 6.2) and the neurotrophic hypertrophic type of arthropathy result in soft-tissue debris, osteosclerosis (Fig. 6.3), dislocation, deformity, and disorganization of the joint.

The atrophic form shows resorption of bone, particularly at the articular surfaces (Fig. 6.4) in the *elbow*. Dislocation may follow (Fig. 6.5). Osteosclerosis, widening of the ulnar notch (Fig. 6.6) soft-tissue debris, and bone disintegration

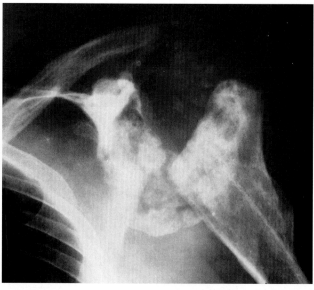

FIGURE 6.2. Neurotrophic arthropathy. Shoulder. Resorption of the humeral head was followed by repair with solid new bone formation at the proximal humerus, and with soft-tissue bony debris.

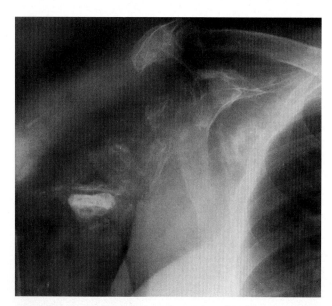

FIGURE 6.1. Neurotrophic arthropathy. Shoulder. There has been resorption of the proximal aspect of the humerus and the glenoid fossa. Soft-tissue debris is noted.

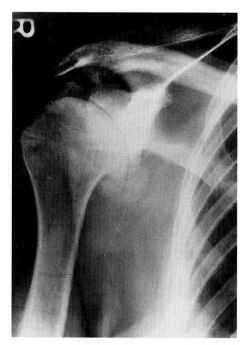

FIGURE 6.3. Neurotrophic arthropathy. Shoulder. There is osteosclerosis of the humeral head and the glenoid. Flattening of the humeral head is seen and large spurs are noted inferiorly. There is narrowing of the joint space and bony debris superiorly.

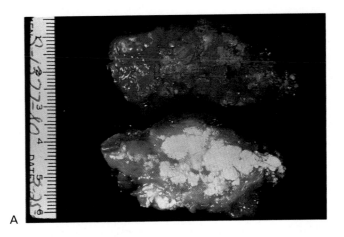

A

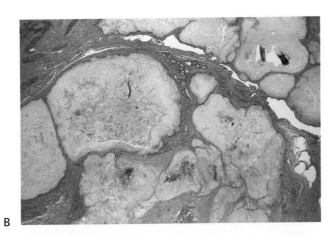

B

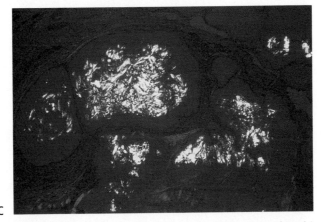

C

FIGURE 10.1. Chronic gout. **A:** Gross appearance of tophi within synovial tissue. **B:** Granulation tissue and multinucleated giant cells surrounding tophi. **C:** Crystals under polarized light.

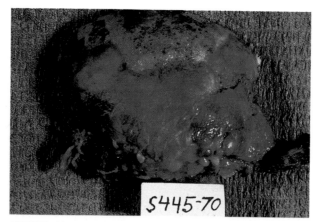

FIGURE 10.2. Osteoarthritis. Gross appearance of degenerated articular surface.

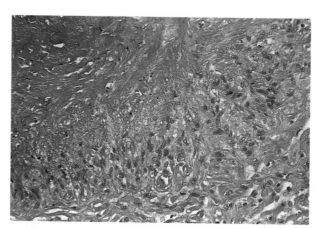

FIGURE 10.3. Rheumatoid arthritis. Palisading nonnecrotizing
granuloma.

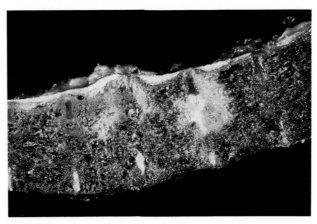

FIGURE 10.4. Ankylosing spondylitis. Fusion of intervertebral joints and spine deformation.

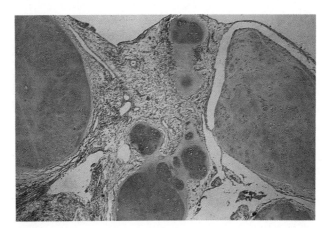

FIGURE 10.5. Synovial chondromatosis. Cartilaginous nodules within the joint.

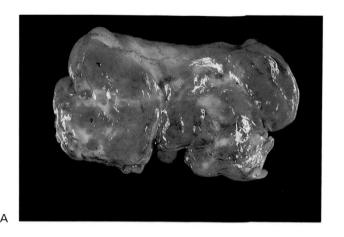

A

B

FIGURE 10.6. Pigmented villonodular synovitis. **A:** Gross appearance of hypertrophic synovium. **B:** Inner aspect (specimen bisected).

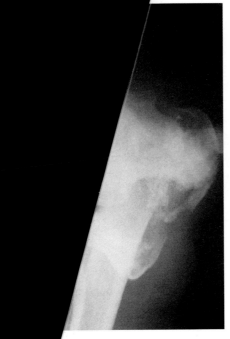

...phic joint. Elbow. Complete disorganiza-...occurred.

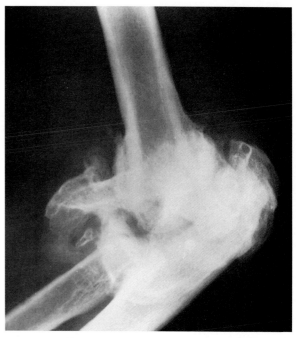

FIGURE 6.9. Neurotrophic joint. Elbow. There is marked hypertrophic change, disorganization, and bony soft-tissue debris.

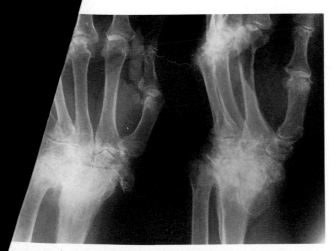

FIGURE 6.10. Neurotrophic joint. Wrist and hand. There has been compression and complete disorganization of the carpus as well as sclerosis of the distal radius and the deformity of the distal ulna. Osteoarthritis of the distal metacarpals with "hooklike" osteophytes are also seen.

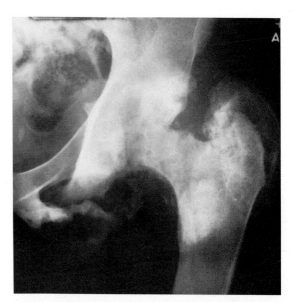

FIGURE 6.11. Neurotrophic joint. Hip. There has been resorption at the femoral head and neck, and at the pubic and ischiac bones. There has been repair with new bone formation, particularly around the greater trochanter.

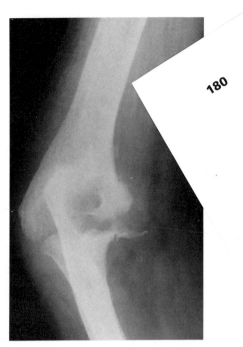

FIGURE 6.4. Neurotrophic joint in a patient with syringomyelia. AP view of the elbow shows resorption at the articular surfaces and at the ulnar notch with a small amount of soft-tissue bony debris.

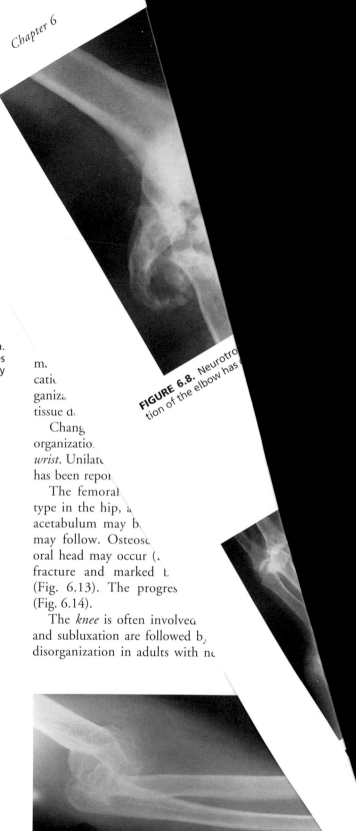

FIGURE 6.8. Neurotro... tion of the elbow has ...

m...
catic...
ganiza...
tissue d...

Chang...
organizatio...
wrist. Unilat...
has been repor...

The femoral...
type in the hip, ...
acetabulum may b...
may follow. Osteos...
oral head may occur (...
fracture and marked t...
(Fig. 6.13). The progres...
(Fig. 6.14).

The *knee* is often involved...
and subluxation are followed b...
disorganization in adults with n...

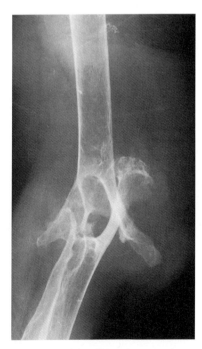

FIGURE 6.5. Neurotrophic elbow in a patient with syringomyelia. There is resorption of bone with a tapered appearance of the proximal radius and dislocation of the ulna.

FIGURE 6.7. Neurotrophic joint. There is dislocation of the ...bow with fixation in an extended position.

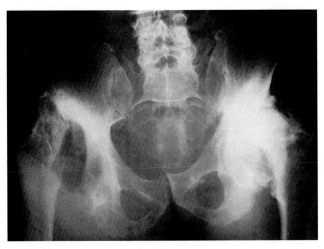

FIGURE 6.12. Neurotrophic joints. Hips. There has been erosion and widening of both acetabula. There has been resorption of the femoral head and dislocation of the femur. Soft-tissue debris is seen. Osteosclerosis around both acetabula is noted. There is deformity and osteosclerosis of the left femoral head.

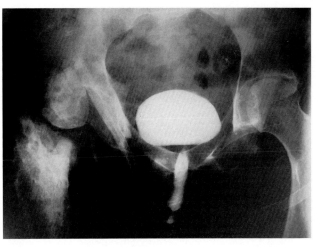

FIGURE 6.13. Neurotrophic joint. Right hip. There has been a fracture of the femoral neck and rotation. Bone production is seen, particularly in the proximal femur. The left hip is not involved.

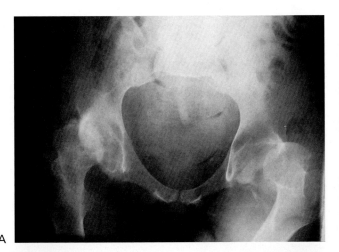

A

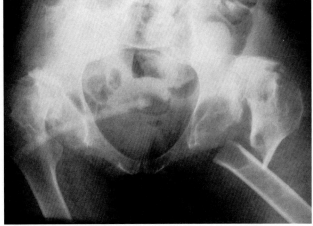

B

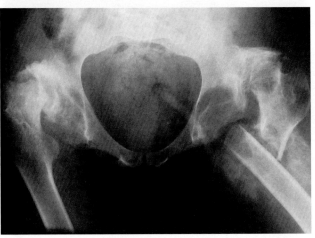

C

FIGURE 6.14. Twenty-eight-year-old paraplegic with rapidly developing neurotrophic hips and pathological fracture. **A:** Initial film. AP view of the pelvis shows subluxation of the right femoral head with a small amount of calcific debris, and dislocation of the left femoral head. There has been resorption of the ischia. **B:** Seven months later. There has been dislocation of the right femoral head with further soft-tissue bony debris and complete dislocation of the left femoral head with formation of a neoacetabulum with hypertrophic changes. A pathological fracture in the subtrochanteric region of the left femur is noted. **C:** One month after **(B)** there is a considerable amount of soft-tissue calcification and callus formation around the fracture site.

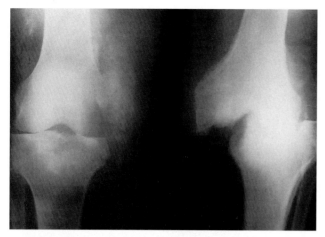

FIGURE 6.15. Neurotrophic arthropathy. Knees. On the right side, sclerosis, fragmentation, and soft-tissue debris are seen as well as narrowing of knee joint space. On the left side, marked erosion of the articular surface is seen with subluxation.

6.16, and 6.17). MRI can show better detail (Figs. 6.18 and 6.19).

Neurotrophic osteonecrosis of the lateral femoral condyle has been reported in children with motor and sensory deficits in the affected limb from several etiologies.[19]

Fragmentation, dislocation, and disorganization also occur in the *ankle* (Fig. 6.20). The most severe changes occur in congenital insensitivity to pain. Early changes may show only as a small amount of fragmentation in the *foot* (Figs. 6.21 and 6.22). Lisfranc's fracture—dislocation with fragmentation at the tarsometatarsal joints occurs later, particularly in patients with diabetes mellitus (Figs. 6.23, 6.24, and 6.25).[20] Fractures and fragmentation of the talus and calcaneus as well as the distal tibia and fibula may occur. Osteomyelitis often complicates

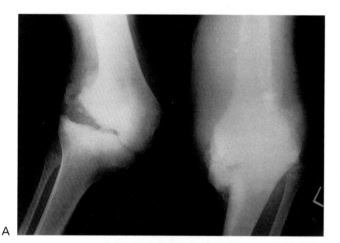
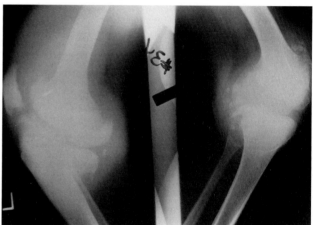

A   B

FIGURE 6.16. Neurotrophic arthropathy. Knees. **A:** AP view of both knees shows disorganization of the knee joint on the left side with marked effusion, and marked erosion and soft tissue debris of the knee on the right side. **B:** Lateral view shows marked flattening of the femoral articular surface and a fracture of the posterior aspect of the tibial plateau, as well as marked effusion. Considerable soft-tissue debris is seen on the right side.

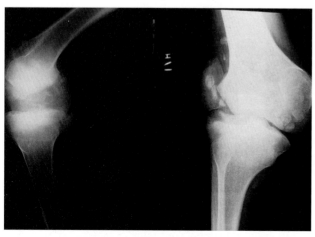
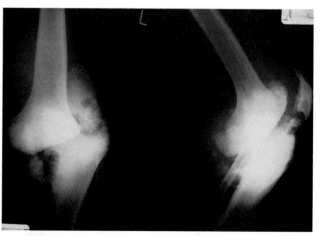

A   B

FIGURE 6.17. Tabes dorsalis. **A,B:** Both knees. AP and lateral views show bilateral fragmentation, subluxation, soft-tissue debris, soft-tissue swelling, and osteosclerosis.

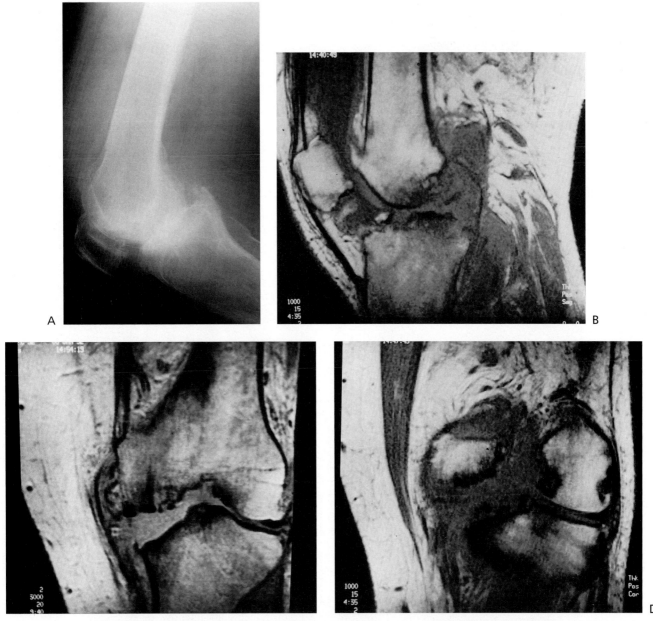

FIGURE 6.18. Neurotrophic joint. Knee. **A:** Lateral view of the knee shows a large effusion in the suprapatellar recess, as well as sclerosis and fragmentation of the articular surface. **B:** MRI (SE 1000/15). Sagittal section shows a large knee joint effusion. Irregularity, fragmentation, and sclerosis of the articular surfaces are seen. **C:** MRI (SE 1000/15). Coronal section reveals articular surface destruction and fragmentation, particularly at the medial tibial plateau. The medial meniscus is destroyed. **D:** MRI (SE 5000/20). Coronal section shows destruction of the medial tibial plateau and details of irregularity of the distal femoral articular surface. Thickening of the medial collateral ligament is also noted.

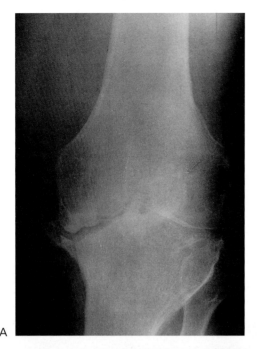

A

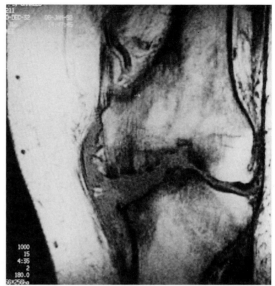

B

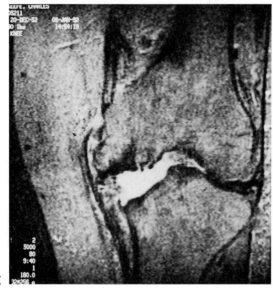

C

FIGURE 6.19. Neurotrophic joint. Knee. **A:** AP view of the knee shows soft-tissue swelling, erosion at the medial tibial plateau, and marked osteophyte formation. **B:** MRI. T1-weighted image showing details of erosion of the medial tibial plateau, and of the medial femoral condyle. Joint effusion is also seen. **C:** MRI. T2-weighted image shows the joint effusion as high signal intensity.

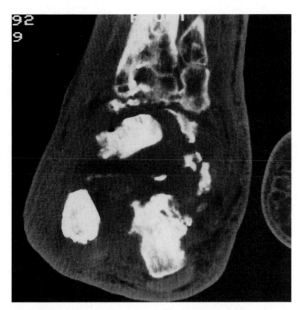

FIGURE 6.20. Neurotrophic joint in a diabetic patient. CT of the ankle. There is complete disorganization of the ankle and tarsal bones, with bony destruction and debris.

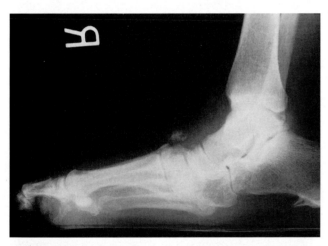

FIGURE 6.22. Neurotrophic foot in a diabetic patient. Lateral view. A small amount of soft-tissue debris is seen at the dorsum of the tarsal bones.

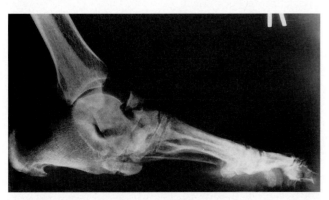

FIGURE 6.24. Diabetes mellitus with neurotrophic arthropathy. Foot and ankle. Fragmentation of the tarsal bones is noted. There is no local osteoporosis. Upward dislocation of the tarsus is seen.

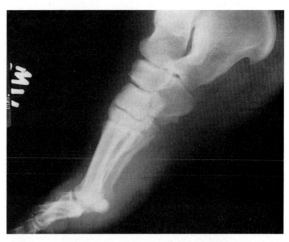

FIGURE 6.21. Early neurotrophic change in the foot of a diabetic patient. Lateral view. There is a small amount of fragmentation at the base of the fifth metatarsal. Soft-tissue swelling is also present.

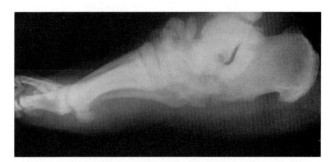

FIGURE 6.23. Lisfranc's fracture with fragmentation of the tarsal bones and flattening of the arch of the foot is noted.

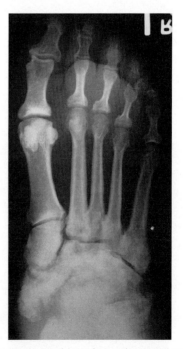

FIGURE 6.25. Neurotrophic arthropathy. AP view of the foot shows disintegration and fragmentation of the tarsus. The proximal metatarsals from 2 to 5 are also involved.

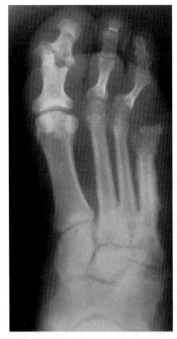

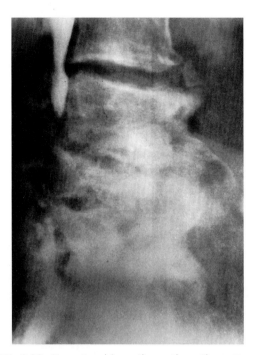

FIGURE 6.26. Neurotrophic arthropathy in the foot complicated by osteomyelitis in a diabetic patient. There has been amputation of the fifth ray and the fourth toe. Dense periosteal new bone formation along the fifth metatarsal is seen. Neurotrophic resorption at the interphalangeal joint of the great toe is present.

FIGURE 6.28. Neurotrophic arthropathy. Charcot's spine. Destruction of L-4. Osteosclerosis and osteophyte formation are seen as well as fragmentation of L-5.

neurotrophic changes in diabetics (Figs. 6.26 and 6.27), and may be impossible to diagnose radiologically in advanced cases. Neuropathic injuries to the lower extremities in children can be seen as long bone fractures, epiphyseal separation, Charcot's joints, and soft-tissue ulceration.[21] Patients with various neuromuscular disorders have been reported to show skeletal changes similar to those seen in juvenile rheumatoid arthritis (JRA) and hemophilia. These include overgrowth of the epiphyses, periarticular osteoporosis,

joint space narrowing, accentuated trabecular pattern, tibiotalar slant, gracile bones, premature epiphyseal fusion, and soft-tissue atrophy.[22]

Central Skeleton. The lumbar and thoracic segments are most frequently affected in the *spine*. This can occur at multiple levels with skip areas in between. Sclerosis and fragmentation of the vertebral bodies occur (Fig. 6.28). Narrowing of the involved intervertebral disc spaces with very marked osteophyte formation is seen (Fig. 6.29). Repair consolidates the fragments, and well-formed osteophytes develop. Paraspinal soft-tissue masses containing ossific debris may be present.

Congenital insensitivity to pain causes severe neurotrophic changes, which may require amputation. The ankle and tarsal bones (Figs. 6.30 and 6.31), knee, and hip (Fig. 6.32) are most often involved. Repair shows areas of well-formed bone in the soft tissues (Fig. 6.33).

Leprosy is caused by infection with *Mycobacterium leprae*.[23] There are two types: lepromatous and neural. Bone changes are seen most often in the neural form but can also be present in the lepromatous type, in which case the bone is directly involved with granulomatous tissue. Neurotrophic arthropathy may be present (Fig. 6.34). The *hands* and *feet* are chiefly affected. There is marked resorption with tapering deformity of the phalanges, similar to but much more severe than other diseases with neurotrophic changes.

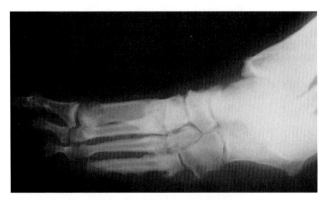

FIGURE 6.27. Diabetic foot following amputation of the fifth ray. Soft-tissue ulceration is present as well as periosteal new bone formation along the fourth metatarsal.

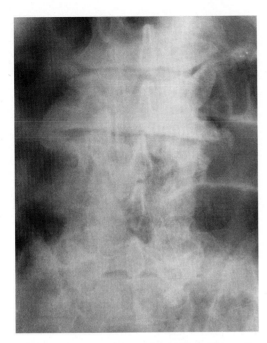

FIGURE 6.29. Neurotrophic arthropathy. Charcot's spine. Lumbar spine. There is sclerosis and marked osteophyte formation. Narrowing of the intervertebral spaces and loss of height of the lower lumbar vertebral bodies are seen.

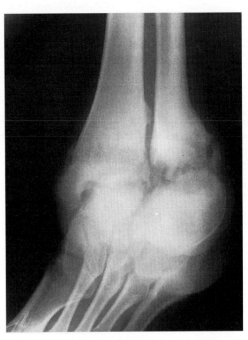

FIGURE 6.31. Congenital insensitivity to pain. Osteosclerosis at the ankle joint in all bones is noted, as well as irregularity of the articular surfaces. Fragmentation and dislocation of the talus and calcaneus, as well as enlargement of the distal fibula is seen.

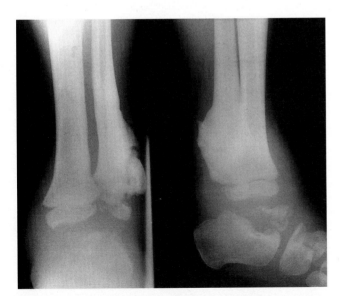

FIGURE 6.30. Congenital insensitivity to pain. Ankle. AP and lateral views showed marked joint effusion and fragmentation at the distal fibula and talus.

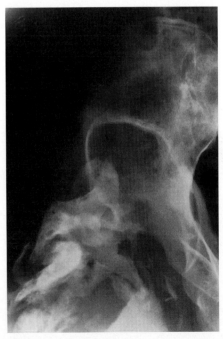

FIGURE 6.32. Congenital insensitivity to pain. Hip. There is destruction and fragmentation of the entire proximal femur. There is marked enlargement of the acetabulum. Bony debris is noted.

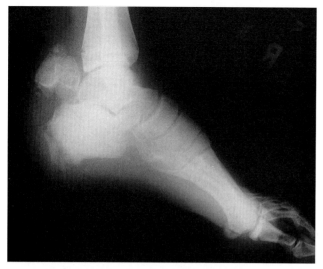

FIGURE 6.33. Congenital insensitivity to pain. Foot. Repair phase. A well-formed bone in the soft tissues is seen posterior to the ankle joint. Fragmentation of the posterior calcaneus is also seen.

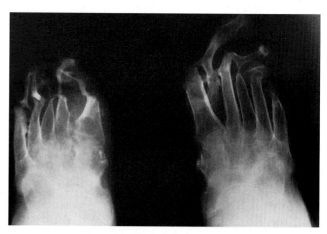

FIGURE 6.35. Leprosy. Feet. Atrophic type. There is neurotrophic resorption at the metatarsophalangeal joints with resorption proceeding in both directions. The distal metatarsals are tapered. Osteoporosis is present.

Cystic changes in the hands and feet may be seen, as well as bone expansion. In severe cases, all of the phalanges of the hands may be completely resorbed and tapering of the distal metacarpals can be seen.

Changes in the feet usually begin at the metatarsophalangeal joints, and destruction and resorption proceed in both directions (Fig. 6.35). There is resorption of the midportion of the shafts of the phalanges, leading to fracture and destruction. Tarsal bone disintegration may occur. Flexion deformities may be present.

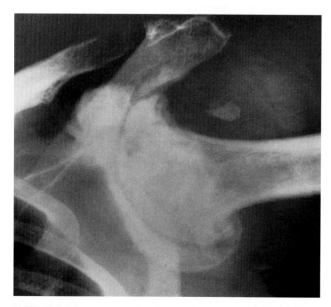

FIGURE 6.34. Leprosy. Shoulder. There is destruction of the glenoid fossa, soft-tissue debris, and osteosclerosis both in the humeral head and the scapula.

REFERENCES

Neuropathic Arthropathy

1. Resnick D. Neuroarthropathy. In Resnick D, Niwayama G, 2nd ed. *Diagnosis of bone and joint disorders.* Philadelphia: WB Saunders, 1981:2,422.
2. Key JA. Clinical observations in tabetic arthropathies (Charcot joints). *Am J Syph* 1932;14:429–447.
3. Pomcranz MM, Rothberg AS. A review of 58 cases of tabetic arthropathy. *Am J Syph* 1941;25:103–119.
4. Jaffe HL. Metabolic degenerative and inflammatory diseases of bone and joints. Philadelphia: Lea & Febiger, 1972:847.
5. Clouse ME, Gramm HF, Legg M, et al. Diabetic osteoarthropathy. Clinical and roentgenographic observations in 90 cases. *AJR* 1974;121:22–34.
6. Gray RG, Gottlieb NL. Rheumatic disorders associated with diabetes mellitus. Literature review. *Semin Arthritis Rheum* 1976;6:19–34.
7. Giesecke SB, Dalinka MK, Kyle GC. Lisfranc's fracture dislocation. A manifestation of peripheral neuropathy. *AJR* 1978;131:139–141.
8. Thornhill HL, Richter RW, Shelton ML, et al. Neuropathic arthropathy (Charcot forefeet) in alcoholics. *Orthop Clin North Am* 1973;4:7–20.
9. Resnick D, Berthiaume M, Sartoris D. Diagnostic tests and procedures in rheumatic disease. In *Kelly's Textbook of Rheumatology,* 4th ed. Philadelphia: WB Saunders, 1993:623.
10. Steinberg CL, Duthic RB, Piva AE. Charcot-like arthropathy following intra-articular hydrocortisone. *JAMA* 1962;181:851–854.
11. Ropes MW, Bauer W. *Synovial fluid changes in joint disease.* Cambridge, MA: Harvard University Press, 1953.

Radiologic Aspects

12. Forrester DM, Brown JC, Nesson JW. *The radiology of joint disease,* 2nd ed. Philadelphia: WB Saunders, 1978.
13. Hollander JL, McCarty DJ. *Arthritis and allied conditions,* 8th ed. Philadelphia: Lea & Febiger, 1972.
14. Allman RM, Brower AC, Kotlyarov EB, et al. Neuropathic bone and joint disease. *Radiol Clin North Am* 1988;26:1373–1381.

15. Brower AC, Allman RM. Pathogenesis of the neurotrophic joint: neurotraumatic vs. neurovascular. *Radiology* 1981;139:349–354.

16. Hollander JL, McCarty DJ. *Arthritis and allied conditions,* 8th ed. Philadelphia: Lea & Febiger, 1972.

17. Forrester DM, Magre G. Migrating bone shards in dissecting Charcot joints. *AJR* 1978;130:133–136.

18. Resnik CS, Reed WW. Hand, wrist, and elbow arthropathy in syringomyelia. *J Can Assoc Radiol* 1985;36:325–327.

19. Citron ND, Paterson FWN, et al. Neuropathic osteonecrosis of the lateral femoral condyle in childhood. *J Bone Joint Surg* 1986;68:96–99.

20. Giesecke SB, Dalinka MK, Kyle GC. Lisfrancs fracture–dislocation: a manifestation of peripheral neuropathy. *AJR* 1978;131:139–141.

21. Schneider R, Goldman AB, Bohne WHO. Neuropathic injuries to the lower extremities in children. *Radiology* 1978;128:713–718.

22. Richardson ML, Helms CA, et al. Skeletal changes in neuromuscular disorders mimicking juvenile rheumatoid arthritis and hemophilia. *AJR* 1984;143:893–897.

23. Enna CD, Jacobson RR, Rausch RO. Bone changes in leprosy. *Radiology* 1971;100:295–306.

INFECTIOUS ARTHRITIS

An infectious agent may involve the joint in several ways. It may be hematogenous. It may be by direct injury and penetration. An adjacent osteomyelitis may penetrate into the joint, or the joint may be involved from contiguous soft tissue infection. Neurovascular changes, common in diabetics, predispose to infection. Involvement of the intervertebral disc occurs in the spine, along with osteomyelitis of the adjacent vertebral bodies.

The agents may be bacterial, tuberculous, or fungal. Viral arthritis and synovitis also occur.

BACTERIAL ARTHRITIS

Clinical Aspects

Joanne Valeriano-Marcet

Clinical Features. The septic joint is acutely painful, red, hot, swollen, and very tender.

Movements are severely restricted by muscle spasm. Eighty to ninety percent of nongonococcal septic arthritis is monarticular; the knee is most commonly affected. Most patients present with a fever, but this may be low grade. Shaking chills are unusual, and more often occur in patients with positive blood cultures.

Diagnosis. When bacterial arthritis is suspected, the most important diagnostic procedures to be performed are arthrocentesis and examination of the synovial fluid. Synovial fluid leukocyte count and differential, although not definitive, can give strong support for the diagnosis of bacterial arthritis. The synovial fluid leukocyte count in bacterial arthritis is usually over 50,000, with more than 80% polymorphonuclear leukocytes (PMNs). Marked synovial leukocytosis can occur in crystal arthritis and rheumatoid arthritis (RA) in the absence of infection, thus requiring Gram stain and culture to make a definitive diagnosis of infectious arthritis. Synovial fluid chemistries, including glucose, protein, and LDH, are not useful in the diagnosis of bacterial arthritis.

Peripheral blood leukocytosis often is present in patients with septic arthritis. The erythrocytes sedimentation rate and other acute phase reactants, such as C-reactive protein (CRP) and amyloid protein AA, are elevated in both infectious arthritis and noninfectious inflammatory states, and thus cannot definitively separate the two possibilities. Other conventional tests for evaluating patients with arthritis, including rheumatoid factor and antinuclear antibodies, are not useful in the diagnosis of septic arthritis. When a patient is suspected of having septic arthritis, blood cultures (at least two) are necessary. Additionally, any possible site of extraarticular infection (e.g., urine or skin lesions) should be examined for Gram stain and culture. These sites may provide clues as to the organism causing the joint infection.

Synovial tissue may be required to confirm the diagnosis of septic arthritis in cases where the synovial fluid is not diagnostic. This technique is particularly valuable in cases where the organism is slow growing (e.g., tuberculous and fungal infections). Synovial tissue can be obtained during open surgical debridement or blind synovial biopsy or arthroscopy. The fresh tissue specimen is transported to the laboratory in a sterile container and processed for bacteriologic and histologic examination.

Plain radiographs may initially be normal; periarticular osteopenia may become evident during the first week of septic arthritis. Evidence of joint space narrowing and erosion may occur within 7 to 14 days. No currently available scintigraphic technique detects the presence of infection; instead all techniques reflect the inflammatory changes or bone reaction associated with infection. Bone scans may detect abnormalities within hours to days of the onset of joint infections; however, the use of technetium phosphate bone scanning cannot differentiate infectious from noninfectious inflammation. Other agents may be used in scanning, either alone or in combination with technetium phosphate bone scanning. Gallium citrate and indium-labeled leukocytes are the currently available agents used for detection of inflammatory processes in bone and soft tissue. Gallium scan may demonstrate joint infection when the technetium phosphate bone scan is normal. Indium-labeled leukocyte scanning is less sensitive than technetium phosphate bone scanning, but is more specific for joint infection. Computed tomography (CT) or magnetic resonance imaging (MRI) scanning may be valuable in evaluating joints that are difficult to evaluate clinically, including hip, shoulder, sternoclavicular, and sacroiliac joints.

Radiologic Aspects

George B. Greenfield

Bacterial arthritis results from invasion of the synovial membrane and joint by any of various microorganisms.[1] The pathway may be hematogenous, posttraumatic, or postsurgical, or it may result from osteomyelitis in an adjacent bone. Common organisms that cause acute pyogenic arthritis are listed in Table 7.1.

An increased incidence occurs in patients with RA, hypogammaglobulinemia, cancer, sickle cell anemia, and neurotrophic arthritis, as well as the elderly, chronically ill, and those taking immunosuppressive medications. Ten to twenty percent of staphylococcal and 75% to 85% of gonococcal arthritis involve two or more joints.

There is a high incidence of *discitis* and osteomyelitis in young adults as a complication of intravenous drug abuse.[10] *Pseudomonas* and *Klebsiella* are common causative organisms. The intervertebral discs, sacroiliac joints, and symphysis pubis are most frequently affected, as well as the sternoclavicular joints and knees.

Acute inflammation with pain, tenderness, swelling, redness, and high fever usually occur clinically in pyogenic arthritis. Some patients, however, may present with minimal signs. Septic arthritis of the hip in infancy and early childhood warrants special attention, because any delay in diagnosis and treatment will cause irreparable damage to the femoral head and triradiate growth plate of the acetabulum.[11,12]

Radiologically, the basic changes in pyogenic arthritis are haziness, joint effusion, loss of the white cortical articular line, synovial thickening, and soft-tissue swelling. Rapid destruction of cartilage and bone follows. Osteoporosis develops rapidly. If osteomyelitis is also present, sequestration and periosteal new bone formation occur. Destructive changes precede osteoporosis in septic arthritis, whereas osteoporosis precedes destruction in tuberculous arthritis. Cartilaginous destruction at contact areas of opposing articular surfaces results in early joint space narrowing, loss of the entire white articular cortical outline on radiographs, and subchondral destruction of bone. Large marginal erosions may also occur. Reactive sclerosis follows. Healing may result in an irregular articular surface or bony ankylosis. Severe and prolonged pyogenic arthritis may result in the presence of dystrophic periarticular calcifications.[13]

Peripheral Skeleton. The knee and hip are affected more often than small joints.

Dislocations of the hip and shoulder are common because of distension of the joint capsule in infants (Fig. 7.1). Swelling of the obturator internus muscle is an early indicator of hip joint involvement in infants (Fig. 7.2).

Fluid in the hip can be excluded if a vacuum sign can be elicited on frog leg view with forced abduction. The apparent dislocation of a hip in an infant prior to ossification of the epiphyseal center may actually result from epiphyseal separation secondary to osteomyelitis.[14,15]

Osteomyelitis may extend into the *joints of the hands*, particularly in sickle cell disease (Figs. 7.3 and 7.4). Soft-tissue swelling of a finger is seen, followed by destruction. Septic arthritis may also result from injuries and penetrating wounds (Figs. 7.5 and 7.6).

The initial plain films may be normal in the *shoulder*; however, subsequent examinations may show osteoporosis and glenohumeral joint space narrowing or widening. Soft-tissue swelling, possibly containing gas collections, destructive foci (Fig. 7.7), and dislocation of the humeral head may follow. Rotator cuff tears are common.[16] The acromioclavicular joint may be involved with widening and bony resorption and destruction (Fig. 7.8). CT not only shows bone changes, but also any associated extension into the soft tissues (Fig. 7.9).

A positive fat pad sign initially may be seen in the *elbow*. Loss of the white articular line and destruction follow.

Septic arthritis of the *hip* may be hematogenous, and result from penetrating injury or a decubitus ulcer.

TABLE 7.1. MICROORGANISMS CAUSING ACUTE PYOGENIC ARTHRITIS[2]

More common
  Diplococcus pneumoniae
  Neisseria gonorrhoeae
  Staphylococcus aureus (most common)
  Streptococcus pyogenes (more common in children)
Less common
  Brucella organisms
  Clostridium bifermentans[3]
  Clostridium welchii[4]
  Coliform organisms
  Corynebacterium pyogenes[5]
  Hamophilus influenzae[6]
  Klebsiella aerobacter
  Propionibacterium acnes[7]
  Proteus organisms[8]
  Pseudomonas aeruginosa
  Pseudomonas pseudomalii
  Salmonellae
  Serratia marcescens[9]

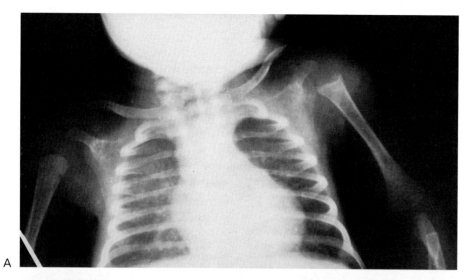

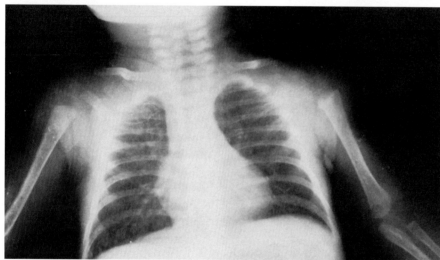

FIGURE 7.1. Septic arthritis. Left shoulder. Ten-month-old girl. **A:** Initial film shows soft-tissue swelling and destructive metaphyseal changes. **B:** One month later. There is dislocation of the left shoulder.

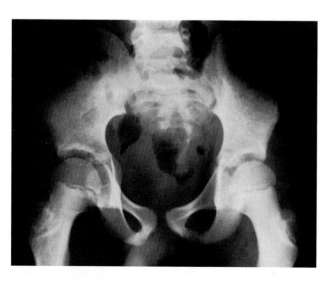

FIGURE 7.2. Early septic arthritis of the left hip. There is internal displacement of the fat plane of the obturator internus muscle indicating edema. This is the obturator sign. There is also slight widening at the triradiate cartilage and edema of the surrounding musculature laterally.

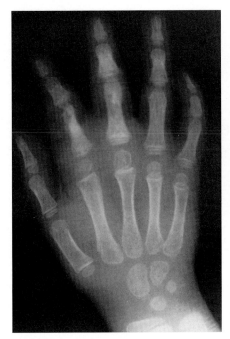

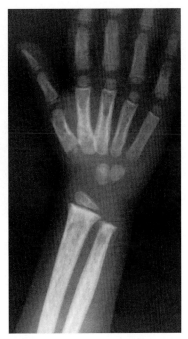

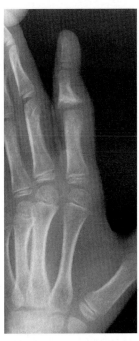

FIGURE 7.3. Osteomyelitis and septic arthritis of the hand. Soft-tissue swelling of the index finger is noted with bony destruction and sclerosis that involves the proximal interphalangeal joint.

FIGURE 7.4. Sickle cell disease with extensive infarctions and oseomyelitis. There is haziness and slight irregularity of the ossification centers of the metacarpophalangeal joints 2, 3, and 4, indicating septic arthritis.

FIGURE 7.5. Septic arthritis following squirrel bite. Index finger. Resorptive and sclerotic changes about the proximal interphalangeal joint are seen associated with soft-tissue swelling.

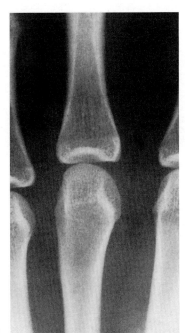

A

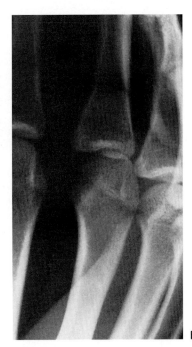

B

FIGURE 7.6. A,B: Septic arthritis of the metacarpophalangeal joint following penetrating injury to the fist on striking a tooth. Note bony resorption.

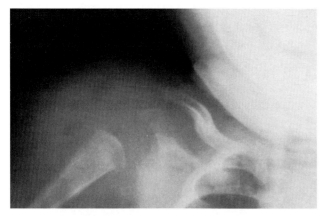

FIGURE 7.7. Septic arthritis in a 2-month-old boy. Shoulder. There is marked soft-tissue swelling and effusion in the right shoulder with soft-tissue air. There is a destructive focus in the medial humeral metaphysis as well as destruction around the glenoid fossa.

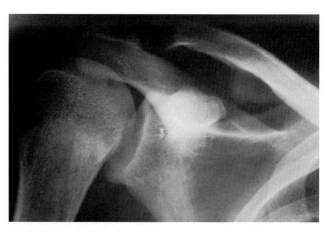

FIGURE 7.8. Septic arthritis of the acromioclavicular joint. There is widening of the acromioclavicular joint with destruction of the distal end of the clavicle.

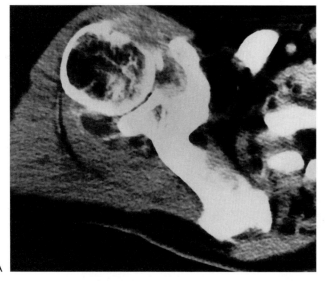

A

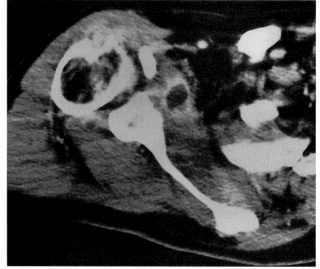

B

FIGURE 7.9. Septic arthritis. Shoulder. CT. **A:** Cortical destruction at the anterior aspect of the humeral head is noted as well as joint effusion, which is seen as low density at the posterior aspect of the joint. **B:** Extension into the subscapularis muscle with enhancement of the wall of an abscess is seen.

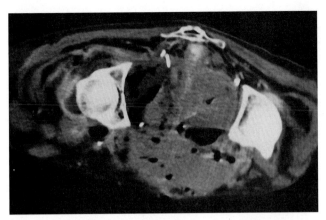

FIGURE 7.10. Septic arthritis. Hip. CT. A left psoas abscess resulting from carcinoma of the bladder has involved the left hip. Gas collections at the left side of the pelvis anterior to the hip joint, within the bone, and small gas bubbles within the joint space are seen. An abscess adjacent to the femoral head is also noted.

Alternatively, it may result from a psoas abscess (Fig. 7.10) or progress to form a psoas abscess. Bone changes range from minimal erosion of the articular surfaces to fragmentation and gross destruction of the proximal femur and acetabulum (Figs. 7.11 through 7.14) .

Effusion, which displaces fat planes, occurs in the knee initially. The patella becomes displaced away from the femur with distension of the suprapatellar space. Haziness of

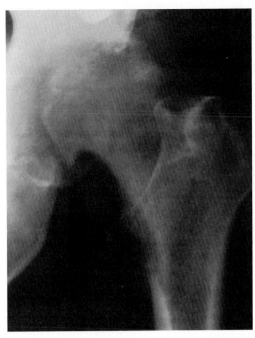

FIGURE 7.12. Septic arthritis. Hip. Irregularity of the joint surface, narrowing of the joint space, a destructive focus in the femoral head, and marked osteoporosis of the proximal femur are noted.

the articular surface and marginal erosions are seen. Joint space widening, followed by narrowing and periarticular osteoporosis occur. Bony destructive changes with sclerosis and irregularity of the articular surface follow. Intraarticular gas may form with certain organisms. A Brodie abscess may

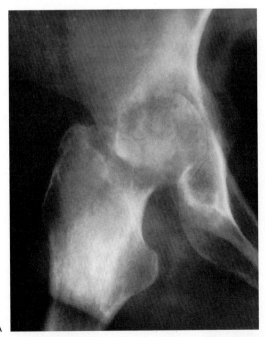
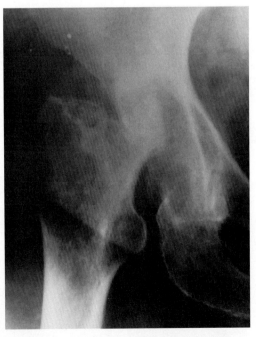

A   B

FIGURE 7.11. Septic arthritis. Hip. **A:** bony destruction at the superior aspect of the femoral head and acetabulum are seen. **B:** Three months later, there has been complete destruction of the femoral head and marked widening of the acetabulum. Osteoporosis is noted to have progressed.

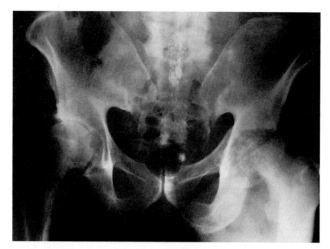

FIGURE 7.13. Septic arthritis of the left hip. Haziness of the articular surfaces and destruction of the femoral articular surface at its superior aspect is seen. The right hip shows osteoarthritis.

affect the knee joint (Figs. 7.15 and 7.16). Chronic multifocal osteomyelitis may also involve the knee joint (Fig. 7.17). The *ankle* and *foot* may also be involved secondary to osteomyelitis of the tarsal bones (Figs. 7.18 and 7.19).

Septic arthritis may be secondary to osteomyelitis in sickle cell disease (Figs. 7.20 and 7.21). This is part of the hand–foot syndrome in sickle cell anemia. Septic arthritis also occurs often in diabetics (Fig. 7.22). Sometimes, restitution of bone can occur following treatment.

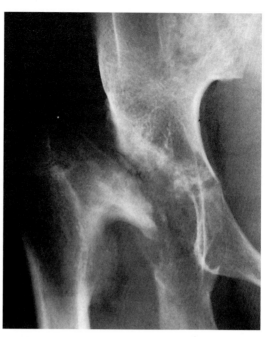

FIGURE 7.14. Septic arthritis. Hip. Destruction of the femoral head and the small bony fragments within the hip joint are noted. Reactive osteosclerosis at the femoral neck and superior aspect of the acetabulum are seen, as well as osteoporosis of the proximal femur.

Central Skeleton. The intervertebral discs are involved early in the *spine*, in contrast to vertebral body involvement in metastatic disease.[17] Any segment may be involved. If the vertebral body is collapsed in a wedgelike fashion with the

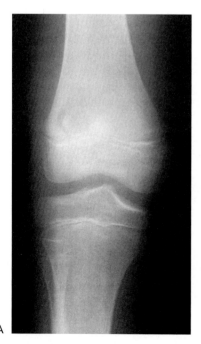
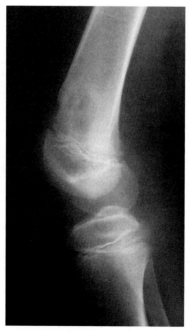

A B

FIGURE 7.15. A: AP view of the knee shows a radiolucency in the distal tibial metaphysis with a sclerotic focus representing a Brodie abscess. Knee joint effusion is also seen. **B:** Lateral view showing a destructive focus anteriorly in the tibial metaphysis as well as centrally. Soft-tissue fullness in the suprapatellar recess is noted, indicating knee joint effusion.

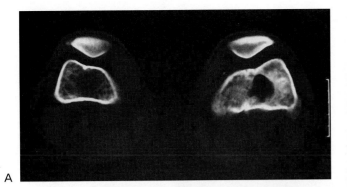

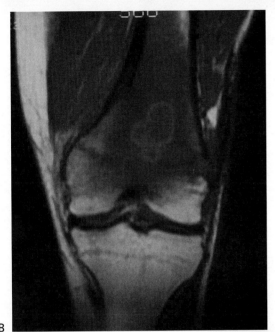

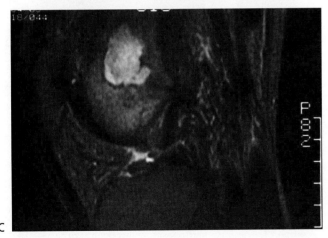

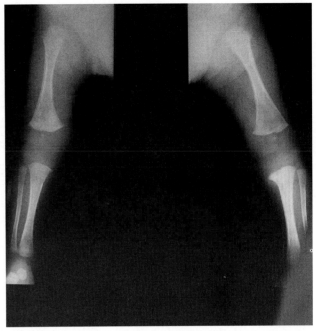

FIGURE 7.17. A 3-month-old infant with chronic multifocal osteomyelitis. The anteroposterior view of the lower extremities shows widespread periosteal new bone formation and destructive changes at the left proximal tibial metaphysis.

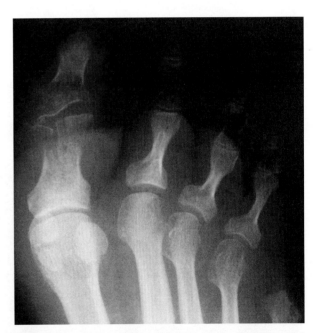

FIGURE 7.16. Osteomyelitis. Brodie abscess in the distal femoral metaphysis. **A:** CT scan shows destruction with a sharp margin. **B:** MRI image (SE 600/20). A large amount of marrow edema extends into the epiphysis and the diaphysis. The margin is outlined by relatively high signal intensity. **C:** MRI image (SE 2700/80). The abscess shows heterogeneous high signal intensity.

FIGURE 7.18. Septic arthritis of the interphalangeal joint of the great toe secondary to osteomyelitis. Periarticular osteoporosis and disruption of the articular surface of the proximal phalanx of the great toe is seen. The articular white line is preserved in this case. The fifth toe has been amputated.

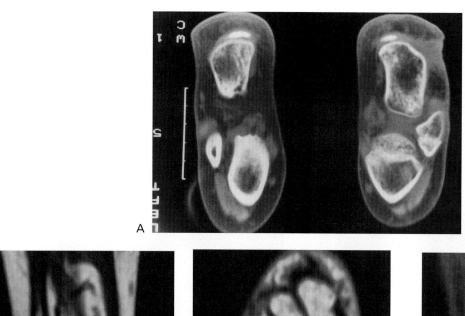

A

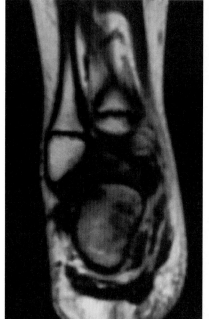

B

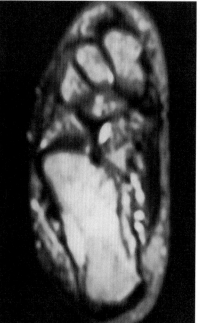

C

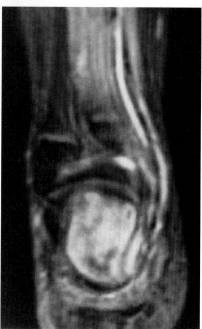

D

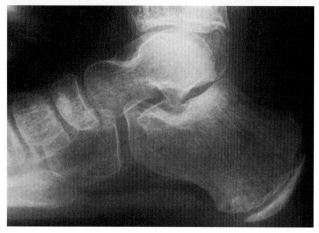

E

FIGURE 7.19. Osteomyelitis of the calcaneus in an 8-year-old girl. **A:** CT scan shows a discrete destructive area in the calcaneus with surrounding soft-tissue reaction. The cortex is intact. Small sequestra are seen. **B:** MRI image (SE 810/15). Heterogeneous signal intensity depicts the calcaneus. **C:** MRI image (SE 2400/80). High signal intensity in the midcalcaneus corresponds to that seen on CT. The fatty marrow signal has been suppressed. High signal intensity is also seen in the surrounding soft tissues. **D:** MRI STIR image. The intense high signal intensity of the calcaneus is shown. **E:** Lateral view of the calcaneus shows only minimal disruption of the trabecular pattern.

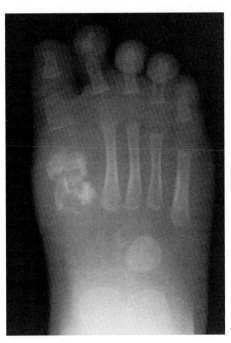

FIGURE 7.20. Osteomyelitis and septic arthritis in a 10-month-old girl with sickle cell disease. Destruction of the first metatarsal bone is noted as well as soft-tissue swelling and involvement of adjacent joints.

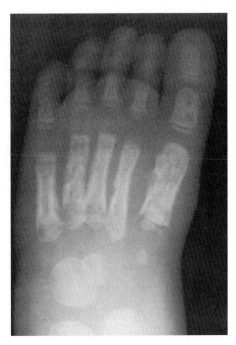

FIGURE 7.21. Sickle cell anemia. AP view of the foot shows changes of bone infarction and osteomyelitis in the metatarsals with destructive changes at the proximal metatarsal bones and septic arthritis of the adjacent joints.

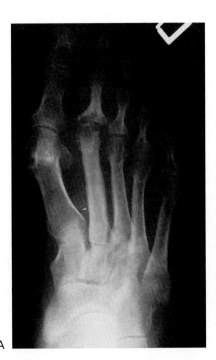

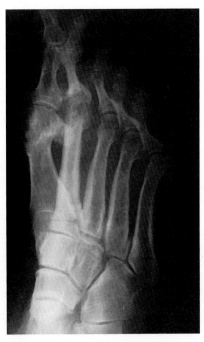

A   B

FIGURE 7.22. Septic arthritis of the first and second metatarsophalangeal joints. **A:** AP view of the foot. **B:** Oblique view of the foot. Bony destruction on both sides of the joint is noted.

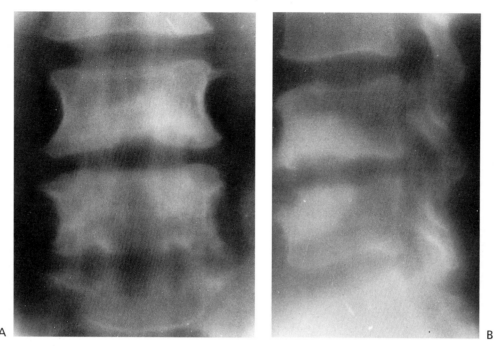

A   B

FIGURE 7.23. Discitis. **A:** AP tomogram. **B:** Lateral tomogram. End plate irregularity, anterior destruction, and osteosclerosis on both sides of the intervertebral disc at L4-5 are noted.

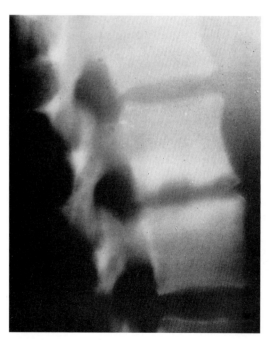

FIGURE 7.24. Discitis. There is narrowing and end plate irregularity along the entire length of the adjacent vertebral bodies. Reactive bony sclerosis is also seen.

discs spared, it is most likely caused by osteoporosis or metastases. If the intervertebral disc is narrowed with end plate irregularity on both sides, it is most likely caused by discitis.

Initially, prevertebral edema is followed by disc space narrowing. Destruction of the vertebral end plates follow (Figs. 7.23 and 7.24). Collapse of vertebral bodies may occur (Fig. 7.25). A paraspinal (Fig. 7.26) or prevertebral abscess may form. Healing is seen as sclerosis, osteophyte formation, and bony fusion (Fig. 7.27).

CT can show details of vertebral body involvement (Fig. 7.28) and soft-tissue extension. The radionuclide bone scan shows a zone or band of increased activity across the entire vertebral body (Fig. 7.29). This can have a similar appearance to vertebral body collapse.

The *sacroiliac joint* may be involved unilaterally, beginning in its lower portion. A slow course is characteristic, with haziness, irregularity, loss of the subchondral cortex, and widening or narrowing of the joint space. Healing results in sclerosis and ankylosis.[18] Pyogenic sacroiliitis frequently occurs in intravenous drug abusers. Radioscintigraphy is useful in early diagnosis when plain films show no abnormality; however, there is normally increased activity in this area making subtle changes difficult to detect.[19]

Sympathetic joint effusion refers to transudate in a joint near the site of an inflammatory or other process. It usually presents as an acute arthritis.[20]

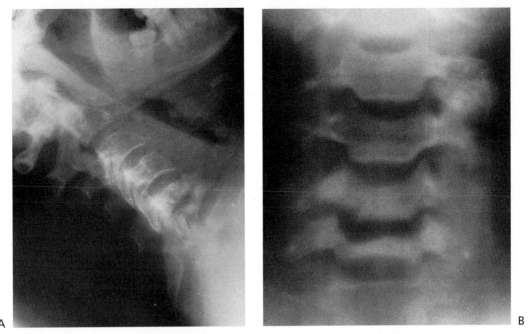

A

B

FIGURE 7.25. Discitis. **A:** Lateral cervical spine shows disc space narrowing at C5-6 with end plate irregularity and destruction of the superior part of the body of C-6. Osteosclerosis is also present. A prevertebral abscess is seen. **B:** AP tomogram shows destruction at C5-6 vertebral bodies.

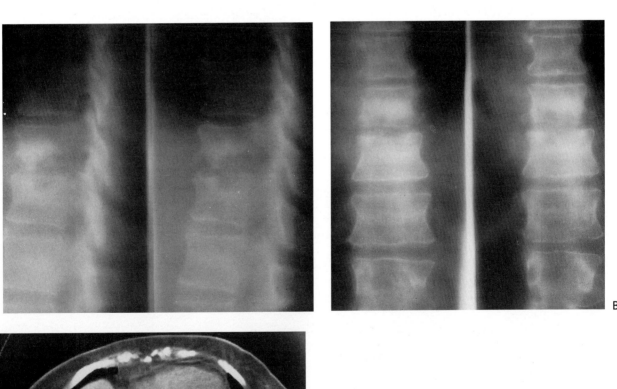

A

B

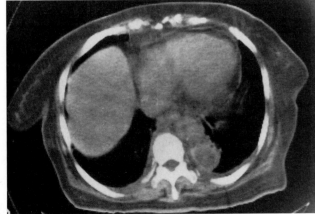

C

FIGURE 7.26. **A:** Lateral tomogram shows marked narrowing of the intervertebral space in the thoracic spine with vertebral end-plate destruction on both sides of the disc. **B:** AP tomogram shows intervertebral space narrowing and end plate destructive and sclerotic changes. **C:** CT shows an enhancing paravertebral abscess on the left side of the thoracic spine.

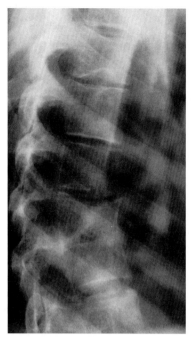

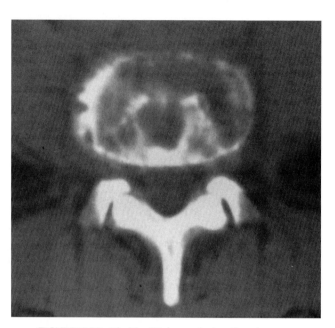

FIGURE 7.27. Discitis in a sickle cell patient. Lateral view of the thoracic spine. There is obliteration of the intervertebral space and bony fusion at the involved site. Typical biconcavity of the vertebral bodies is seen in the upper thoracic spine.

FIGURE 7.28. Discitis. CT shows destructive changes.

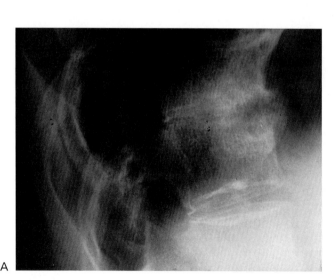

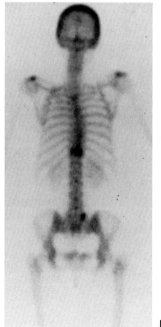

A   B

FIGURE 7.29. Discitis. **A:** Lateral view at the T-11,T-12 level shows discitis with intervertebral space narrowing, end plate irregularity, and reactive osteophyte formation. **B:** Radionuclide bone scan shows a zone of increased activity across the entire width of the spine at that level.

TUBERCULOUS ARTHRITIS

Clinical Aspects

Joanne Valeriano-Marcet

Mycobacteria may be responsible for chronic bone and joint infections. The clinical presentation usually evolves slowly.[21] The local inflammatory processes produced by mycobacteria are insidiously destructive and may spontaneously exacerbate and remit. An average of 19 months elapses from the onset of symptoms until the time of diagnosis in the case of *Mycobacterium tuberculosis*.

Pain is the most common presenting symptom. Systemic symptoms are often absent. Tuberculous joint involvement is usually monarticular, involving weight-bearing joints, hip, knee, and ankle in descending order of frequency.[12–14]

Diagnosis. Chest radiographs are normal in more than one-half of the cases of osteoarticular tuberculosis (TB). Tuberculin skin testing is usually positive. The definitive diagnosis is established when *M. tuberculosis* is detected in synovial fluid or involved tissue obtained by open or closed biopsy. Biopsy of bone and joint lesions that are clinically and radiographically consistent with TB may not be necessary in cases where there is microbiologic proof of extraskeletal TB. Synovial fluid analysis reveals positive for acid fast bacillos (AFB) smears in 20% and positive cultures in 80% of cases of tuberculosis arthritis. Synovial fluid WBC counts are variable, ranging from fewer than 1,000 cells/mm³ to more than 100,000 cells/mm³, with an average of 10,000 to 20,000/mm³. Open synovial biopsies are diagnostic in more than 90% of cases. Radiographic changes usually take months to develop. Weight-bearing joints and subchondral erosions are followed by sequestration of subchondral bone, with joint space narrowing occurring late in the course of the infection. Osteomyelitis may develop secondarily in association with tuberculosis. Osteomyelitis may lead to a septic joint. The radiographic changes may be indistinguishable from other chronic joint infections or rheumatoid arthritis in some cases.

Appendicular osteomyelitis may occur in the absence of joint involvement. It typically presents as an isolated lesion, most commonly involving the metaphysis of long bones (e.g., fibula, tibia, ulna). Plain radiographs reveal lytic lesions with various degrees of sclerosis and periosteal reaction.

Vertebral TB (Pott's disease) comprises 50% of all skeletal involvement. The thoracolumbar spine is more commonly involved than the cervical or acral regions. Infection may be confined to a single vertebra, but commonly extends by direct spread to adjacent vertebrae. Associated soft-tissue infections include psoas or paraspinal abscesses and sinus tract formation. Neurologic compromise may result when abscess or granulation tissue encroaches on the spinal cord. The radiographic appearance of the bone lesions vary from well-defined lytic lesions to a mixed lytic sclerotic picture.

CT may help to define the extent of vertebral and paravertebral involvement.[22] Seven to nine percent of skeletal TB cases involve the sacroiliac joints. Involvement is usually unilateral. Radiographic findings include pseudo-widening, erosions, and sclerosis.

Radiologic Aspects

George B. Greenfield

Tuberculous arthritis and spondylitis occur in 1% of patients with tuberculosis.[21,23,24] Of those, 50% have spinal involvement, 30% have hip or knee disease, and 20% have involvement of other joints. The early symptoms are mild, and the arthritis progresses very slowly. It usually involves only one large joint. The route may be hematogenous or a direct extension from tuberculous osteomyelitis. About one-half of patients with skeletal tuberculosis do not show active pulmonary TB. *Pathologically,* caseating granulomatous synovitis occurs. There is late cartilaginous destruction owing to lack of proteolytic enzymes. *Mycobacterium tuberculosis* of the human strain is causative in most cases. The *bovine* strain and *atypical mycobacteria* may affect some patients.

Peripheral Skeleton. Radiologically, the classic *Phemister triad* of local osteoporosis, late joint space narrowing, and marginal erosions has long been the hallmark in the peripheral skeleton. Osteoporosis is severe and may also be present distal to the involved joint. A hazy appearance of the articular surface is seen in the early stages. Osteoporosis develops slowly and occurs before destructive changes (Fig. 7.30). This is in contrast to acute pyogenic arthritis, where destruction appears before osteoporosis. In children, localized hyperemia may cause premature appearance and enlargement of the epiphyseal ossification centers, similar to JRA and hemophilia.

Articular cartilage in contact with its opposing member is involved relatively late. The bare marginal areas are eroded first. It is later that the articular cartilage is uniformly destroyed and joint space narrowing occurs. The subchondral bone then becomes involved with destructive foci. These tend to lie directly opposite each other at points of contact. Irregularity and sequestration occur here along with subchondral sclerosis. Sequestration in opposing articular surfaces in contact, called "*kissing sequestra,*" can be seen (Fig. 7.31). Fractures may be present. Little or no periosteal reaction is present.

The initial destruction is widespread in the *shoulder* because of a small surface contact area of articular cartilage.

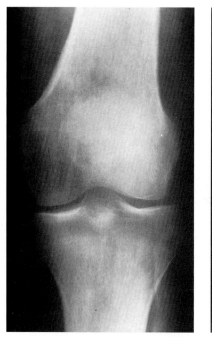
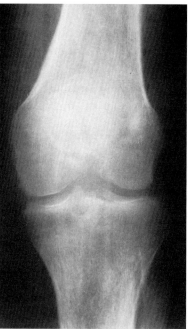
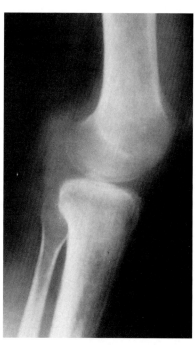

A   B   C

FIGURE 7.30. Tuberculous arthritis. Knee. **A:** A large erosion at the lateral margin of the distal femur is noted as well as osteoporosis. **B:** Three months later. AP view. There has been marked progression of osteoporosis and an erosion is seen at the intercondylar notch of the distal femur, and a small sequestrum is seen at the midportion of the tibial articular surface. Periosteal new bone formation along the lateral aspect of the distal femur is also seen. **C:** Lateral view at the same time as **(B)**. A large knee joint effusion is present. There is marked osteoporosis of the patella and distal femur.

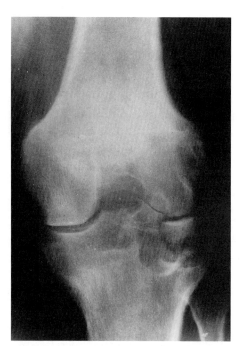

FIGURE 7.31. Knee. The subchondral bone shows destructive foci, which lie directly opposite each other at points of contact. Irregularity and sequestration are seen along with subchondral sclerosis. Sequestration in opposing articular surfaces in contact, so-called *"kissing sequestra"* are present. No periosteal reaction is present.

The appearance in the humeral head is that of multiple large erosive and destructive lesions. Effusion is minimal. The classic description is "dry caries."

Osteoporosis, uniform joint space narrowing, and articular surface erosions occur (Fig. 7.32) in the *hip*. Involvement of the greater trochanter may also be seen (Fig. 7.33). Any joint, including the sternoclavicular joint 494.1 may be affected (Fig. 7.34). The adjacent bone may be involved with tuberculous osteomyelitis, which may show a destructive or expansile appearance.

The *ankle* (Fig. 7.35) may show bony fragmentation at the tibiotalar joint with soft-tissue swelling. CT is helpful to delineate bony details.

Central Skeleton. The *spine* is the most common site of involvement, leading to destruction of intervertebral discs and vertebral bodies. This results in vertebral collapse, kyphosis with gibbus formation, reactive sclerosis, and a paraspinal soft-tissue mass (Fig. 7.36), which may be calcified (Figs. 7.37 and 7.38). This may extend to form a psoas abscess. This is the classic Pott's disease. Atlantoaxial subluxation may also occur. Rarely, a tuberculous psoas abscess can be seen without visible vertebral lesions. MRI with gadolinium infusion may demonstrate the communication of vertebral and paravertebral components. Rarely, the anterior aspects of the vertebral bodies may be

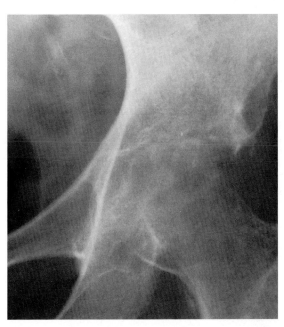

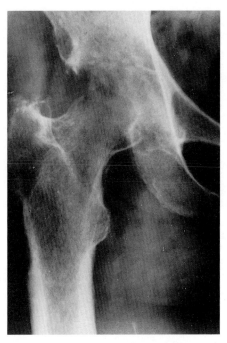

FIGURE 7.32. Tuberculous arthritis. AP view of the hip shows osteoporosis, uniform joint space narrowing, and erosions of the articular surface.

FIGURE 7.33. Tuberculous arthritis. AP view of the hip shows uniform joint space narrowing and erosions of the articular surface. A destructive lesion in the greater tuberosity is seen.

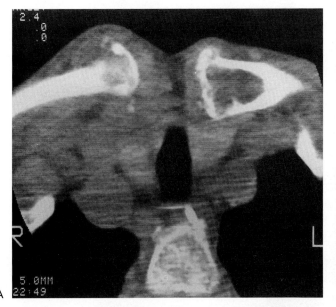

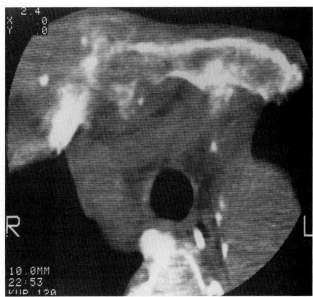

FIGURE 7.34. Tuberculous arthritis. Sternoclavicular joints. CT. **A:** Destruction at the distal aspect of the right clavicle and expansion at the distal aspect of the left clavicle are seen. **B:** Destructive changes involving the manubrium particularly at the right side are seen.

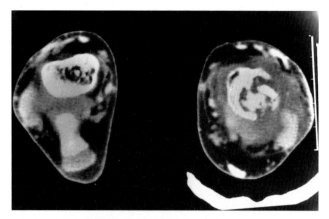

FIGURE 7.35. Tuberculous arthritis. Ankle. CT. Destructive changes and a soft-tissue mass are seen on the left side at the tibiotalar region.

eroded. This may occur with a tuberculous abscess in the retropharyngeal and retrotracheal regions, and may be involved with anterior destruction associated with an anterior cold abscess, but without vertebral collapse.

Tuberculosis of the vertebral pedicles occurs in about 2% of spinal cases. The pedicles may be destroyed unilaterally or bilaterally, at one or multiple levels. Large paravertebral abscesses are present, and paraplegia may result from spinal cord involvement.

Unilateral involvement with widening, sclerosis, destruction, or joint obliteration may occur (Fig. 7.39) in the *sacroiliac joints*. There is a lack of osteoporosis. Bilateral involvement (Fig. 7.40) sometimes may be seen.

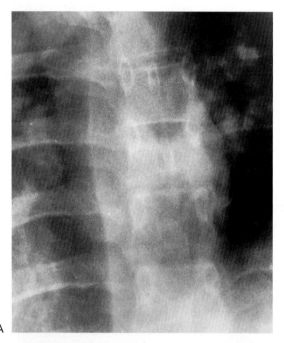

A

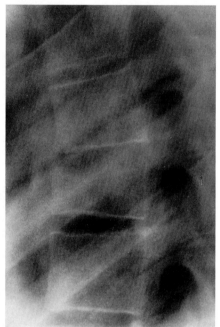

B

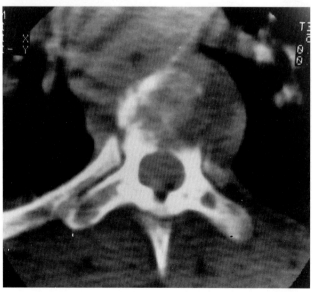

C

FIGURE 7.36. Tuberculosis. Spine. **A:** AP view showing destruction of the superior end plate of the body of T-8. **B:** Lateral view confirming findings. **C:** CT showing marked destruction of the vertebral body with bony fragmentation and a large paraspinal mass on both sides.

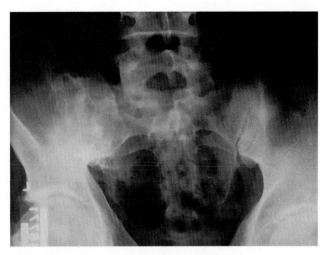

FIGURE 7.39. Tuberculous arthritis of the right sacroiliac joint. AP view of the pelvis shows obliteration of the right sacroiliac joint both in the upper third and lower two-thirds. Reactive sclerosis is also present. There is lack of osteoporosis.

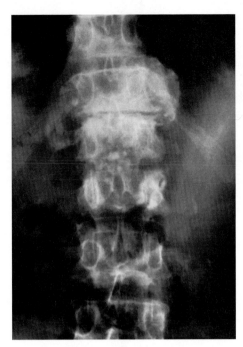

FIGURE 7.37. Tuberculosis. Spine. End plate irregularity and sclerosis is seen.

Healing occurs with increased bony sclerosis, and may be accompanied by extensive soft-tissue calcification. There may be fibrous ankylosis, in which case the articular cortex appears irregular, or total bony ankylosis may follow. Secondary pyogenic infection may complicate the picture.

If tuberculous arthritis is first seen in a chronic stage where healing has begun, the predominant appearance may be that of osteosclerosis rather than osteoporosis.

CT shows destructive bony changes associated with adjacent soft-tissue masses that show rim enhancement. Soft-tissue calcification is usually present.

Miliary tuberculosis may involve the skeleton. Multiple areas of increased activity on the radionuclide bone scan may mimic metastases. Some of the lesions may become photopenic on antituberculous therapy.

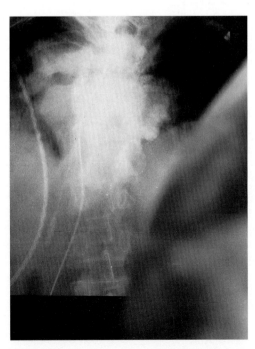

FIGURE 7.38. Pott's disease. A calcified tuberculous abscess involves the major portion of the thoracic spine with marked kyphosis. Calcification tracks are seen down the right psoas margin.

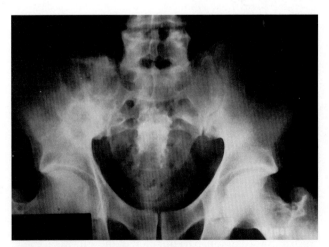

FIGURE 7.40. Tuberculous arthritis. Sacroiliac joints. There is obliteration and osteosclerosis at the right sacroiliac joint. A destructive area at the inferior aspect of the left sacroiliac joint on the iliac side is seen.

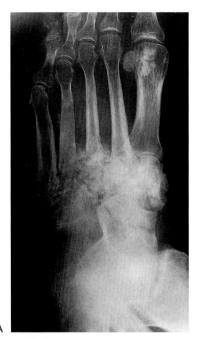
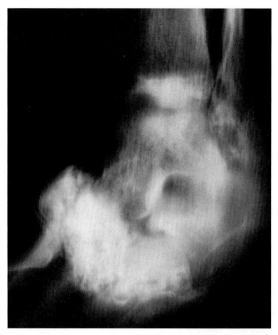

FIGURE 7.41. Sporotrichosis. Foot. **A:** AP. **B:** Linear tomogram. There is reactive sclerosis of the tarsal bones and cystic radiolucencies in the distal fibula. The subtalar joint is widened and the intertarsal joints are narrowed with erosions at their articular surfaces.

FUNGAL AND PARASITIC ARTHRITIS

George B. Greenfield

Fungal arthritis may be caused by coccidioidomycosis, histoplasmosis, blastomycosis, cryptococcosis, and sporotrichosis (Fig. 7.41), with frequency depending on geographic location.[22,25] Coccidioidomycosis may present in the spine with a picture similar to Pott's disease, or as a purely destructive lesion. Candida arthritis and osteomyelitis in infants may be seen. *Sporothrix schenckii* may show joint involvement. Radiologically, synovial involvement may resemble pigmented villonodular synovitis, and a destructive type of arthritis may occur. The knees, elbows, wrists, and small joints of the hands are most often involved. Actinomycosis may also involve the spine and joints. Acute guinea-worm synovitis of the knee joint has been reported. Yaws osteitis has been reported to result in concentric bone atrophy and "doigt-en-lorgnette" deformity.

VIRAL SYNOVITIS AND ARTHRITIS

George B. Greenfield

Viral synovitis and *arthritis* result in acute transient polyarthritis with little tendency toward chronicity. Rubella is a common cause. Polyarthritis involving the small joints of the hands is common. The duration of the arthritis averages 9 days. Mumps, variola, and serum hepatitis are other viral diseases associated with transient arthritis. Acute monarticular herpetic arthritis has been reported, as have sclerotic and destructive metaphyseal lesions associated with destructive arthritis after rubella vaccination.[26,27]

LYME ARTHRITIS

George B. Greenfield

Lyme arthritis is a component of a syndrome characterized by a skin rash, severe systemic manifestations, and nondeforming oligoarthritis.[28–32] It is caused by infection with the spirochete *Borrelia burgdorferi,* which is transmitted by the deer tick or a related ixodid tick. It is prevalent during the summer months, presenting with a skin rash accompanied by influenzalike or meningitislike symptoms. Neurologic and cardiac abnormalities may develop later. Arthritis may develop weeks to years later. Migratory arthritis involving the knees, shoulders, and elbows occurs. This may be followed by recurrent episodes of oligoarthritis separated by periods of complete remission. Initially, joint effusion combined with soft-tissue swelling involving the periarticular regions, infrapatellar fat pad, and the entheses are seen. The entheses may be thickened, calcified, or ossified. Inflammatory arthritis may follow, with juxtaarticular osteoporosis, joint space narrowing, and bone erosions.

REFERENCES

Infectious Arthritis

1. Kelly PJ, Martin WJ, Coventry MB. Bacterial (suppurative) arthritis in the adult. *J Bone Joint Surg [Am]* 1970;52: 1595–1602.

Septic Arthritis
2. Hollander JL, McCarty DJ. *Arthritis and allied conditions,* 8th ed. Philadelphia: Lea & Febiger, 1972.

Microorganisms Causing Acute Pyogenic Arthritis
3. Nolan B, Leers WD, Schatzker J. Septic arthritis of the knee due to *Clostridium bifermentans:* report of a case. *J Bone Joint Surg [Am]* 1972;54:1275–1278.
4. Kelly PJ, Martin WJ, Coventry MB. Bacterial (suppurative) arthritis in the adult. *J Bone Joint Surg [Am]* 1970;52:1595–1602.
5. Norenberg DD. *Corynebacterium pyogenes* septic arthritis with plasma-cell synovial infiltrate and monoclonal gammopathy. *Arch Intern Med* 1978;138:810–811.
6. Wale JJ, Hunt DD. Acute hematogenous pyarthrosis caused by *Hemophilus influenzae. J Bone Joint Surg [Am]* 1968;50:1657–1662.
7. Yocum RC, McArthur J, Petty B, et al. Septic arthritis caused by Propionibacterium acnes. *JAMA* 1982;248:1740–1741.
8. Hardin JG. Occult chronic septic arthritis due to *Proteus mirabilis. JAMA* 1978;240:1889–1890.
9. Rogala EJ, Cruess RL. Multiple pyogenic arthritis due to *Serratia marcescens* following renal homotransplantation. Report of case. *J Bone Joint Surg [Am]* 1972;54:1283–1287.
10. Kido D, Bryan D, Halpern M. Hematogenous osteomyelitis in drug addicts. *AJR* 1974;118:356–363.
11. Nade S. Acute septic arthritis in infancy and childhood. *J Bone Joint Surg [Br]* 1983;65:234–241.
12. Wientroub S, Roberts GCL, Fraser M. The prognostic significance of the triradiate cartilage in suppurative arthritis of the hip in infancy and early childhood. *J Bone Joint Surg [Br]* 1981;63:190–193.
13. Shawker TH, Dennis JM. Periarticular calcifications in pyogenic arthritis. *AJR* 1971;113:650–654.
14. Glassberg GB, Ozonoff MB. Arthrographic findings in septic arthritis of the hip in infants. *Radiology* 1978;128:151–155.
15. Kay JJ, Winchester PH, Freiberger RH. "Neonatal septic dislocation" of the hip: true dislocation or pathological epiphyseal separation. *Radiology* 1975;114:671–674.
16. Armbuster TG. Extra-articular manifestations of septic arthritis of the glenohumeral joint. *AJR* 1977;129:667–672.

17. Griffiths HED, Jones DM. Pyogenic infection of the spine. *J Bone Joint Surg [Br]* 1971;53:383–391.
18. Konstantinov VD. Verlauf der Purulenten Sakroileitis im Röntgenbild. *Fortschritte Gebeit Röntgenstrahlen* 1984;140:195–199.
19. Guyot DR, Manoli A II, et al. Pyogenic sacroiliitis in IV drug abusers. *AJR* 1987;149:1209–1211.
20. Baker SB, Robinson DR. Sympathetic joint effusion in septic arthritis. *JAMA* 1979;240:1989.

Tuberculosis Arthritis
21. Berney S, Goldstein M, Bishko F. Clinical and diagnostic features of tuberculous arthritis. *Am J Med* 1972;53:36–42.
22. Greenfield GB. *Radiology of bone diseases,* 5th ed. Philadelphia: JB Lippincott, 1990:956.
23. Goldblatt M, Cremin BJ. Osteoarticular tuberculosis: its presentation in coloured races. *Clin Radiol* 1978;29:669–677.
24. Versfeld GA. A diagnostic approach to tuberculosis of bone and joints. *J Bone Joint Surg [Br]* 1982;64:446–449.

Fungal and Parasitic Arthritis
25. Rajah R. Case report 513. *Skeletal Radiol* 1989;17:601–602.

Viral Synovitis and Arthritis
26. Brna JA, Hall RF Jr. Acute monoarticular herpetic arthritis. *J Bone Joint Surg [Am]* 1984;66:623.
27. Peters ME, Horowitz S. Bone changes after rubella vaccination. *AJR* 1984;143:27–28.

Lyme Arthritis
28. Culp RW, Eichenfield AH, et al. Lyme arthritis in children. *J Bone Joint Surg* 1987;69:96–99.
29. Dryer RF, Goellner PG, Carney AS. Lyme arthritis in Wisconsin. *JAMA* 1979;241:498–499.
30. Lawson JP, Liu YM. Pinemoth caterpillar disease. *Skeletal Radiol* 1986;15:422–427.
31. Lawson JP, Steere AC. Lyme arthritis: radiologic findings. *Radiology* 1985;154:37–43.
32. McLaughlin TP, Zemel L, et al. Chronic arthritis of the knee in Lyme disease. *J Bone Joint Surg* 1986;68:1057–1060.

OTHER CONDITIONS

GEORGE B. GREENFIELD

Certain conditions and tumors are unique to joints, whereas others involve joints secondarily. Several of these are described in this chapter.

PIGMENTED VILLONODULAR SYNOVITIS AND VILLONODULAR TENOSYNOVITIS

Pigmented villonodular synovitis (PVS) and villonodular tenosynovitis (giant cell tumors or xanthomas of synovium and tendon sheaths) are uncommon chronic proliferations of the synovia of the joints, bursae, and tendons.[1-5] Young adults are most commonly affected, with intermittent pain and swelling of a joint. Hemarthrosis may occur. The disease usually diffusely affects the entire synovium. A localized form also exists, often in the knee (Fig. 8.1).[6] This disease is usually considered to be inflammatory or reactive. Rare cases with metastases have been observed.[7] A malignant counterpart also exists.

Radiologically, joint swelling with lobular soft-tissue masses are seen. They may extend beyond the capsule, or they may rarely be entirely extracapsular. These do not calcify but may appear dense, because of hemosiderin deposits. The disease is usually monarticular and most commonly occurs in the knee, with lesser frequency the hip, ankle, shoulder, and hand.

Erosion or invasion of bone occurs in about one-half of cases, affecting both subchondral and marginal areas (Figs. 8.2–8.4). Cystlike defects of varying sizes may be present, with sharp and sclerotic margins. The larger erosions may be lobulated. Erosive narrowing of the femoral neck may occur. Some cases may progress to joint destruction. Joint space narrowing and regional osteoporosis are relatively absent. The disease may involve the synovium of a tendon sheath, in which case erosions are seen away from a joint (Fig. 8.5). It is then called *pigmented villonodular tenosynovitis.* Calcifications and osteophytes are not formed in this disease.

Involvement of a lumbar vertebral facet joint has been reported. An extradural mass behind the vertebral body and displacing the dural sac on a myelogram was reported, associated with destructive changes of the facet joint.[8] Another site of possible involvement is the infrapatellar fat pad.[9] The lesions are usually monarticular; however, biarticular involvement has been reported.[10,11] Temporomandibular joint involvement may also occur.[12] Polyarticular disease has also been reported in six separate joints.[13]

Ultrasound can demonstrate synovial thickening, joint effusion, and echogenic villous projections.[14] Radionuclide bone scanning may show increased activity. CT shows soft-tissue masses focally eroding bone (Fig. 8.6), which enhance following intravenous infusion of contrast material.

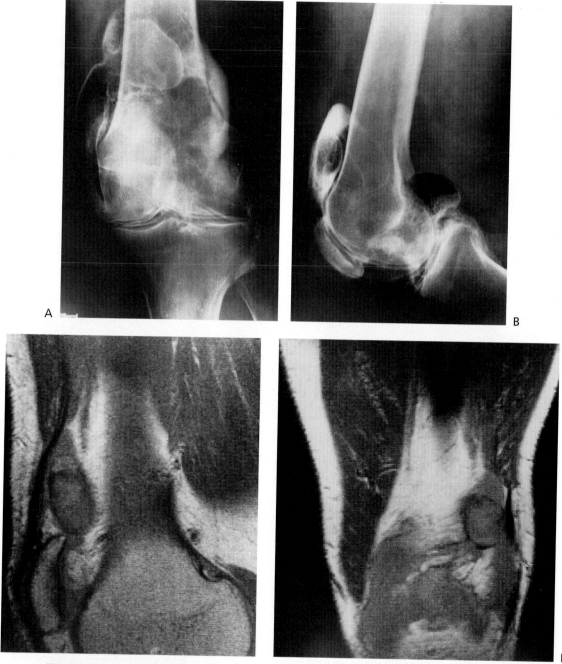

FIGURE 8.1. Focal pigmented villonodular synovitis. **A,B:** Arthrogram of the knee shows a well-circumscribed mass in the suprapatellar region. **C,D:** MRI. T1-weighted images show an intermediate heterogeneous signal intensity mass.

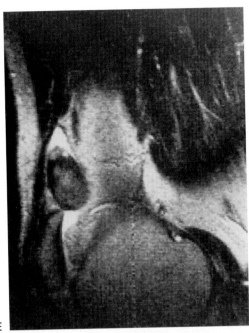

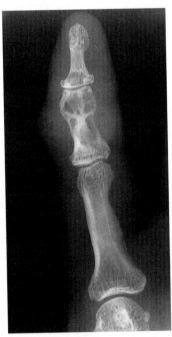

E

FIGURE 8.1. *(continued)* **E:** T2-weighted image shows heterogeneous signal intensity with central high signal.

FIGURE 8.3. Pigmented villonodular synovitis. Finger. Lobulated soft-tissue swelling is seen as well as bony erosion, particularly in the subchondral region in the middle phalanx. There is no osteoporosis.

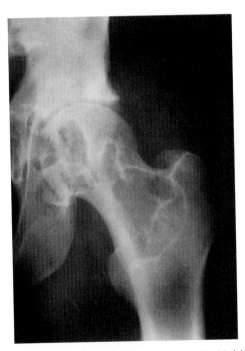

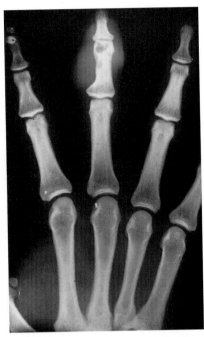

FIGURE 8.2. Pigmented villonodular synovitis. Hip. Multiple erosions are seen. The joint space is preserved.

FIGURE 8.4. Pigmented villonodular tenosynovitis. Finger. A soft-tissue mass causing erosions in the middle phalanx and the base of the proximal phalanx is seen.

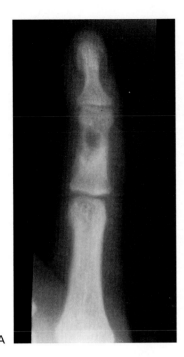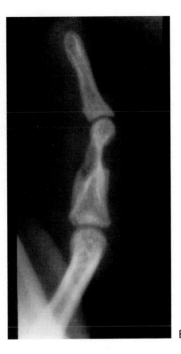

A   B

FIGURE 8.5. Pigmented villonodular tenosynovitis. Finger. **A:** AP view showing an erosion in the midportion of the middle phalanx away from the joint. **B:** Lateral view showing that this is localized to the dorsal surface.

MRI, on T1-weighted images shows the synovium as intermediate in signal intensity. T2-weighted images show the synovium as areas of increased signal interspersed with decreased signal. Hemosiderin deposition accounts for the low signal intensity, whereas increased signal results from fluid and inflamed synovium.[15,16]

Arthrography demonstrates capsular distention and multiple nodular filling defects of various sizes, either sessile or pedunculated. This is termed *cobblestoned synovium.*[17]

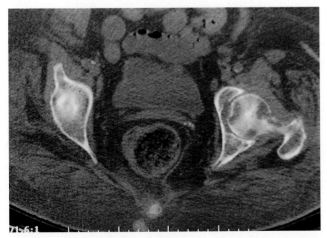

FIGURE 8.6. Pigmented villonodular tenosynovitis. Left hip. Erosion of the femoral neck is seen.

SYNOVIAL OSTEOCHONDROMATOSIS

Synovial osteochondromatosis is a condition in which foci of cartilage develop in synovial membrane through chondrometaplasia.[18–20] Cartilage fragments become detached and float free in the joint cavity. They increase in size, nourished by synovial fluid. The cartilage eventually becomes calcified and ossified. It is usually monarticular, occurring in young adults or middle-aged persons. Men are affected more frequently than women. It is rare in children.[21,22] The disease may be classified as primary if no cause is identified or secondary to trauma, degenerative disease, or inflammatory etiology.

Radiologically, the most frequent sites of involvement are the knee, hip, elbow, and shoulder. Extraarticular location adjacent to joints may occur rarely. Bursae may be involved as well as periarticular tendons.[23,24] Involvement of the ankle, knee, wrist, hand, and temporomandibular joint have been reported.[25–29] The last may extend into the middle cranial fossa, which can be demonstrated by CT or MRI.[30]

The characteristic finding is multiple small to large calcified or ossified opacities within the joint capsule (Figs. 8.7 and 8.8). They may also be in a Baker's cyst (Fig. 8.9). The cartilage bodies may not be calcified in a smaller percentage of cases. Osteoporosis is usually absent. Joint space narrowing and osteophytes may be seen at times. Rarely, joint effusion may be present. The calcifications range from small to large, with more uniformity in primary disease. They are round or oval, with smooth margins. Extensive erosions of bone and destruction may occur.[31,32] Pathological fracture

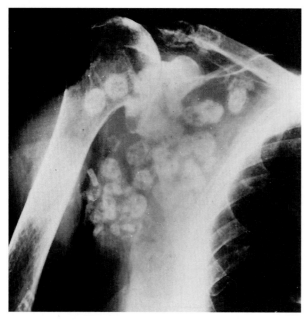

FIGURE 8.7. Synovial osteochondromatosis. Multiple calcific densities of various sizes in a distended joint capsule are seen.

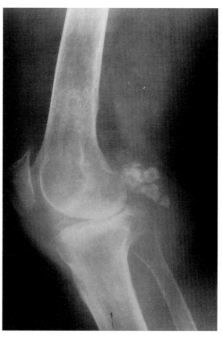

FIGURE 8.9. Synovial osteochondromatosis with loose bodies in a Baker's cyst. Narrowing of the knee joint with subchondral sclerosis is also seen.

and an intrapelvic mass have been reported as presenting features in the hip.[33,34]

Fewer and larger intraarticular calcifications and ossifications are more likely to result from trauma, neuropathic arthropathy, or osteochondrosis dissecans (Fig. 8.10). The lesions of osteochondromatosis tend to increase in size after

incomplete synovectomy. The lesions may be well demonstrated by CT (Fig. 8.11). Ultrasound is also useful in diagnosis.[35] Malignant transformation of synovial chondromatosis to a chondrosarcoma has been reported as a rare complication.[36,37]

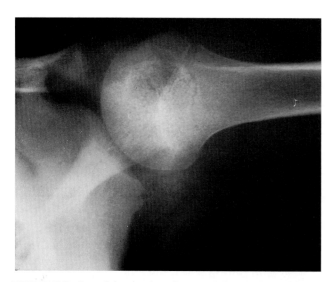

FIGURE 8.8. Synovial osteochondromatosis in a 13-year-old girl. Shoulder. Very fine and small calcific bodies seen within the glenohumeral joint.

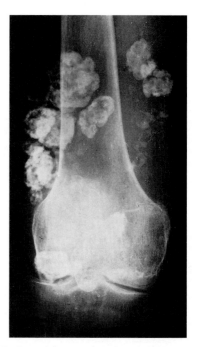

FIGURE 8.10. Synovial osteochondromatosis. Knee. Large synovial osteochondromata are seen. There is distention of the joint capsule. Osteoarthritis of the knee is seen with joint space narrowing.

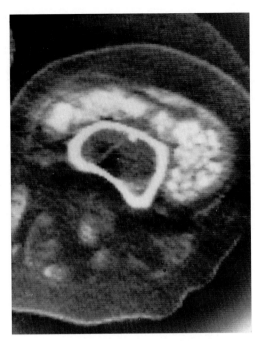

FIGURE 8.11. Synovial osteochondromatosis. Knee. CT. Large ossific bodies are seen within the joint capsule.

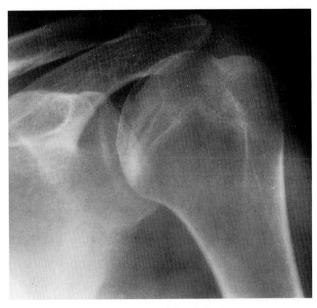

FIGURE 8.13. Avascular necrosis. Shoulder. A subchondral radiolucent fracture line of the humeral head is seen.

AVASCULAR NECROSIS (ISCHEMIC NECROSIS)

Avascular necrosis (AVN; ischemic necrosis) is important with respect to joint manifestations. There are many etiologies, but the more common ones are steroid administration, trauma, sickle cell disease, collagen disease, and pancreatitis; it may be idiopathic also. The most important joints that can be involved are the hip and shoulder. The process starts subchondrally with sclerosis of the femoral head and preservation of the joint cartilage. A subtle radiolucent subchondral line then follows. This is called the "crescent sign" and is a fracture line. This may be seen before the sclerosis. Collapse and deformity of the femoral head follow in the superolateral aspect. Osteosclerosis, radiolucencies, and sequestration then ensue (Figs. 8.12–8.15). Computed

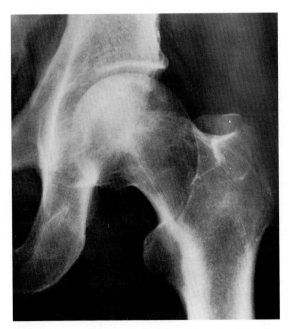

FIGURE 8.12. Avascular necrosis. Hip. Sclerosis of the femoral head is seen.

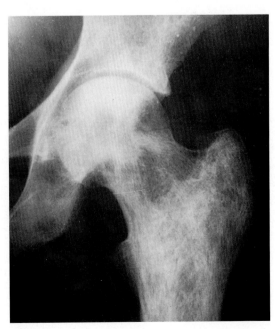

FIGURE 8.14. Avascular necrosis. Hip. Sclerosis and small cysts are noted in the femoral head.

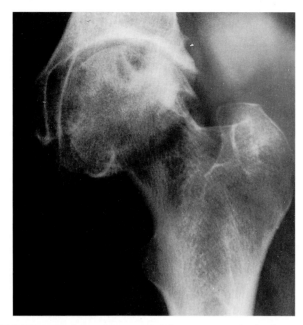

FIGURE 8.15. Avascular necrosis. Hip. Larger cysts in the femoral head are present along with osteoarthritis.

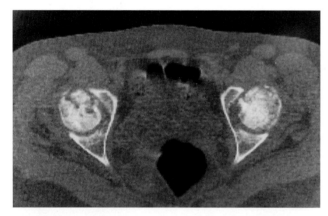

FIGURE 8.16. Avascular necrosis. Hips. CT shows fragmentation of the femoral heads.

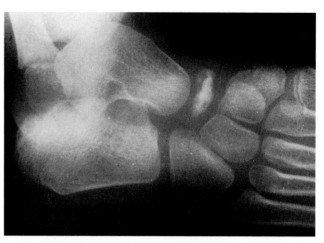

FIGURE 8.18. Koehler's disease. Foot. Flattening and sclerosis of the tarsal navicular bone is seen.

tomography (CT) can show the preceding changes (Fig. 8.16).

Magnetic resonance imaging (MRI) in earliest stages shows a segmental decreased marrow signal on T1-weighted images in the involved area (e.g., femoral head). It can show details of advanced changes.[38] The necrotic segment is demarcated from normal bone by a low signal intensity band on all pulse sequences, and an adjacent high signal intensity band on T2-weighted images (Fig. 8.17). Radionuclide bone scan shows increased activity in early stages and focal photopenia later.

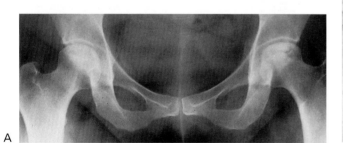
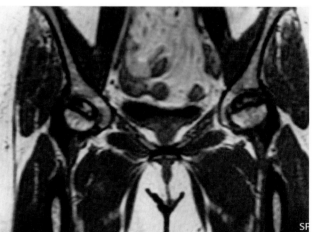

FIGURE 8.17. Avascular necrosis. Hips. **A:** AP view shows avascular necrosis in both hips with osteosclerosis and deformities of the femoral heads. **B:** MRI. T1-weighted image. Segmental low signal intensity of the superior aspects of the femoral heads are seen interspersed with patches of normal marrow signal. There is a low signal intensity band demarcating the involved segments.

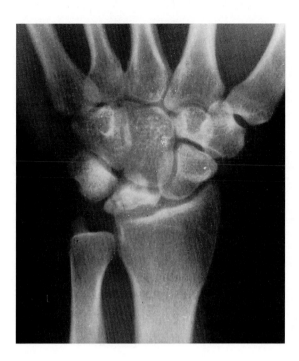

FIGURE 8.19. Kienböck's disease. Hand. There is flattening and sclerosis as well as fragmentation of the lunate. There is negative ulnar variance (shortening of the ulna within the radiocarpal joint). This is thought to be an etiologic factor.

Any joint may be involved, as well as the tarsal navicular (Koehler's disease) (Fig. 8.18), lunate (Kiembock's disease) (Fig. 8.19), and proximal portion of the scaphoid following fracture. Bone infarcts may extend to a joint (Fig. 8.20).

OTHER CONDITIONS

Trevor's disease (dysplasia epiphysealis hemimelica) is a rare, unilateral, asymmetric growth of epiphyses resulting in swelling, deformity, and functional impairment of the involved joints.[39] The knees and ankles are most commonly involved. The clinical findings include limitation of motion, genu varus and valgus, and pes planus.

Radiologically, there is early intraarticular cartilaginous overgrowth and irregular ossification, usually limited to one-half of the epiphysis. The affected limb may be longer or shorter than normal. The knee may have a varus or valgus deformity. The most frequent sites of involvement are the talus, distal femur, and distal tibia (Figs. 8.21–8.23). Bony overgrowth from a fracture may simulate Trevor's disease (Fig. 8.24).

Multiple epiphyseal dysplasia shows generalized irregularity of the ossification centers (Fig. 8.25).

Osteochondritis dissecans causes osteochondral defects at the articular surfaces. Loose bodies may become detached (Fig. 8.26). MRI can show this condition to good advantage (Fig. 8.27).

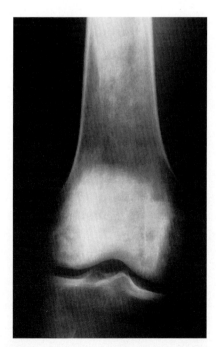

FIGURE 8.20. Bone infarction secondary to pancreatitis. Knee. AP view. Patchy osteosclerosis in the distal femur is seen, with a well-demarcated radiolucency in the lateral condyle.

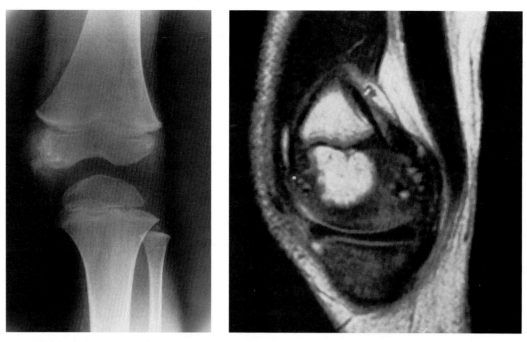

A   B

FIGURE 8.21. Trevor's disease. **A:** AP view of the knee shows soft-tissue swelling with calcification, medially at the distal femoral epiphysis. **B:** MRI. T2-weighted image. The low signal intensity of the enlarged nonossified distal femoral epiphysis is seen containing calcifications. This is an early stage.

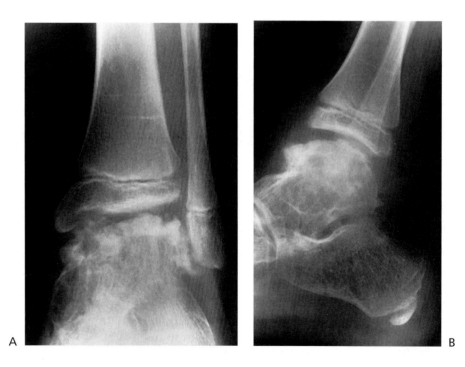

A   B

FIGURE 8.22. Trevor's disease. Ankle. **A,B:** Later stage. AP and lateral views of the ankle show irregularity and calcification at the talar dome.

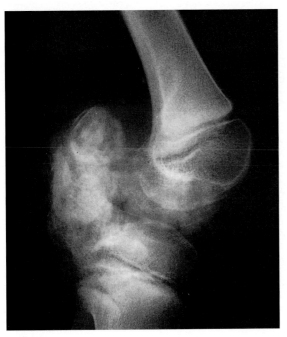

FIGURE 8.23. Trevor's disease. Knee. A large fused bony mass is seen posteriorly.

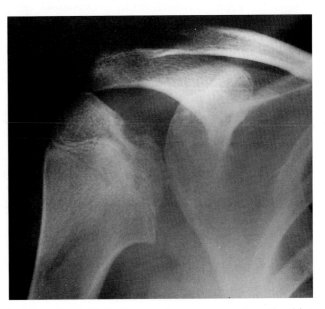

FIGURE 8.25. Multiple epiphyseal dysplasia. Shoulder. Irregularity of the humeral capital epiphysis is noted.

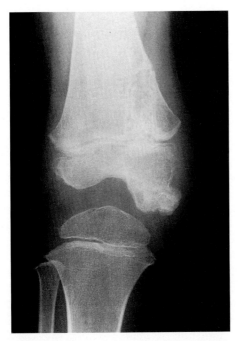

FIGURE 8.24. Healed fracture of the medial epiphysis and metaphysis with bony overgrowth simulating Trevor's disease.

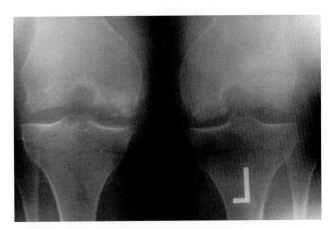

FIGURE 8.26. Osteochondritis dissecans. Knees. Bilateral loose bodies are seen at the medial condyles.

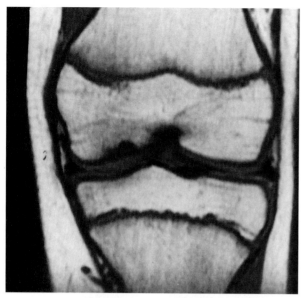 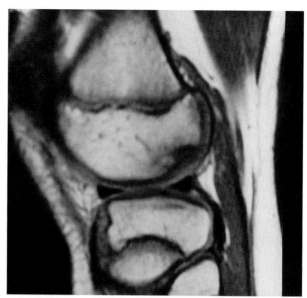

FIGURE 8.27. Osteochondritis dissecans. Knee. MRI. **A,B:** T1-weighted images show an osteochondral defect at the posterior medial condyle at low signal intensity.

Capsular constriction of the hip, or adhesive capsulitis, is a condition analogous to frozen shoulder and may be diagnosed by arthrography.[40] The normal capacity of the hip joint capsule varies from 14 to 20 mL in adults. Significant reduction in this capacity occurs. Symptoms include pain and limitation of motion. It has also been reported in the ankle.[41] Adhesive capsulitis of the wrist can be diagnosed best by arthrography. Findings include decreased capacity, small volar and styloid recesses, and adhesions.[42]

MYOSITIS OSSIFICANS

Myositis ossificans is a benign, heterotopic, soft-tissue ossification that may result from several different causes. The pathogenesis is unknown, and there is no primary inflammation of skeletal muscle, despite the name. The condition is a metaplasia of intramuscular connective tissue. Young adults are usually affected; it is rare in children. It is not premalignant. The ectopic bone may lie longitudinally along the axis of muscle and may also be attached to the bone. The adjacent periosteum may react. A radiolucent zone of soft-tissue separates the lesion from the underlying periosteal reaction and cortex in the early stages. Bone erosion and blending of the new bone with the cortex may occur.

MYOSITIS OSSIFICANS CIRCUMSCRIPTA

Myositis ossificans circumscripta is localized ossification after direct acute or chronic trauma.[43,44] The symptoms are a persistent soft-tissue mass, pain, and tenderness after an injury. It begins as an ill-defined cloud of calcifica-

tion 2 to 6 weeks after the onset of symptoms. Flocculent densities within the mass and local periosteal reaction are seen after about 1 month. After 6 to 8 weeks, a lacy pattern of bony trabeculation appears that is circumscribed by a cortex. At about 6 months, it matures to a bony appearance, and the mass reduces in size. The ectopic bone may lie parallel to the bone. Localized myositis ossificans must be differentiated from parosteal sarcoma, which also has a thin, radiolucent line separating tumor from cortex, except at its origin from bone. The hallmark is that more mature bone is seen peripherally in myositis ossificans.

Myositis ossificans is common around the elbow joint. An example caused by chronic trauma is rider's bone, or ossification of the adductor longus muscle. Drug-induced myositis ossificans circumscripta caused by injections into the antecubital vein has been reported.[45] Hemophiliacs may develop myositis ossificans resulting from intramuscular hematomas.[46]

Arteriography during the active stage shows a diffuse blush of fine vessels. The lesions are avascular in the mature stage.[47]

CT shows the progress of ossification from an early attenuation value lower than muscle to a calcific density. The zone phenomenon is demonstrated, with ossification around the periphery of the mass and central decreased attenuation, usually seen after 4 to 6 weeks. Later, complete ossification may be seen.[48] Ultrasound can demonstrate calcification within a soft-tissue mass.[49]

Radionuclide bone scan with technitium phosphate, using the three-phase bone scan technique, may show regional soft-tissue hyperemia in the flow study, increased activity in an early blood pool image, and generalized increase in soft-tissue activity in the involved region on static images.[50]

The MRI appearance depends on the age and maturation of the lesion.[51,52] Acute and subacute lesions may display a mass effect or no changes on T1-weighted images, or they may produce a pattern of edema and hemorrhage with high signal intensity on T2-weighted images. Fluid-fluid levels secondary to hemorrhage sometimes may be seen. Adjacent bone marrow edema also may be revealed. Mature lesions show low signal intensity margins corresponding to the calcific zone seen on plain films. The calcifications are of low signal intensity on T1- and T2-weighted images. The central pattern varies, sometimes showing the signal characteristics of fat and sometime producing intermediate signal intensity. Mature lesions may be seen as an irregular signal void on all sequences (Fig. 8.28) sometimes with areas con-

taining fat. Active lesions enhance with gadolinium infusion.

Myositis ossificans may also result from neurologic disease and may be caused by a variety of conditions, including diseases of the brain, spinal cord (including trauma), compression of the cauda equina, peripheral neuropathy, and tetanus.[53] Extensive soft-tissue ossification, particularly in the paraarticular regions, leads to joint ankylosis. Disuse osteoporosis and bone erosions are seen. The ossification may blend with the cortex. Ossification may form rapidly. Myositis ossificans develops below the level of the neurologic lesion. Pressure erosions develop at bony prominences, such as the trochanters and ischia in paraplegics, and should not be confused with a trochanterectomy, which is sometimes performed to alleviate decubitus ulcers. Increased radionuclide uptake occurs in the heterotopic osseous tissue.

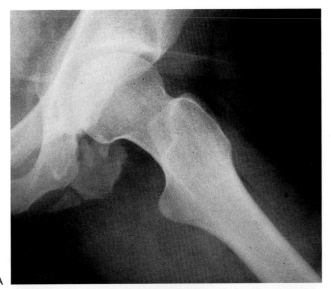

A

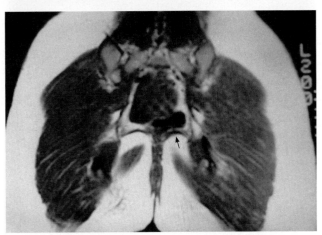

B

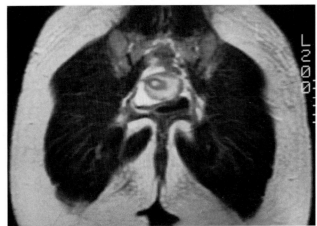

C

FIGURE 8.28. Myositis ossificans in a 16-year-old girl. **A:** A lateral view of her left hip shows mature myositis ossificans in the region of the ischiac bone. **B:** MR image (SE 650/16). The ossification is seen as a signal void. **C:** MR image (FSE 4000/102 Ef). The ossification remains as a signal void.

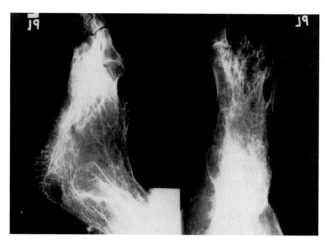

FIGURE 8.29. Myositis ossificans progressiva. Extensive ossification of the soft tissues of the foot has occurred.

FIBRODYSPLASIA OSSIFICANS PROGRESSIVA

Fibrodysplasia ossificans progressiva (myositis ossificans progressiva) is a mesodermal disorder in which congenital anomalies, such as hypoplasia of the thumbs, and inflammatory foci in the fascia and ligaments occur. These foci progress to fibrosis and ossification, which may be extensive (Fig. 8.29).

TUMORS INVOLVING JOINTS

Tumors, both benign and malignant, of bone and soft tissue, may affect joints and their surroundings. Their symptoms may overlap those of arthritis. Clinically, pain, swelling, redness, and heat may be experienced in both tumors and arthritis. Radiologically, destruction, expansion, osteosclerosis, local osteoporosis, soft-tissue calcification, and joint effusion are imaging signs that are common to both types of conditions.

Certain tumors arise from synovium. Some arise in the vicinity of a joint. These include synovioma (synovial sarcoma). Another tumor that has overlapping symptoms of arthritis in the spine is chordoma. Certain tumors typically involve the epiphysis, which may give rise to joint symptomatology. These are giant cell tumor (GCT), chondroblastoma, aneurysmal bone cyst (ABC), and clear cell chondrosarcoma. Osteoid osteoma may be intracapsular or be in the vicinity of a joint giving rise to joint symptomatology. Finally, certain tumors incidentally may involve the joints.

Malignant Tumors That Principally Affect Joints

Malignant tumors that *principally* affect joints and their vicinity include malignant tumors of the synovium. They are most often synovial sarcoma (synovioma), and very rarely synovial chondrosarcoma. Benign conditions include pigmented villonodular synovitis (PVS) and synovial osteochondromatosis (discussed in the preceding).

Synovial Sarcoma

Synovial sarcoma (synovioma) is a highly malignant, fibroblastic, common soft-tissue tumor. The lower extremities are most often involved. Only 10% of these tumors are located within a joint capsule. The majority arise near a joint or from a tendon sheath along a limb. The buttocks, back, neck, chest, hands, feet, hips, abdominal wall, and orbits are other reported sites. They may occur in unusual locations and have even been reported in the oropharynx.[54] The peak age of incidence is between 18 and 35 years. Patients usually present with a mass associated with pain and tenderness.

A large lobulated soft-tissue mass usually is seen on conventional radiographs, with calcification in about 30% of cases, with possibly more than one bone involved.[55] The adjacent bone may show invasion with irregular destructive changes. Local osteoporosis is present. CT may demonstrate calcification within a mass.[56] MRI shows the tumor with low signal intensity on T1-weighted images and higher signal intensity on T2-weighted images, usually as a heterogeneous, septated mass with infiltrative margins, possibly with hemorrhage near a joint.[57] Fluid-fluid levels may be seen. The pattern and extent of the calcification cannot be accurately depicted on MRI. The tumor may cause destruction or erosion of several adjacent bones (Fig. 8.30). The tarsal tunnel may be involved (Fig. 8.31). Angiography shows marked vascularity. The tumor may involve the carpal or tarsal tunnel (Fig. 8.32). This tumor can be demonstrated to be markedly vascular by angiography.

Chordoma

Chordoma is an uncommon tumor derived from notochordal remnants or rests.[58,59] It is malignant, with local invasiveness, but distant metastases are rare. Most chordomas develop in the sacrum and at the base of the skull in the sphenoid-occipital area, with approximately 10% of cases occurring elsewhere along the spine. Men are affected more than women. The usual age distribution for patients is 30 to 70 years. Benign notochordal rests in the occipital-occipital region also occur and must be differentiated from malignant tumor. Chordomas are painful and are associated with neurologic symptoms and usually with a palpable mass. Distant metastases occur rarely, most commonly involving lymph nodes, liver, and lungs. Chordoma has also been reported in the posterior mediastinum.[60]

This tumor most often appears as a large midline mass, causing bone destruction at the base of the skull or in the caudal region, particularly the sacrum. It usually originates in the vertebral body. Bony destruction and cortical expan-

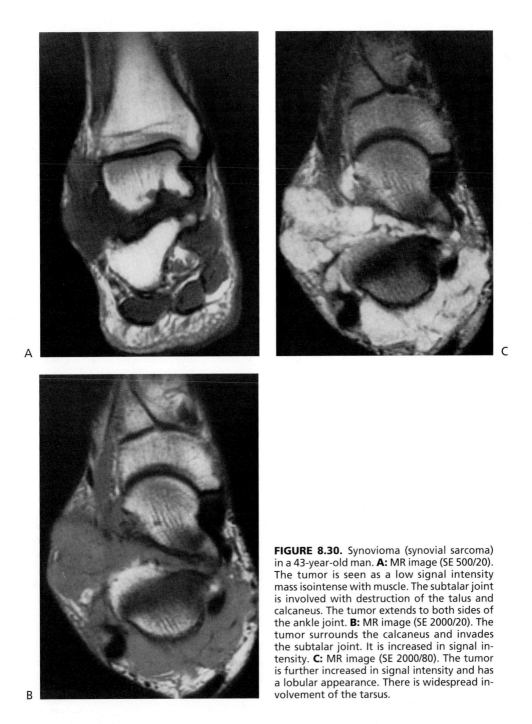

FIGURE 8.30. Synovioma (synovial sarcoma) in a 43-year-old man. **A:** MR image (SE 500/20). The tumor is seen as a low signal intensity mass isointense with muscle. The subtalar joint is involved with destruction of the talus and calcaneus. The tumor extends to both sides of the ankle joint. **B:** MR image (SE 2000/20). The tumor surrounds the calcaneus and invades the subtalar joint. It is increased in signal intensity. **C:** MR image (SE 2000/80). The tumor is further increased in signal intensity and has a lobular appearance. There is widespread involvement of the tarsus.

sion may be seen, as well as a soft-tissue mass with flocculent calcifications. Osteosclerosis may be pronounced.[61]

Intracranial lesions may present as sella turcica tumors, with erosion of the clivus, calcification, or extensive destruction. A nasopharyngeal mass is present in one-third of these cases. Rarely it may not be in the midline.

Sacral tumors are seen as midline destructive and expansile lesions, accompanied by a large soft-tissue mass, with or without calcification or osteosclerosis. In the later stages, the tumor need not be confined to the midline, and may involve the sacroiliac joint. Bone destruction with or without destruction of the intervertebral disc may occur in spinal involvement, and two or more vertebrae may be affected. A paraspinal soft-tissue mass containing calcification is often present.[58] Chordoma of the cervical spine has been reported with intervertebral foramina enlargement resembling neurofibroma.[62]

CT is more accurate than conventional x-ray films, because it can better define an associated soft-tissue mass and calcific debris.[63] It can show better detail, providing cross-

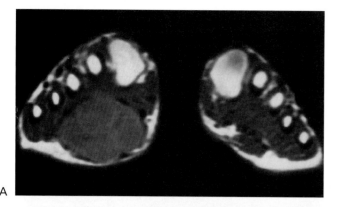

A

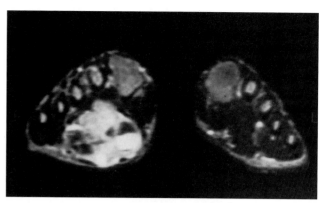

C

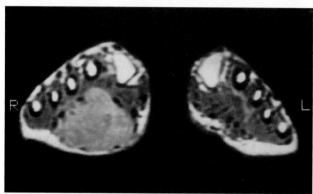

B

FIGURE 8.31. Synovial sarcoma. **A:** MR image (SE 750/20). A large low signal intensity soft-tissue mass is seen at the plantar aspect of the right foot, which appears fairly homogeneous. **B:** MR image (SE 2000/20). The mass has increased in signal intensity and retains its fairly homogeneous appearance. **C:** MR image (SE 2000/80). The mass shows high signal intensity. The various tendons are of low signal intensity. (From Greenfield GB, Arrington JA, Kudryk BT. MRI of soft-tissue tumors. *Skeletal Radiol* 1993;22:77–84, with permission.)

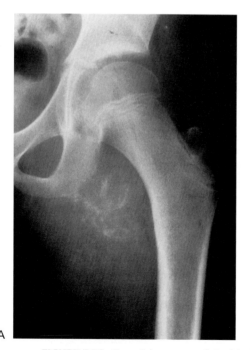

A

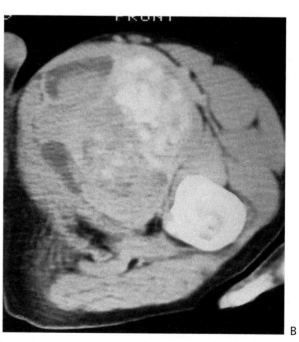

B

FIGURE 8.32. Synovial sarcoma of the hip in a 10-year-old boy. **A:** Anteroposterior view of the left hip shows a large soft-tissue mass containing multiple small calcifications. These calcifications do not have the linear or circular pattern of cartilage calcifications. **B:** The CT scan shows a large soft-tissue mass with calcifications and necrotic areas. The posterior aspect of the bony cortex is minimally involved.

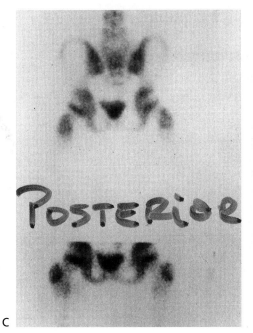

C

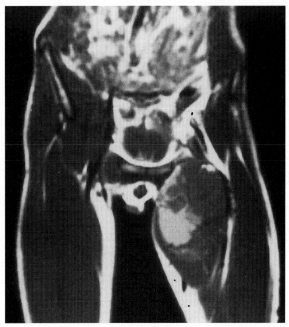

D

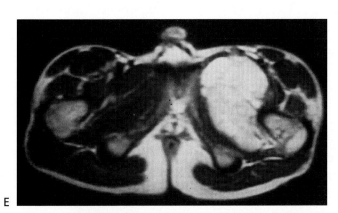

E

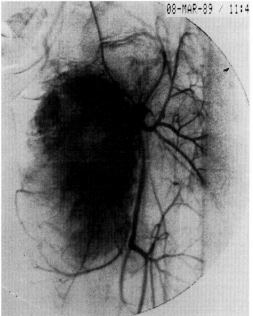

08-MAR-89 / 11:4

F

FIGURE 8.32. *(continued)* **C:** The radionuclide bone scan shows minimally increased activity in the left subtrochanteric region. **D:** MR image (SE 600/20). A large inhomogeneous mass in the soft tissues adjacent to the hip extends down the medial thigh. **E:** MR image (SE 2500/80). The mass is of high signal intensity and has irregular margins and internal septations. **F:** Digital subtraction angiography shows the mass to be markedly hypervascular, displacing the major vessels. Early venous filling is also depicted.

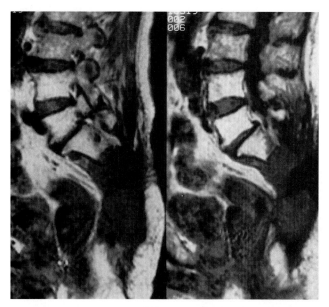

FIGURE 8.33. Chordoma. MR images (SE 700/20). A large tumor is destroying a major portion of the sacrum. The tumor is of low signal intensity.

sectional anatomy at the base of the skull and in the sacrum. The extent of intrapelvic involvement can be ascertained.

MRI provides superior contrast with surrounding soft tissues and intrapelvic viscera, defining the precise extent of the tumor.[64] Chordoma may be seen as a low signal intensity or as a mixed signal intensity tumor on T1-weighted images, with increased or inhomogeneous signal intensity seen on T2-weighted images (Figs. 8.33 and 8.34).

Bone Tumors That May Affect Joints

Aneurysmal Bone Cyst

Aneurysmal bone cyst is a lesion characterized by a highly expansile appearance.[66,67] There are two types: A primary cyst occurs without an associated lesion, and a secondary cyst occurs in association with a bone tumor. The radiologic appearance of a secondary aneurysmal bone cyst is most often that of the associated bone lesion. The ratio of primary to secondary lesions is 2 to 1.

The bone lesions that occur with an aneurysmal bone cyst are presented in the following in order of frequency:

Giant cell tumor
Osteosarcoma
Solitary bone cyst
Nonossifying fibroma
Fibrous dysplasia[68]
Metastatic carcinoma
Chondromyxoid fibroma

Hemangioendothelioma
Osteoblastoma
Chondroblastoma
Fibromyxohemangioma
Fracture[69]

The histologic appearance is of interconnecting cavernous spaces separated by fibrous septa filled with unclotted blood that may show thin bone formation. An endothelial lining of the blood spaces and numerous multinuclear giant cells may be seen. A solid portion of fibroblastic, fibrohistiocytic, and osteoblastic proliferation with osteoid production also is evident. Rarely, the latter portion predominates, and the tumor is devoid of cavernous spaces. This has been called a solid aneurysmal bone cyst. Its radiologic appearance may include an osteolytic lesion with a wide zone of transition, cortical expansion, and destruction with soft-tissue invasion.[70,71]

Older children and young adults are most often affected, with complaints of mild, local pain, swelling, and impairment of function of a contiguous joint of several months' duration. If a vertebral body is involved, pathologic fracture often ensues, sometimes with neurologic symptoms. Females are affected more often than males.

The femur is the most common site of involvement (Fig. 8.35). In most cases, the lesion is found in a segment of the long bones or spine, including the bodies and neural arch.[72] Any bone may be involved, including the flat bones, and can extend to a joint (Fig. 8.36), ribs, calvarium, orbits, small bones, calcaneus, pubis, and zygoma.[73,74] Multiple aneurysmal bone cysts in a 3-month-old infant have been reported.[75]

The origin is usually in the metaphysis in the tubular bones, but it may later involve the entire epiphysis. The lesion has been reported to extend into an unfused epiphyseal ossification center.[76]

The typical appearance is a radiolucency off of the central axis with marked ballooning of a thinned cortex. Light trabeculation within the lesion usually is seen. It may be in a subperiosteal location, in which case it presents as a bone blister. Periosteal new bone is usually limited to the margins, where a periosteal buttress sometimes is seen. The long axis of the lesion is parallel to the long axis of the bone, and it may be as long as 8 cm. The thin outer cortical shell may not be seen on conventional radiographs. There may be a thin sclerotic zone of transition, and pathologic fracture may occur.

Vertebral involvement is seen as an expansile, lightly trabeculated lesion that may attain large size. The body, arch, transverse, and spinous processes (Fig. 8.37) are affected alone or in combination. The vertebral body may collapse.

An expansile lesion with thin or thick margins may be seen in flat bones. It may present as a large, intrathoracic mass in the ribs.[77] These lesions may present as a pelvic mass.

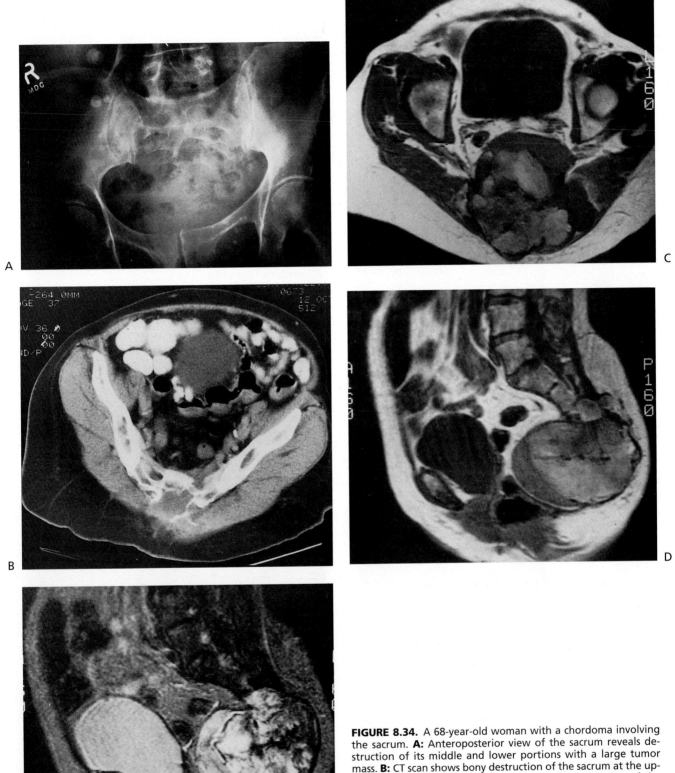

FIGURE 8.34. A 68-year-old woman with a chordoma involving the sacrum. **A:** Anteroposterior view of the sacrum reveals destruction of its middle and lower portions with a large tumor mass. **B:** CT scan shows bony destruction of the sacrum at the upper aspect of the tumor. **C:** MR (SE 600/20) axial section of the pelvis at a slightly lower level shows a large inhomogeneous tumor mass with loculated high signal intensity, which may represent hemorrhage. **D:** MR (650/20) sagittal section shows the entire intrapelvic and extrapelvic extent of the tumor. **E:** MR image (SE 2000/90). The tumor increases in signal intensity and shows greater heterogeneity in this T2-weighted image.

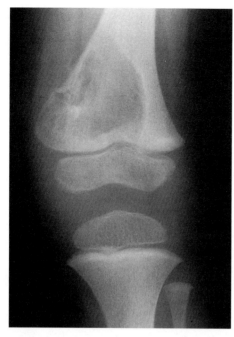

FIGURE 8.35. Aneurysmal bone cyst. Anteroposterior view. Knee. An expansile lesion in the distal femoral metaphysis with a thin outer margin located off of the central axis is seen. The lesion is well defined but has no sclerotic margin with the bone. The epiphyseal ossification center has not as yet fused, and there is no involvement of the epiphysis.

The occipital bone is most frequently involved in the calvarium. Aneurysmal bone cysts have been described in the sacrum, where it had radiographic appearances similar to a simple bone cyst, both with significant exophytic components.[78]

CT may show fluid-fluid levels with the proper window and level settings if the patient is immobilized long enough.[79,80] This is the result of blood layering in blood-filled spaces of various sizes (Fig. 8.38).

A radionuclide bone scan shows increased uptake of isotope.[81] Some patients show an extended uptake beyond the margins of the lesion. Angiographically, the lesion is hypervascular, with large vascular spaces.[82]

MRI findings are characteristic.[83] Internal septations; cystic loculations, occasionally with fluid-fluid levels of various signal intensities; and an expanded low signal intensity rim surrounding the lesion are seen. Portions of the lesion have high signal intensity on T1- and T2-weighted images. Fluid-fluid levels may also be seen in telangiectatic osteosarcoma, giant cell tumor, synovioma, cystic chondroblastoma, and tumoral calcinosis.

Chondroblastoma

Chondroblastoma is an uncommon bone tumor originating from chondroblasts in the epiphyseal cartilage plate.[85–88] Generally it is considered to be benign.

Microscopically, the cells are moderate-sized polyhedral cells with little intercellular connective tissue. Focal areas of calcification, necrosis, and giant cells may be seen. Differentiation from clear cell chondrosarcoma may be difficult.[89]

The age distribution peaks between 10 and 25 years of age, with a range of 8 to 59 years. The symptoms are joint pain, tenderness, heat, swelling, limitation of motion, weakness, numbness, and muscle atrophy.

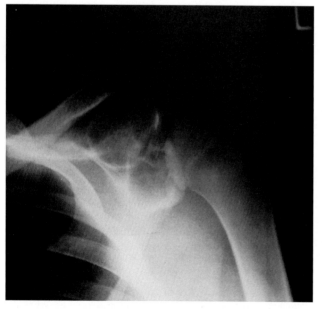

A

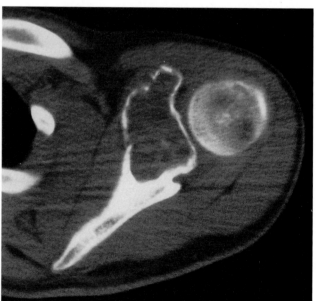

B

FIGURE 8.36. Aneurysmal bone cyst showing expansion. Shoulder. **A:** Conventional radiograph of the left shoulder shows expansion of the glenoid with thinning of the cortex and small cortical discontinuities superiorly. **B:** An axial CT scan similarly shows expansion of the glenoid, thinning of the white cortical stripe, and small disruptions of the medial and anterior cortex. .

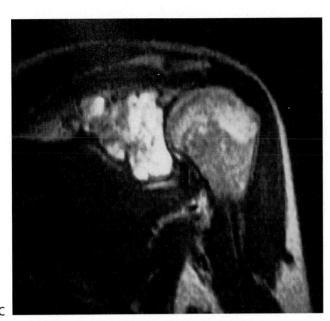

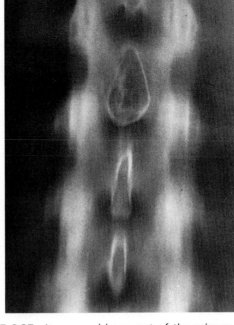

FIGURE 8.36. *(continued)* **C:** A coronal oblique MR image (SE 500/20) demonstrates the expanded glenoid and an intact but thinned black cortical stripe with superior cortical disruptions. The image also shows blood pools within the expansile lesion (bright signal on T1-weighted image).

FIGURE 8.37. Aneurysmal bone cyst of the spinous process. Seventeen-year-old girl with back pain. An expansile appearance of the spinous process is seen with a thin cortical shell in this conventional tomogram.

The tumor arises in the epiphyseal cartilage plate and extends into the epiphysis (Fig. 8.39), sometimes involving the adjacent metaphysis, but to a lesser extent. Rarely, it may be confined to the metaphysis, abutting the epiphyseal cartilage plate.[90] The sites of most frequent involvement are the lower femur, upper tibia, upper humerus, lower tibia, femoral head and greater trochanter, calcaneus, astragalus, ilium, and ischium. It has also been reported in the patella, finger, rib, scapula, proximal fibula, and distal radius and more rarely in the manubrium, capitate,

metatarsal, vertebra, mandibular condyle, calvarium, and mastoid.[91–94] The hands, feet, and tarsals may also be involved, with a predilection for the calcaneus and talus. Tumors in the pelvis tend to arise from the triradiate cartilage. Extensive osteolysis with an intrapelvic soft-tissue mass has been reported.[95]

This tumor typically presents as a well-demarcated oval or round that is usually between 3 and 6 cm in diameter. It may eccentrically expand the cortex.[96] A thin, sharply demarcated sclerotic bony margin is usually part of the picture

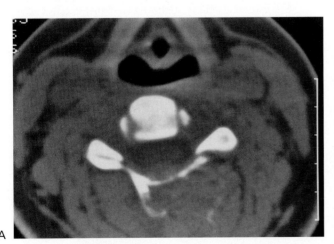

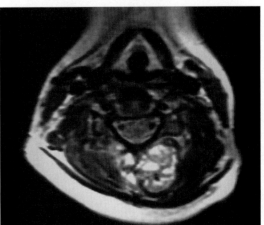

FIGURE 8.38. Aneurysmal bone cyst. **A:** CT scan shows an expanded neural arch. **B:** Gradient echo MR image. Fluid-fluid levels are seen within the lesion.

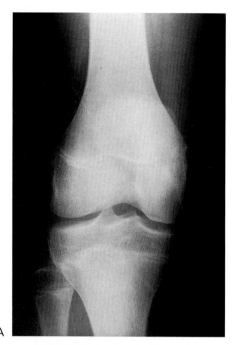

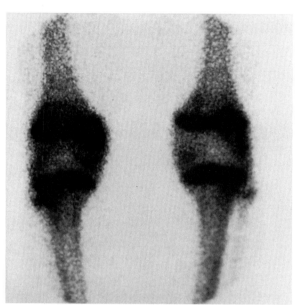

A

B

FIGURE 8.39. Chondroblastoma. **A:** AP view of the right knee shows a radiolucency at the medial margin of the femoral condyle with involvement of the metaphysis and to a greater extent the epiphysis. **B:** Radionuclide bone scan showing greater activity at the right medial femoral condyle than at the left.

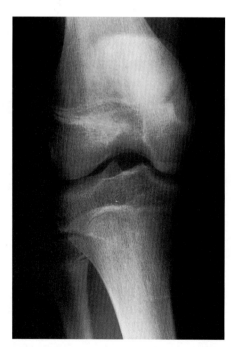

FIGURE 8.40. Chondroblastoma. Knee. Anteroposterior view. A radiolucent lesion is seen in the medial aspect of the distal femoral epiphysis. The major portion lies in the epiphysis, and a smaller portion lies in the metaphysis. The outer cortex is eroded. A sclerotic margin is seen only in the epiphyseal portion of the tumor.

and occasionally is scalloped. The metaphyseal portion of the tumor may not show this sclerotic rim. The outer cortex may be eroded (Fig. 8.40). Surrounding nonuniform reactive bone sclerosis may be seen at a slight distance from the tumor. A thick, solid periosteal reaction that extends distally along the shaft has been reported in about one-half of all chondroblastomas.[97] There is amorphous, spotty calcification reflecting its cartilaginous origin in a minority of cases. Pathologic fracture is rare, but synovitis and effusion of the adjacent joint may occur (Fig. 8.41).

Radionuclide bone scan shows increased activity but is not useful in differentiating benign from malignant forms. CT is most useful for defining the bony extent and location of the tumor. It can also demonstrate matrix calcification.

MRI can identify the tumor, which shows low to intermediate signal intensity on T1-weighted images with variable to high signal intensity on T2-weighted images. Extensive bone marrow edema may be seen with low signal intensity on T1-weighted images, which increases on T2-weighted images. This area may enhance after gadolinium infusion. The adjacent soft-tissue may show edematous changes with low signal intensity on T1-weighted images and high signal intensity on T2-weighted images. An effusion may affect an adjacent joint (Fig. 8.42).[97,98] Cystic chondroblastoma may show fluid(fluid levels.

Angiography shows a low degree of vascularity. Chondroblastoma must be differentiated from giant cell tumor and, in the femoral head, from ischemic necrosis.[99] Complications include the formation of a secondary

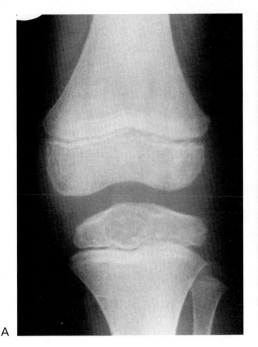

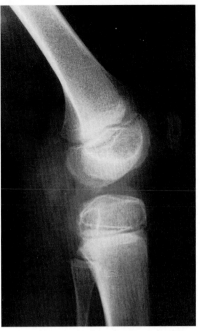

FIGURE 8.41. Chondroblastoma. Proximal tibial epiphysis. **A:** AP view. A thin shell outlines the lesion in the proximal tibial epiphysis. A knee joint effusion is noted medially. **B:** Lateral view showing knee joint effusion with increased soft-tissue bulging posteriorly and anterior displacement of the patella.

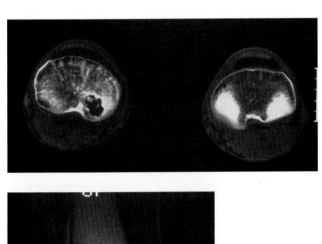

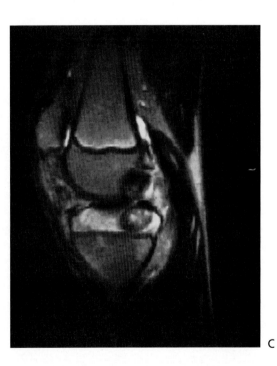

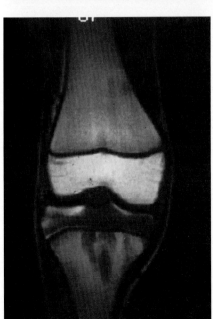

FIGURE 8.42. Chondroblastoma in a 16-year-old boy involving the proximal tibial epiphysis. **A:** CT scan shows a well-defined, low density lesion with sclerotic margins that contains several calcifications in the epiphysis. **B:** MR image (SE 700/17). The low signal intensity of the proximal tibial epiphysis extends down to the metaphysis in a streaky fashion. This represents bone marrow edema. **C:** The sagittal MR (SE 2500/90) section shows the low signal intensity chondroblastoma within the epiphysis, containing high signal intensity cartilage. The high signal intensity of the remainder of the epiphysis indicates edema. Soft-tissue edema and joint effusion are of high signal intensity.

aneurysmal bone cyst, development of a malignant chondroblastoma, and fibrosarcoma after radiation therapy.[100] Malignant chondroblastomas of bone have been reported.[102] These may represent a variant of chondrosarcoma or clear cell chondrosarcoma.

Osteoid Osteoma

Osteoid osteoma is a common benign lesion of bone.[103–105] The lesion is 1 cm or smaller in diameter and is called the nidus. This nidus, initially uncalcified, later may develop calcification, which can range from minimal to complete. If located in the cortex, the lesion evokes a great deal of reactive sclerosis with cortical thickening, periosteal new bone, and a possible reactive soft-tissue mass. The degree of reactive new bone formation varies according to the location of the nidus. The nidus consists of osteoid within a highly vascular stroma with giant cells, and it is sharply demarcated from the surrounding reactive sclerosis.

The clinical hallmark of this lesion is local pain, which is worse at night and relieved by activity and aspirin. It has been shown that prostaglandins, which have been recovered in large amounts in this tumor, are probably responsible for the pain. Prostaglandin inhibitors provide some relief. The duration of symptoms before presentation usually ranges from 6 months to 2 years. The pain may be referred to a nearby joint, and it later increases in severity. Focal soft-tissue swelling, point tenderness, and limitation of motion also occur. Heat and erythema do not occur. If in the lower extremities, limp, weakness, muscle atrophy, and depressed deep tendon reflexes are seen. With spinal involvement, osteoid osteoma produces a painful, rigid scoliosis causing nerve irritation simulating a neurologic lesion.[106] Scoliosis and back pain may result from osteoid osteoma of a rib.[107] Radicular pain and torticollis may occur in a cervical spinal location.[108] There are no systemic symptoms. Rarely, a lesion may not be painful.[109] The tumor has presented with symptoms of carpal tunnel syndrome in the capitate bone.[110] It may present with osteosclerosis, joint effusion, and a periosteal reaction in the elbow.[111] Leg-length discrepancy with tibial osteoid osteoma has been reported.[112] Joint pain occurs with a juxtaarticular lesion.[113,114] Osteoarthritis has developed in one-half of the patients with intraarticular hip lesions.[115]

Ninety percent of patients are seen before the age of 25 years. The lesion is rare in patients younger than 2 years of age or older than 50 years of age, but it has been reported in the tibia of an 8-month-old boy.[116] The ratio of males to females is 2 to 1. One-half of the lesions are in the femur and tibia. Other common sites are the fibula, humerus, and vertebral arch, but any bone may be involved, including the tarsals, metatarsals, and skull.[117–119] The nidus may be intracortical, intramedullary, subperiosteal, or within a joint capsule. Double and triple nidi have been reported, as have osteoid osteomas in adjacent bones.[120–123]

The typical imaging appearance is that of a small, radiolucent intracortical nidus less than 1 cm in diameter, surrounded by a large, dense, sclerotic zone of cortical thickening (Fig. 8.43). There may be a solid or, rarely, laminated or spiculated periosteal reaction. The dense sclerotic reaction may obscure the nidus on conventional films, and CT may be necessary for its demonstration. The nidus may be uncalcified, partially calcified, or have its center calcified, which presents radiologically as a radiolucent halo within the sclerotic zone. The nidus is not always centrally located within the area of sclerosis but may be eccentrically placed or even at the edge. Synovitis may occur in an adjacent joint not involved by an intracapsular lesion.[124,125] An intramedullary nidus causes little bone sclerosis and may cause endosteal thickening.

A subperiosteal nidus is less common. It presents as a small, radiolucent bulge of the contour of the bone. A thin margin and variable cortical thickening are seen.

A common location for an intramedullary osteoid osteoma is in the femoral neck, where it results in local osteoporosis and possible growth disturbances. Lymphofollicular synovitis and soft-tissue inflammation has been reported for intraarticular osteoid osteoma. The findings include uniform narrowing of the joint space and subperiosteal bone formation involving the affected bone and adjacent bones.[126]

The neural arch is usually affected by osteoid osteoma in the spine. There may be enlargement of the adjacent transverse process with lamina involvement. The appearance is similar to that seen in other bones involved with osteoid os-

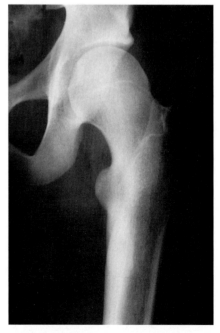

FIGURE 8.43. Osteoid osteoma. Proximal femur. AP view of the left hip shows cortical thickening below the lesser trochanter. A radiolucent nidus is seen within the area of osteosclerosis.

teoma. Conventional radiographs were normal for all patients in one series of spinal osteoid osteomas. Bone scans were positive and useful in localizing the lesion and directing CT to the appropriate level. In all cases, CT accurately demonstrated the location, nidus, and other diagnostic radiographic features of osteoid osteoma.[127]

The lesion may often be seen well only on CT scans, which are particularly valuable in diagnosing osteoid osteoma of the femoral neck (Fig. 8.44). The nidus is usually readily identified unless it is completely calcified. Rarely, a spiculated periosteal pattern may be seen on CT. Deformity of the femoral neck with widening and shortening and with flattening of the femoral capital epiphysis may occur if the diagnosis of an intracapsular lesion is delayed.[128]

Radioscintigraphy is of particular value for osteoid osteomas in the spine, joints, and small bones of the foot. On the triple-phase flow scan, an osteoid osteoma produces a discretely localized blush.[129] A characteristic pattern of uptake of this lesion is called the "keyhole" or "double-density" sign.[130] A smaller, more intense focus of activity is superim-

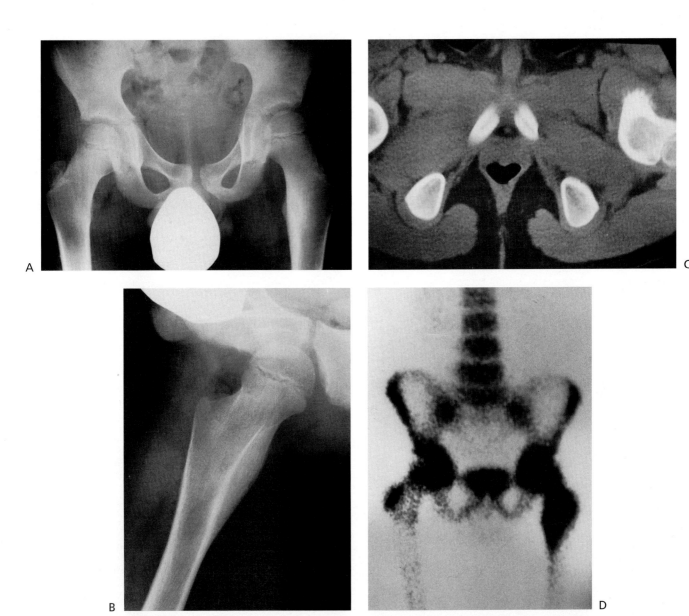

FIGURE 8.44. Osteoid osteoma involving the left proximal femur in an 8-year-old girl. **A:** Anteroposterior view of the pelvis shows marked cortical thickening medially. This is centered at the level of the lesser trochanter. **B:** Lateral view of the left proximal femur shows marked cortical thickening and layered periosteal new bone formation blending with the cortex. **C:** CT shows the nidus within an area of cortical thickening medially. CT scan at a higher level shows cortical thickening with spiculated periosteal new bone formation anteriorly. **D:** Radionuclide bone scan shows increased activity in the left hip and proximal femur to the subtrochanteric region.

posed on a lesser increase in activity of a larger area of bone (Fig. 8.45). A bone scan is particularly helpful in assessing intracapsular osteoid osteomas of the femoral neck, because it can provide guidance for CT planning.

The radionuclide scan is also useful in the operative management of the patient. The specimen can be evaluated by autoradiography to determine whether the nidus has been removed.[131]

MRI demonstrates abnormalities in all cases of osteoid osteoma. The nidus may not be identified or may show signal intensity characteristics from low to intermediate on all pulse sequences.[132] Mild to inhomogeneous enhancement after gadolinium infusion may occur in the nidus, and the adjacent bone marrow may be enhanced. This area also shows low signal intensity on T1-weighted images, which increases on T2-weighted images. A thickened cortex is seen as a signal void. Peritumoral edema and a reactive soft-tissue mass adjacent to the nidus also occurs. This is fairly well defined but varies in size. It may have inhomogeneous low to high signal intensity on T1-weighted images and increased signal intensity on T2-weighted images (Fig. 8.46).[133,134]

Angiographically, osteoid osteomas are hypervascular, with an intense, uniform vascular stain located only in the nidus. The feeding vessels to the nidus arise from surrounding soft-tissues and completely opacify it. They are best seen on subtraction films. Tumor stain usually persists late into the venous phase.

The differential diagnosis includes an intracortical abscess, which may present a similar imaging appearance. Enhancement on postinfusion CT of the nidus correlating with the histologic vascular stroma in osteoid osteoma can aid in the differentiation. A necrotic abscess cavity demonstrates no such finding. If the nidus is not seen, differentiation from osteosarcoma must be made.

An osteoid osteoma may recur as an osteoblastoma if it is incompletely excised.[135]

Giant Cell Tumor

Giant cell tumor (GCT, osteoclastoma) is an uncommon tumor derived from skeletal connective tissue, accounting for about 5% of all primary bone tumors.[136–143] It is not possible to predict histologically or radiologically the future behavior of most of these lesions. Even histologically benign-appearing GCT can metastasize to the lungs.[144] The incidence of malignancy has been estimated at about 20%.

Most of these lesions occur in patients between the ages of 20 and 40. It has rarely been reported in children and in one patient 80 years of age.[145] This is one of the very few bone tumors that have a female predominance. The patients complain of an intermittent dull ache, sometimes associated with a palpable, tender mass. Symptoms in a contiguous joint often develop, and pathologic fracture may occur. The tumor may recur after excision or metastasize to the lungs. Malignant transformation into fibrosarcoma or osteosarcoma after radiation therapy also is known to occur. GCT also may rarely be associated with Paget's disease.

When the diagnosis of GCT is considered, it is imperative to determine the serum calcium, phosphorus, and alkaline phosphatase levels, because a brown tumor of hyperparathyroidism may simulate this lesion radiologically and histologically.

The most common locations are the distal femur, proximal tibia, and the distal radius. The lesion has been reported

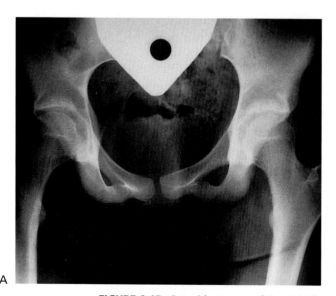

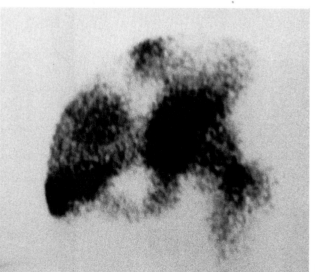

A

B

FIGURE 8.45. Osteoid osteoma of the right femoral neck. **A:** AP view of the pelvis. Local osteoporosis of the right femoral head and neck is noted with a small sclerotic area in the femoral neck. **B:** Radionuclide bone scan. There is increased activity in the femoral head and neck with a strong focus of increased activity at the base of the femoral neck.

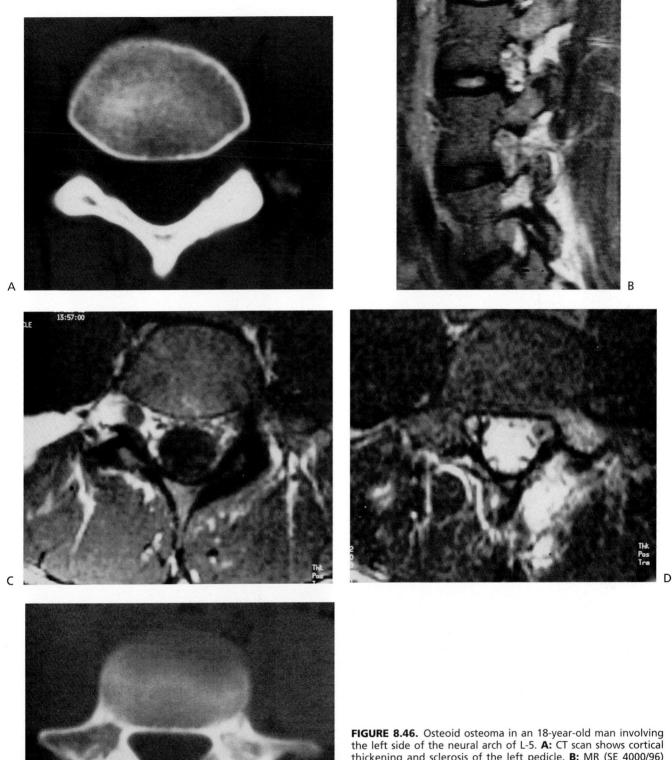

FIGURE 8.46. Osteoid osteoma in an 18-year-old man involving the left side of the neural arch of L-5. **A:** CT scan shows cortical thickening and sclerosis of the left pedicle. **B:** MR (SE 4000/96) sagittal image shows high signal intensity in the left pedicle of L5. **C:** MRI (SE 800/15). Axial section shows cortical thickening corresponding to that seen on the CT scan of the left lamina. The soft-tissue fat planes are obliterated on the left side but not on the right. **D:** MRI (SE 2000/80). The soft tissues adjacent to the left lamina show an increase in signal intensity. The well-circumscribed appearance somewhat suggests a mass. This represents soft-tissue reaction. No tumor or organism was found in the soft-tissues on biopsy. **E:** CT scan shows a nidus at the junction of the left lamina and pedicle.

in almost all tubular bones, as well as a rib, the patella, talus, calcaneus, hamate, and ischium.[146–148] It extends to the articular cortex, and usually is eccentric with respect to the central axis. The true origin is metaphyseal, attested to by the principal metaphyseal location of the rare giant cell tumor that arises in a young patient before fusion of the epiphyseal cartilage plate.[149–151] The tumor may then be limited by the cartilage plate or extend into the epiphysis. The epiphysis is not involved if the growth plate is still open. Epiphyseal involvement increases with age in children and adolescents.[152] This lesion may rarely not quite extend to the articular surface, extend down the shaft, or be located in the shaft in an adult.[153,154] Locations other than the long bones occur in about 15% of patients. Mandibular involvement is rare. GCT of the spine is rare, except in the sacrum. It may involve the body, pedicle, or the rest of the neural arch. The pelvis, ribs, or scapula rarely may be involved. Multicentric giant cell tumors are rare and difficult to differentiate from primary giant cell tumors that have metastasized.

The classic appearance is a roundish, moderate-sized, expansile, radiolucent lesion off the central axis of the bone extending to the articular surface (Fig. 8.47). Light trabeculation often occurs. The tumor may also involve the entire diameter of the bone (Fig. 8.48). The lesion also may be elongated (Fig. 8.49). Pathologic fracture may occur. Occasionally, no trabeculations are seen. Heavy trabeculation or margination (Fig. 8.50) suggests posttreatment change or recurrence. The tumor margin is fairly well de-

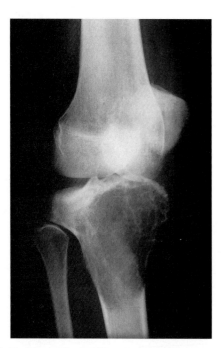

FIGURE 8.48. Knee. Giant cell tumor. The lesion extends to the articular surface and involves both sides of the bone. There is a wide zone of transition between the distal margin of the lesion and the normal bone.

fined. There is usually neither a sclerotic rim nor a wide zone of transition. The cortex is expanded and thinned (Fig. 8.51), and segments may not be seen on plain x-ray films because it is too thin to be visible. There is typically no periosteal new bone formation, even with a pathologic frac-

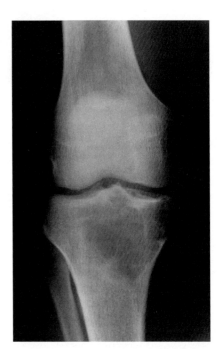

FIGURE 8.47. The classic appearance of a giant cell tumor. A rounded, medium-size, expansile, radiolucent lesion off of the central axis of the bone is seen.

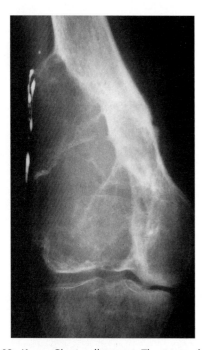

FIGURE 8.49. Knee. Giant cell tumor. The tumor has an elongated appearance and extends down to the articular surface at the lateral aspect of the distal femur.

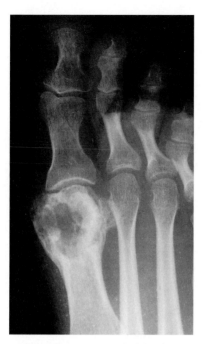

FIGURE 8.50. Giant cell tumor. Head of the first metatarsal. The lesion extends to the articular surface. This patient had a previous curettage and now has a thick sclerotic margin surrounding the lesion.

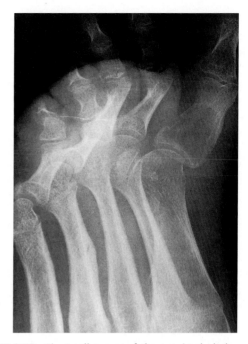

FIGURE 8.52. Giant cell tumor of the proximal phalanx of the great toe, showing expansion and extension to the articular surface. The cortex is interrupted at its inferior aspect. The tumor is well marginated.

ture. The cortex may be destroyed with soft-tissue invasion. Short tubular bone involvement shows changes similar to that of a long bone (Fig. 8.52).

The flat bones may also be involved with GCT (Fig. 8.53).

CT is of value to determine any soft-tissue component, assess the intraosseous extent, demonstrate the integrity of the cortex, and evaluate postoperatively.[155] Contrast-enhanced CT scans provide useful information about soft-tissue extent and relation to major vessels.

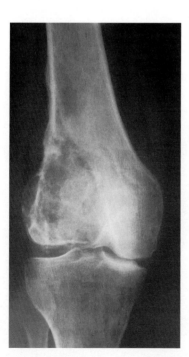

FIGURE 8.51. AP view of the knee. Giant cell tumor. The lesion extends to the articular surface. There is an expansile appearance of the lateral femoral condyle.

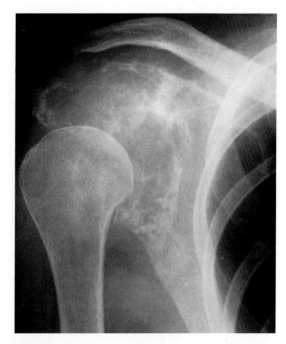

FIGURE 8.53. Giant cell tumor involving the scapula with an expansile appearance about the glenoid fossa and showing light trabeculation.

MRI is crucial in defining the extent of bone marrow replacement, inhomogeneity within the tumor, and soft-tissue invasion.[156,157] MRI provides the ability to evaluate the joint. It can show destruction of articular cartilage and demonstrate tumor spread into the subchondral cortex and within the joint. T1-weighted images show diminished signal intensity, and T2-weighted images show isointense or hyperintense signal intensity of tumor compared with uninvolved marrow (Fig. 8.54). Irregular tumor margins may rarely be seen.[153] Fluid-fluid levels are occasionally detected.

Radioscintigraphy of giant cell tumors show increased uptake, usually more intense at the periphery than at the center. Intense uptake beyond the true tumor limits may be seen.[158] Bone scan may not detect soft-tissue tumor extension. Gallium scans are unreliable in assessing this condition.[159]

The following section illustrates tumors that can incidentally affect joints and their vicinity, and the various imaging modalities that can detect them. The radionuclide bone scan is the most facile means of detecting these lesions. Conventional film radiography is sufficient for tumors in the peripheral skeleton, whereas CT is useful in the central skeleton. MRI can show detail in the bone marrow and soft tissues, including the joint.

Metastases

All malignant extracranial tumors may metastasize to bone, with random involvement of the vicinity of a joint. This may give rise to symptomatology that can overlap that of arthritis.

Metastases may be osteoblastic, osteolytic, or mixed. Osteolytic lesions may sclerose after therapy.

The most common osteoblastic metastases in an untreated adult male results from carcinoma of the prostate (Figs. 8.55 and 8.56). Osteolytic metastases most commonly result from carcinoma of the lung, and of the female breast (Figs. 8.57 and 8.58). Carcinoma of the kidney and thyroid yield bony metastases with an expansile appearance. Mixed metastases show both osteolytic and osteoblastic features (Fig. 8.59).

Osteosarcoma

Osteosarcomas are classified with respect to cell type and to central or surface location.[160,161] Osteosarcoma (e.g., central osteosarcoma) is a primary malignant tumor of bone in which tumor cells directly form osteoid matrix.[162–164] Conventional osteosarcomas have traditionally been divided into three groups: osteoblastic, chondroblastic, and fibroblastic. About one-half are osteoblastic, in which large amounts of osteoid are formed and the appearance is usually osteosclerotic. About one-fourth are chondroblastic. These usually show a cartilaginous pattern of calcification. The rest are fibroblastic with minimal osteoid, giving an osteolytic appearance.

Osteosarcomas may be grouped by location into central

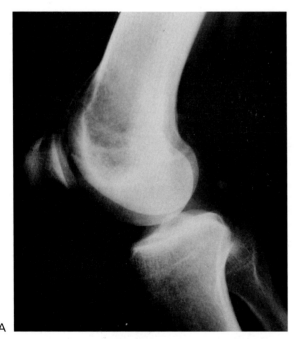
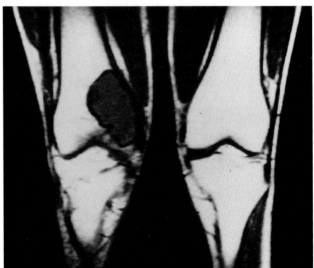

A   B

FIGURE 8.54. Giant cell tumor. Knee. **A:** Lateral view. A radiolucent expansile lesion in the distal femur is seen extending to the articular surface of the patella. **B:** MRI. T1-weighted image showing a low-signal intensity lesion at the medial aspect of the right distal femur. The lesion is well demarcated from the normal bone marrow.

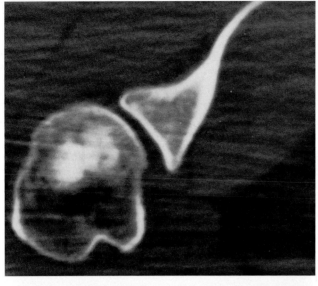

A

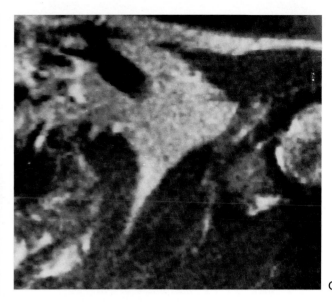

C

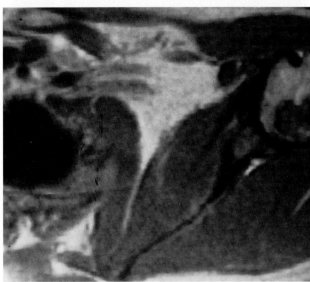

B

FIGURE 8.55. Osteoblastic metastases to the left humeral head from carcinoma of the prostate in a 60-year-old man. **A:** CT scan shows a dense osteosclerotic focus in the humeral head. **B:** MR image (SE 3000/25). The metastatic focus is of low signal intensity replacing high signal intensity marrow fat. **C:** MRI (SE 3000/80). The metastatic focus remains of low signal intensity, and the marrow fat is decreased in signal intensity.

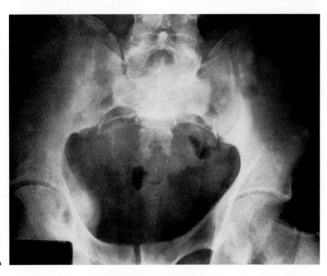

A

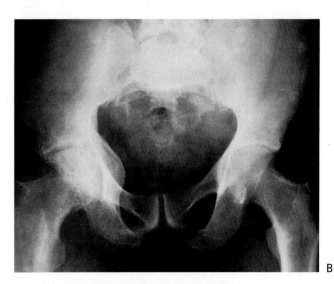

B

FIGURE 8.56. Osteoblastic metastases from carcinoma of the prostate. **A:** A large osteosclerotic mass with a spiculated margin is seen medial to the right acetabulum. Smaller osteosclerotic patches scattered throughout the pelvis are seen. **B:** Following a course of treatment, the bony mass adjacent to right acetabulum has consolidated and a cortex is now seen. This simulates acetabular protrusion.

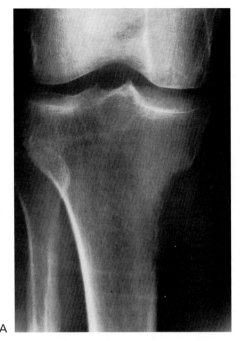
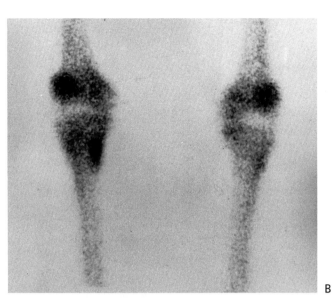

A

B

FIGURE 8.57. A 38-year-old woman with carcinoma of the breast. **A:** Anteroposterior view of the right knee shows a cortical or subperiosteal metastasis destroying the medial tibial metaphyseal cortex. **B:** Radionuclide bone scan shows increased activity at the site of destruction.

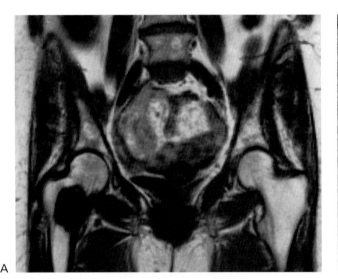
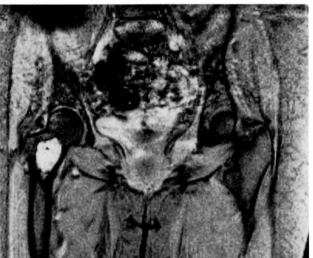

A

B

FIGURE 8.58. A 71-year-old woman with metastasis to the proximal femur from carcinoma of the breast. **A:** T1-weighted MR image shows a low signal intensity area in the intertrochanteric region of the right femur. **B:** T2-weighted MR image shows an increase in the signal intensity of the lesion.

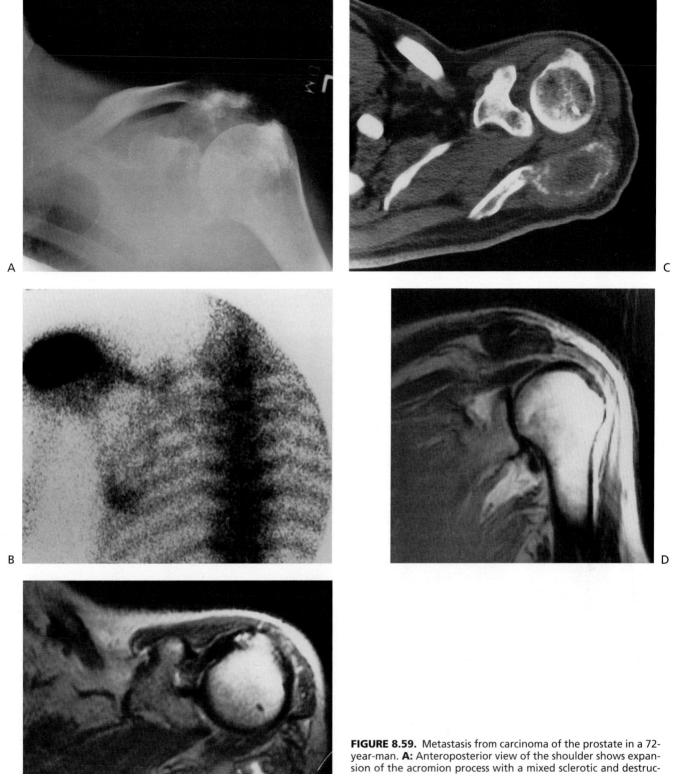

FIGURE 8.59. Metastasis from carcinoma of the prostate in a 72-year-man. **A:** Anteroposterior view of the shoulder shows expansion of the acromion process with a mixed sclerotic and destructive appearance. **B:** Radionuclide bone scan shows increased activity in the left shoulder region. **C:** CT scan shows an expanded acromion process with a thin, permeated outer shell. **D:** MR image (SE 600/20). The low signal intensity of the metastatic tumor at the acromion process is shown. **E:** MR image (SE 2500/80). The tumor is heterogeneous in signal intensity, with increased signal intensity in its central portion.

osteosarcomas and surface osteosarcomas, which include parosteal sarcoma. There is also soft-tissue osteosarcoma.

About 75% of the tumors are conventional osteosarcomas. The remainder are classified into various subtypes. One such type is telangiectatic osteosarcoma, which is osteolytic throughout and radiographically may simulate Ewing's sarcoma. These tumors are bloody and necrotic, and the prognosis is poor. Parosteal osteosarcoma arises on the surface of the bone and is less aggressive than the conventional type.

Osteosarcoma is the second most common primary sarcoma of bone, after multiple myeloma. The ratio of affected males to females is about 2 to 1. Most tumors arise in the 10- to 25-year age group. They can even occur in a 3-year-old child. A smaller peak incidence occurs in older age groups. Osteosarcomas in older age groups may be associated with Paget's disease (Fig. 8.60), postirradiated bone, or osteochondromas. They may also arise de novo. Osteosarcoma most often involves the tubular bones in younger patients. When it occurs in older persons, the flat bones are often involved.

The tumor metastasizes by way of the bloodstream in most instances. The most common site of metastasis is the lung. Nodular pulmonary densities, best seen on CT scans, may ossify or cavitate. Skeletal metastases, usually involving the spine or pelvis, may be seen. Skip metastases along the shaft in the long bones also occur and are best demonstrated by MRI.

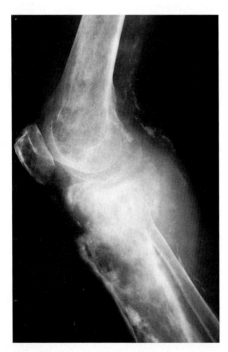

FIGURE 8.60. Osteosarcoma in Paget's disease. Knee. Lateral view. Paget's disease in the tibia is noted with destructive changes proximally at a large soft-tissue mass posteriorly, which involves the joint.

The chief symptom is pain at the tumor site, which begins insidiously and progresses to severe constancy. A palpable mass develops, with inflammation and local venous dilatation. Systemic symptoms follow. Effusion in a contiguous joint is common. Pathologic fracture may occur. The duration of symptoms before diagnosis averages several months. The serum alkaline phosphatase level is usually slightly elevated in the case of a large tumor.

The areas most frequently involved in conventional osteosarcoma are the distal femur (Figs. 8.61 and 8.62) and the proximal tibia. This occurs in about 75% of tubular bone involvement. The proximal humerus, the distal radius, and the pelvis (Fig. 8.63) are not uncommon sites, and there may be involvement of the femoral shaft, maxilla, sternum, ribs, pelvis, spine, and skull, or almost any bone in the body, including the patella.

The plain film findings in early osteosarcoma are subtle. There may be only minimal increase in bone density. CT can show increased marrow attenuation and calcification and subtle cortical and periosteal changes. Radionuclide bone scanning is more sensitive than CT, and MRI is most sensitive to early changes. Conventional x-ray films are the primary imaging means of diagnosis of a peripheral skeletal lesion. They are most accurate in demonstrating calcific patterns. Osteosarcoma most often originates in the tubular bones in the metaphysis. The epiphysis is commonly involved, with a reported incidence of 80%, and is more readily seen on MR images. The thickness of the epiphyseal cartilage plate is a factor in preventing transepiphyseal spread of tumor in younger patients and the tumor readily crosses the cartilage plate after or near the time of epiphyseal fusion. The joint cartilage forms an effective barrier against transarticular spread until the tumor becomes very large.

Primary osteosarcoma of the spine occurs in less than 2% of patients.[165] The findings may include osteolytic, mixed, expansile, or sclerotic lesions, which progress to compression and destruction of the vertebral body, and involvement of the neural canal and arch. Osteosarcoma of the pelvis occurs less often than in the long bones, and this tumor is rare in the ribs.

Periosteal new bone formation is seen as delicate filiform spicules radiating from a central point, called a sunburst pattern. A long-segment pattern of parallel spiculation may occur in other cases. Simple, laminated, and mixed types of periosteal reaction may occur, and there may be a transition from one type to another.

Spiculated periosteal reaction may also be seen in metastatic tumors, particularly carcinoma of the prostate, and in benign conditions, such as healed fractures, osteomyelitis, and thyroid acropachy. Malignant spicules tend to be long, thin, filiform, and delicate, but benign spicules are short and squat.

A Codman's triangle is often apparent. Pathologic fractures are common. Cortical destruction and invasion of the soft tissues is characteristic of osteosarcoma. The soft-tissue

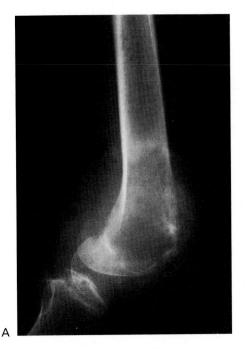

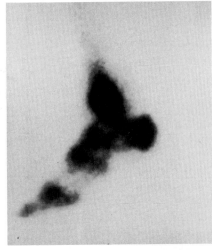

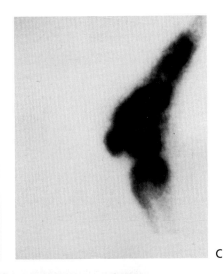

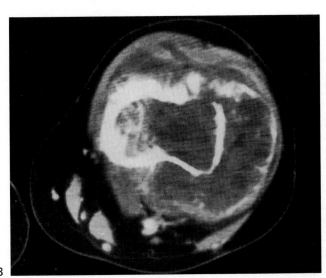

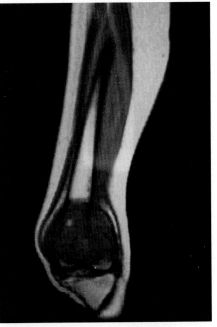

FIGURE 8.61. A 19-year-old woman with osteosarcoma of the left distal femur. **A:** Lateral view shows destruction of the distal femoral metaphysis, a large adjacent soft-tissue mass, and spiculated periosteal new bone formation anteriorly along with cortical destruction. **B:** CT scan shows a large soft-tissue mass surrounding the bone on its lateral aspect along with cortical destruction. **C:** Radionuclide bone scan. Increased activity in the distal femur is seen. There is also activity in the proximal tibia, the distal tibia, and the tarsal bones, although there is no tumor involvement at these sites. **D:** MR (SE 800/20) sagittal section. The tumor is seen in the metaphysis with considerable soft-tissue extension into the popliteal fossa. A small skip area replaces the marrow signal posteriorly, proximal to the tumor.

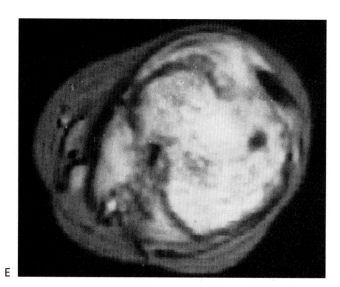

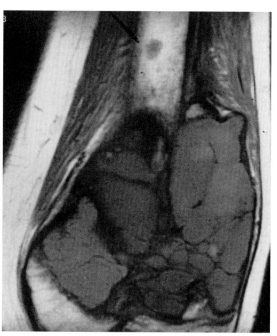

E

F

FIGURE 8.61. *(continued)* **E:** T2-weighted MR image. The large soft-tissue mass involves the popliteal artery. **F:** MR (SE 600/20) image taken after 3 months of treatment. The soft-tissue mass has a lobulated appearance, and it is marginated by a thin, low signal intensity shell. There is a small skip lesion proximal to the main tumor.

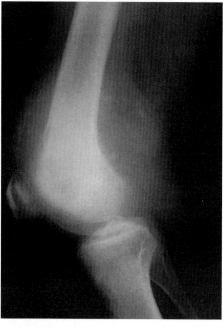

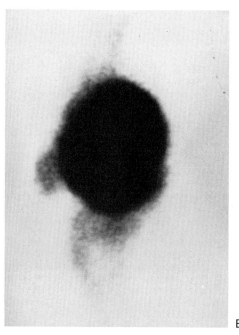

A

B

FIGURE 8.62. Osteosarcoma of the distal femur in an 18-year-old woman. **A:** Lateral view of the right femur shows sclerosis of the distal femoral metaphysis extending to the epiphysis with a large, calcified, adjacent soft-tissue mass representing an osteosarcoma. **B:** Radionuclide bone scan shows increased uptake in the distal femur and in the soft-tissue component of the tumor.

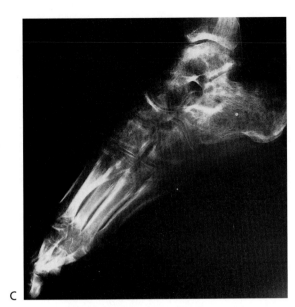

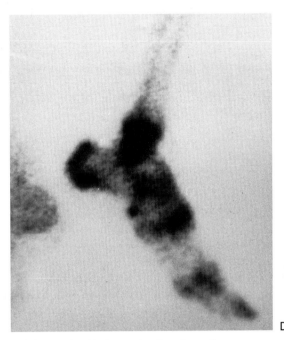

C

D

FIGURE 8.62. *(continued)* **C:** Lateral view of the right foot and ankle 2 months after chemotherapy. Marked patchy osteoporosis is seen. **D:** Radionuclide bone scan of the right foot and ankle shows multiple areas of increased activity. No tumor was evident.

mass may be very large. Areas of ossification or amorphous calcification may be present in the mass, and there may be an apparent alignment of calcific densities radiating outward from the central tumor. The amount of new bone formation in the soft tissues may exceed that in the intraosseous component.

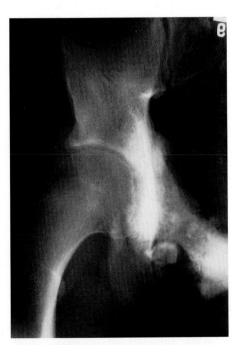

FIGURE 8.63. Osteosarcoma of the pelvis in a 19-year-old man. AP view of the left hip shows bony sclerosis adjacent to the acetabulum and the pubis with spiculated periosteal new bone formation.

Chondroblastic osteosarcoma has a predominant chondroid differentiation. This may be reflected as a cartilaginous pattern of calcification inside the medullary cavity or in the surrounding tumor mass. This pattern is composed of amorphous, stippled, linear, circular, or popcornlike calcification. It can be seen on conventional films, CT scans, or MR images and can sometimes be extensive.

CT offers several imaging advantages, particularly in assessing the central skeleton.[166,167] It can determine the extent of the soft-tissue component, but not as accurately as MRI. Intravenous contrast enhancement is useful for determining the vascularity and the relation of the soft-tissue mass to major vessels. Calcification within the tumor can be detected more readily with CT than with conventional films. It can show bony detail in the central skeleton and calcification and new bone formation in the marrow cavity and soft tissues that are not seen using MR spin echo techniques. CT can determine intramedullary extension and can best assess the response of the bony portion of the lesion to chemotherapy.[168]

MRI is most important and is more accurate than CT in defining the extent of and staging of osteosarcoma.[169] The tumor extent is sharply demarcated from normal muscle. Its relation to vessels, tendons, compartments, joints, and other structures can be assessed. Joint effusion can be seen. Marrow edema may simulate tumor involvement.

Radionuclide bone scans of osteosarcoma demonstrate increased uptake by the tumor, but osteosarcoma is usually evident on conventional x-ray films at presentation. The chief uses of radionuclide bones scans are to detect bony metastases.

Parosteal osteosarcoma arises at the surface of the bone at a single site, and then grows around the bone without destroying the periosteum. The resulting radiolucent line between the bone and tumor is called the "string sign" (Fig. 8.64). A large calcified mass may be seen in the soft tissues adjacent to bone or joint. It may dedifferentiate into a more aggressive form.

Ewing's Tumor

Ewing's tumor is a distinctive small, round cell, primary sarcoma, probably arising from undifferentiated mesenchyme.[170,171] Ewing's tumor occurs less frequently than myeloma, osteosarcoma, or chondrosarcoma. The peak age incidence is 15 years, with a usual range between 5 and 30 years. It is rare in Blacks. Males are more often affected than females. Clinically, local pain occurs, usually of several months' duration, which increases in severity. The duration of the pain is important in differentiating this tumor from osteomyelitis, which may present with similar clinical and imaging findings but with a history of pain of only a few weeks' duration. A soft-tissue mass, tender but not warm, and dilated veins are usually present. Malaise, fever as high as 105°F (40.5°C), leukocytosis, anemia, and a rapid erythrocyte sedimentation rate are seen. The tumor spreads to the surrounding soft tissues by permeating through the cortex. It produces early hematogenous metastases to the lungs and other bones.

The site of involvement varies with the age of the patient because of the different sites of red marrow conversion at various ages. The tubular bones are most often involved in younger patients, but in patients older than 20 years of age,

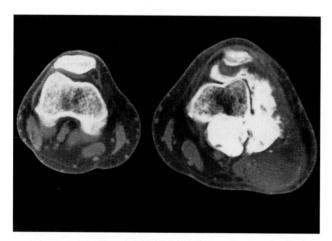

FIGURE 8.64. A 38-year-old man with parosteal sarcoma of the left distal femoral metaphysis. A densely calcified soft-tissue mass originates from the posterior cortex and extends around the anterior aspect of the bone. There is a radiolucency between the calcified mass and the cortex of the bone laterally and anteriorly. This corresponds to the periosteum and has been referred to as the "string sign." The medullary cavity is free of tumor.

the flat bones are the most common sites. These can involve the shoulder and hip (Fig. 8.65). Of the long bones, the femur followed by the tibia are affected most commonly. The most frequent site in the flat bones is the innominate bone. Tumors may develop in the hands and feet.[172–174] The os calcis may also be involved.

The classic appearance of this tumor in the long bones probably accounts for much less than one-half of cases. This pattern consists of a permeative area of bone destruction involving a large segment of the diaphysis, associated with delicate laminated periosteal new bone formation. There is a large soft-tissue component with a relatively intact cortex. There is no tumor bone, only reactive bone formation or debris.

Ewing's tumor in the flat bones has a characteristic appearance of mottled destruction and patchy reactive bone sclerosis. The cortex may be destroyed or thickened, and thin delicate laminations may be present. The os calcis has a similar appearance when involved with this tumor. This appearance resembles osteomyelitis.

An expansile lesion in the short tubular bones of the hands (Fig. 8.66) or feet with a thinned cortex but without periosteal new bone formation is a common appearance when these sites are involved.[175] Bone sclerosis may range from minimal to prominent, and it may be patchy or take the form of thickened trabeculae. Pathologic fractures occur in 5% to 10% of patients. Vertebral body collapse, sclerotic reaction, and a paraspinal or extradural soft-tissue mass may be present in the spine.[176] More than one segment may be involved, with spread to the intervertebral spaces and contiguous vertebral bodies. Expansion of the neural arch and a calcified paravertebral mass have been reported.[177] Sacral involvement has been reported as presenting with spondylolisthesis.[178] The ribs are involved in about 10% of patients.[179] They usually show a fusiform, expansile lesion without periosteal reaction, but it may be sclerotic. An extrapleural soft-tissue mass and pleural effusion are frequently observed.[180]

MRI is the method of choice for demonstrating soft-tissue, joint (Fig. 8.67), and bone marrow involvement. It can precisely define tumor extent. It can show cortical permeation by small, high signal intensity foci in the cortex on T2-weighted and PD-weighted images.

Chondrosarcoma

Chondrosarcoma is a primary malignant tumor of cartilage.[181,182] It accounts for slightly more than 10% of all malignant bone tumors. It is slow growing and may range in size from small to large. It is rare in the distal extremities. Chondrosarcomas originating within a bone are central chondrosarcomas. One originating outside of the cortex is either a peripheral or a juxtacortical chondrosarcoma. A central chondrosarcoma may be primary or secondary. Peripheral chondrosarcoma is a secondary lesion.[183]

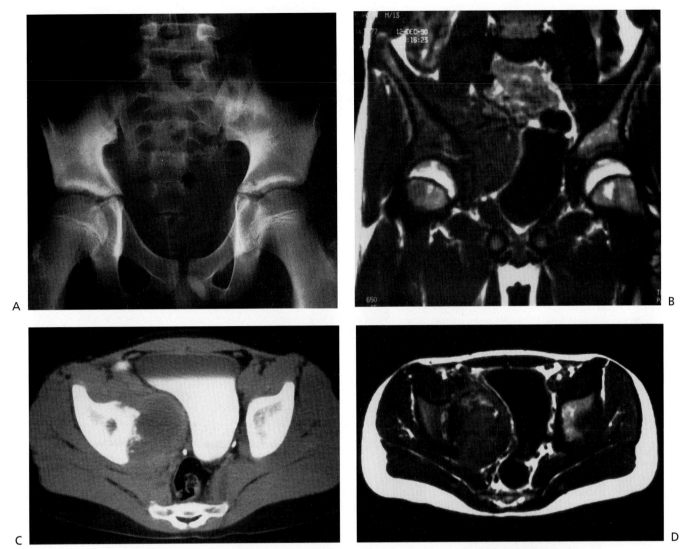

FIGURE 8.65. A 15-year-old boy with Ewing's tumor involving the right iliac bone. **A:** Anteroposterior view of the pelvis shows cortical thickening of the right iliac bone and reactive periosteal new bone formation. This film does not demonstrate involvement of the medulla of the bone. **B:** T1-weighted MR image shows a large low signal intensity tumor mass displacing the pelvic viscera, and marrow replacement of the entire iliac bone and acetabulum. **C:** CT scan shows a large intrapelvic soft-tissue mass displacing the bladder, sclerosis of the iliac bone, and reactive bone in the soft tissues. **D:** T1-weighted MR image corresponding to **(C)**. A large, mixed signal intensity soft-tissue mass displaces the bladder, and there is cortical thickening. Marrow replacement in the iliac bone is seen as low signal intensity.

Central chondrosarcoma is more common than peripheral chondrosarcoma, and primary chondrosarcomas are much more common than secondary ones. Secondary chondrosarcomas occur in a younger age group.

The age range of distribution for patients with central chondrosarcoma is that of adulthood to old age, with more than one-half of the patients older than 40. Men are slightly more affected than women. The most frequent complaint is dull pain, with an average duration of several years. Local swelling without inflammatory signs and involvement of a contiguous joint may also be present. The tumor is slow growing and usually metastasizes late, hematogenously.

Cartilage is recognized on conventional x-ray films and CT scans by amorphous, punctate, small, linear, circular, flocculent, dense, or irregular calcifications, which range from sparse to heavy. This finding is seen in approximately two-thirds of central chondrosarcomas. A large segment of the shaft of a long bone may be affected.

The tumor may present as an osteolytic, well-marginated, expansile lesion with cortical thickening or

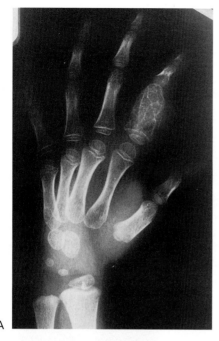

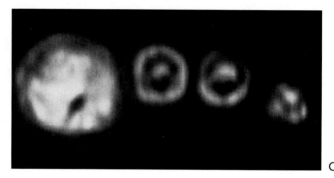

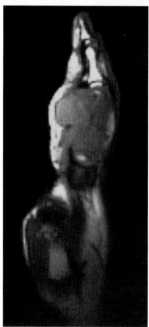

FIGURE 8.66. A 3-year-old girl with Ewing's tumor involving the proximal phalanx of the index finger. **A:** Anteroposterior view of the hand shows an expansile trabeculated proximal phalanx with an intact cortex. **B:** T1-weighted MR sagittal image. The soft-tissue component is seen at the palmar aspect. **C:** T2-weighted axial image shows a high signal intensity tumor involving the soft tissue surrounding the bone.

thinning (Fig. 8.68). It may not be possible to differentiate this appearance from an enchondroma, but a large size or a location in the proximal skeleton should raise the suspicion of malignancy (Fig. 8.69). Deep endosteal scalloping is a sign of malignancy. There may be simple periosteal elevation or, rarely, fine spiculation or lamination. A large, bulky, soft-tissue tumor mass containing calcifications associated with bone destruction is characteristic of advanced chondrosarcoma. Cortical thickening along the medial femoral neck and intertrochanteric area, remote from where the tumor is, may sometimes be seen with a

proximal femoral tumor. Rarely, it may present as a sclerotic lesion.

It may occur in the spine as a purely destructive process of the body with involvement of the lamina or other portions of the neural arch.[184] A case of primary chondrosarcoma of the proximal tibia with transarticular spread to the distal femur has been reported.[185]

Peripheral chondrosarcoma refers to tumors resulting from the malignant change of multiple or solitary osteochondromas.[186] The average age of patients with peripheral chondrosarcoma is lower than that of patients having the

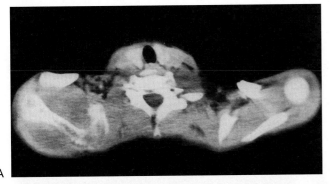

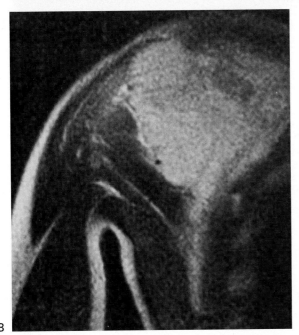

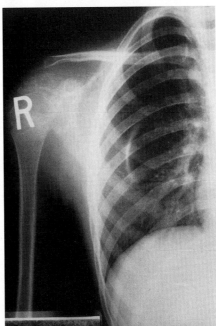

FIGURE 8.67. An 8-year-old boy with Ewing's tumor involving the right scapula. **A:** CT scan shows a large, low density tumor mass surrounding the scapula, which is expanded with a thin cortex. **B:** MR image (SE 2000/80) shows a high signal intensity soft-tissue component of the tumor about the scapula. **C:** Anteroposterior view of the right shoulder shows bony destruction and a soft-tissue mass.

central type. The most frequent areas of involvement are the pelvic and shoulder girdles, upper femur, and humerus.

Non-Hodgkin's Lymphoma of Bone

Primary non-Hodgkin's lymphoma (NHL) of bone is a rare, round cell malignant tumor.[187–189] This is considered by many investigators to be a separate entity distinct from generalized lymphoma involving bone. It previously was called reticulum cell sarcoma, a name that is still used by some. The criteria for primary NHL include initial involvement of a single bone and at least 6 months' duration before the appearance of distant metastases without generalized NHL. Pain and swelling of long duration at the tumor site are usually present, whereas systemic symptoms are usually absent.

Pathologic fractures occur. The usual age range of patients is between 25 and 40 years. The ratio of male to female involvement is 2 to 1. About one-half of the lesions occur in the lower extremities, especially the femora, with the remainder in the humeri, scapulae, vertebrae, pelvis, and other bones. In the long bones, the shaft or the metaphysis may be involved.

The principal imaging finding is permeative bone destruction in separate areas that coalesce to a moth-eaten appearance. The cortex is broken through, and pathologic fracture frequently occurs. Periosteal reaction of a simple or laminated type and cortical expansion may be seen rarely. Cortical thickening and reactive bone sclerosis may be present, as well as a geographic destructive area. Sequestration, single or multiple, has been reported in 11% of cases in one

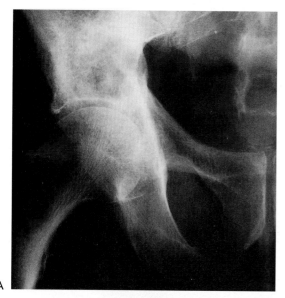

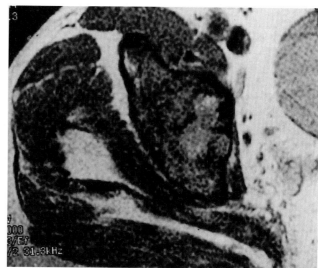

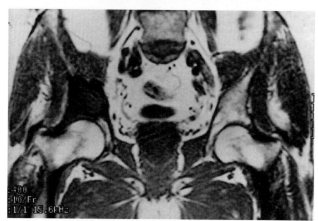

FIGURE 8.68. Chondrosarcoma in the right supra-acetabular region abutting the articular surface. **A:** AP view of the right hip shows an expansile lesion superior to the acetabulum containing several calcifications. **B:** MRI T1-weighted image. The lesion is seen as low signal intensity containing several signal void strands reflecting calcification. **C:** MRI T2-weighted image showing a heterogeneous signal with lobular high signal intensity foci.

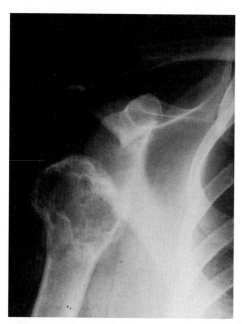

FIGURE 8.69. Chondrosarcoma of the humeral head. AP view of the shoulder shows an expansile trabeculated appearance of the humeral head.

series of 246 primary bone lymphomas.[155] A localized osteolytic lesion in the epiphysis with surrounding sclerosis has been reported.[156] An associated soft-tissue mass may be present. CT or MRI can demonstrate the extent of the mass. Synovitis and effusion may occur with a tumor near a joint. Generalized NHL may also involve joints (Fig. 8.70).

Multiple Myeloma

Multiple myeloma is a primary malignant tumor of bone marrow, characterized by malignant proliferation of a single clone of plasma cells.[190] It is the most common primary malignant neoplasm involving bone. The annual incidence is 3 per 100,000 members of the population. The tumors tend to remain confined to bone. The disease is most often generalized but may be localized to a single osseous focus, called a solitary myeloma or solitary plasmacytoma. About three-fourths of patients are between the ages of 50 and 70 years at the time of diagnosis. The male-to-female ratio is 2 to 1. The symptoms initially are vague complaints, fever, and symptoms resulting from the accompanying anemia. Bone

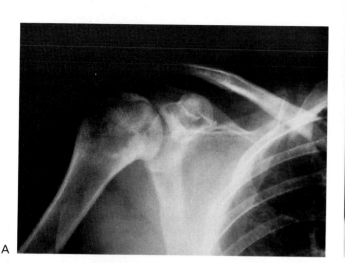
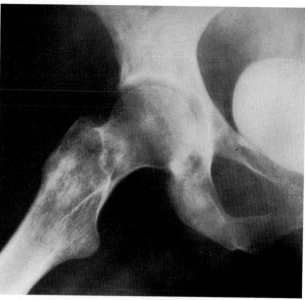

FIGURE 8.70. A 48-year-old woman with intermediate grade, large cell non-Hodgkin's lymphoma. **A:** Anteroposterior view of the right shoulder shows patchy osteosclerosis of the proximal humerus and around the glenoid fossa. **B:** Lateral view of the left hip shows patchy osteosclerosis around the proximal femur, the ischium, and the iliac bone.

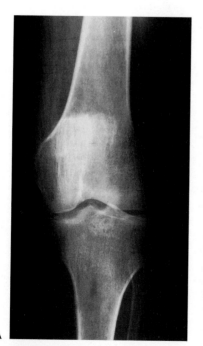
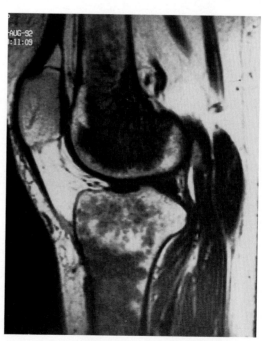

FIGURE 8.71. A 73-year-old woman with multiple myeloma. **A:** Anteroposterior view of the left knee shows diffuse osteopenia and a radiolucency in the midproximal tibia. **B:** MR (SE 400/15) sagittal section of the knee. Marrow replacement in the distal femur and in the proximal tibial metaphysis by tumor is seen. A patchy appearance of fatty marrow in the proximal tibial epiphysis is also seen.

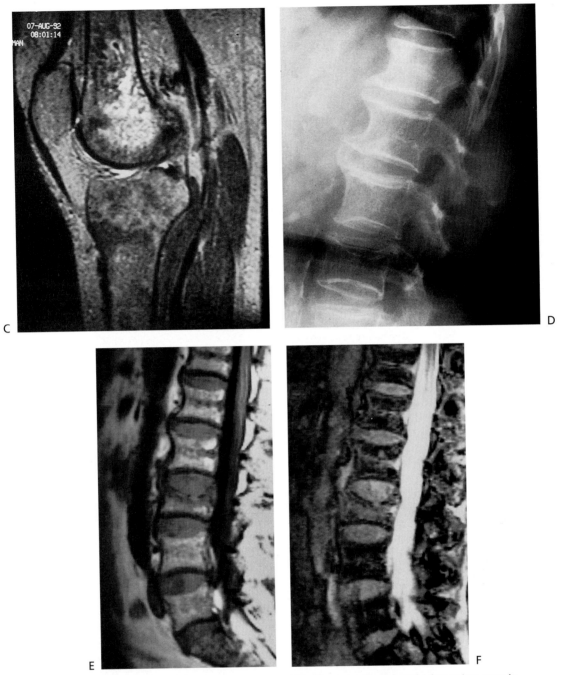

FIGURE 8.71. *(continued)* **C:** MR image (SE 2700/80). The tumor in the distal femur increases in signal intensity, but the tumor in the proximal tibia does not. **D:** Lateral view of the lumbar spine shows a partial collapse of the third lumbar vertebral body and osteopenia in all of the vertebral bodies. **E:** MR image (SE 650/15). Collapse of the third lumbar vertebra is seen with a spotty marrow pattern in all of the vertebral bodies. **F:** T2-weighted MR image. Partial collapse of the third lumbar vertebral body has occurred with a slightly higher signal intensity than the remainder of the vertebral bodies. There has been no general increase in signal intensity in the vertebral bodies.

pain is progressive in severity and usually occurs in the lower back. This can be complicated by pathologic compression fracture of the vertebral bodies, resulting in severe pain and paraplegia. Amyloid deposits are common.

Multiple myeloma characteristically is associated with a monoclonal increase of immunoglobulins, arising from a single clone of antibody-forming cells. The monoclonal proteins are designated as M components. They are normal immunoglobulins present in abnormal quantities. Nonsecretory myeloma does not show an M protein peak.

Radiologically, the findings of myeloma vary. The hallmark of this disease is the sharply circumscribed, punched-out lesion. These lesions are multiple, round, sharply marginated, and purely osteolytic, without a sclerotic rim. They may involve the endosteal surface of the cortex, causing scalloping or involve both surfaces. They vary in size and may coalesce, destroying large segments of bone. The bones most commonly involved are the skull and long bones. The distal clavicle and the acromion are frequently involved, as are the ribs, glenoid, and pelvis. Pathologic fractures are common. The terminal phalanges rarely may be involved. A joint may also be involved (Fig. 8.71), including the sacroiliac joint (Fig. 8.72). Expansion of bone is a common feature. Periosteal reaction is sparse.

Radionuclide bone scanning in myeloma is unreliable, because many lesions do not provoke enough bone repair to cause uptake. Soft-tissue invasion commonly occurs and can often be seen as a paraspinal or extrapleural mass.

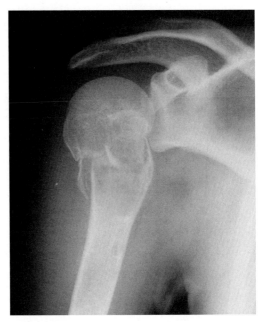

FIGURE 8.73. Unicameral bone cyst. AP view of the shoulder. A bone cyst in the proximal humerus is seen with a pathological fracture in the metaphysis involving the neck of the humerus.

Bone Cyst

A unicameral bone cyst is typically in the metaphysis. It can cause joint problems, particularly if there is a pathologic fracture (Fig. 8.73). Very rarely, the cyst may penetrate into the epiphysis (Fig. 8.74).

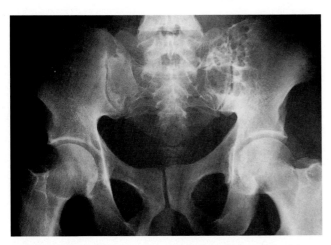

FIGURE 8.72. Multiple myeloma. AP view of the pelvis. A large multilocular expansile lesion in the left sacroiliac region is noted.

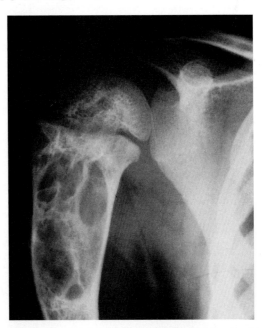

FIGURE 8.74. Unicameral bone cyst. AP view of the shoulder reveals a bone cyst in the metaphysis that has penetrated into the epiphysis. This is an extremely rare finding.

REFERENCES

PVS and Pigmented Villonodular Tenosynovitis

1. Davis S, Lawton G, Lowy M. Pigmented villonodular synovitis: bone involvement of the fingers. *Clin Radiol* 1975;26: 357–361.
2. Flandry F, Hughston JC, et al. Current concepts review: pigmented villonodular synovitis. *J Bone Joint Surg* 1987; 69:942–949.
3. Jergesen HE, Mankin JH, Schiller AL. Diffuse pigmented villonodular synovitis of the knee mimicking primary bone neoplasm: a report of 2 cases. *J Bone Joint Surg [Am]* 1978;60: 825–829.
4. Kindblom LG, Gunterberg G. Pigmented villonodular synovitis involving bone: a case report. *J Bone Joint Surg [Am]* 1978; 60:830–832.
5. Lin J, Jacobson JA, Jamadar DA, et al. Pigmented villonodular synovitis and related lesions: the spectrum of imaging findings. *AJR* 1999;172:191–197.
6. Goldman AB, DiCarlo EF. Pigmented villonodular synovitis diagnosis and differential diagnosis. *Radiol Clin North Am* 1988; 26:1327–1347.
7. Spanier S. Case 46. Presented at the meeting of the International Society, Stockholm, 1992.
8. Campbell AJ, Wells IP. Pigmented villonodular synovitis of a lumbar vertebral facet joint. *J Bone Joint Surg [Am]* 1982; 64: 145–146.
9. Lowenstein MB, Smith JRV, Cole S. Infrapatellar pigmented villonodular synovitis: arthrograph detection. *AJR* 1980; 135:279–282.
10. Crosby EB, Inglis A, Bullough PG. Multiple joint involvement with pigmented villonodular synovitis. *Radiology* 1977; 122:671–672.
11. Eisenberg RL, Hedgecock MU. Bilateral pigmented villonodular synovitis of the hip. *Br J Radiol* 1978;51:916.
12. Lapayouker MS, Miller WT, Levy WM, et al. Pigmented villonodular synovitis of the temporomandibular joint. *Radiology* 1973;108:313–316.
13. Wagner ML, Spjut HJ, Dutton RV, et al. Polyarticular pigmented villonodular synovitis. AJR 1981;136:821–823.
14. Gagneri F, Taillan B, et al. Three cases of pigmented villonodular synovitis of the knee. *Fortschritte Gebeit Röntgenstrahlen* 1986;145:227–228.
15. Kottal RA, Vogler JB, et al. Pigmented villonodular synovitis: a report of MR imaging in two cases. *Radiology* 1987; 163:551–553.
16. Spritzer CE, Dalinka MK, et al. Magnetic resonance imaging of pigmented villonodular synovitis: a report of two cases. *Skeletal Radiol* 1987;16:316–319.
17. Goldman AB, DiCarlo EF. Pigmented villonodular synovitis diagnosis and differential diagnosis. *Radiol Clin North Am* 1988; 26:1327–1347.

Synovial Osteochondromatosis

18. Milgram JW. Synovial osteochondromatosis: a histopathological study of 30 cases. *J Bone Joint Surg [Am]* 1977; 59:792–801.
19. Prager RJ, Mall JC. Arthrographic diagnosis of synovial chondromatosis. *AJR* 1976;127:344–346.
20. Jaffe HL. *Tumors and tumorous conditions of the bones and joints.* Philadelphia: Lea & Febiger, 1958.
21. Carey RPL. Synovial chondromatosis of the knee in childhood. *J Bone Joint Surg [Br]* 1983;65:444–447.
22. Pelker RR, Drennan JC, Ozonoff MB. Juvenile synovial chondromatosis of the hip. *J Bone Joint Surg [Am]* 1983;65: 552–554.

23. Pope TL Jr, Keats TE, et al. Idiopathic synovial chondromatosis in two unusual sites: inferior radioulnar joint and ischial bursa. *Skeletal Radiol* 1987;16:205–208.
24. Lynn MD, Lee J. Periarticular tenosynovial chondrometaplasia: report of a case at the wrist. *J Bone Joint Surg [Am]* 1972;54: 650–652.
25. Bauer M, Johsson K. Synovial chondromatosis of the ankle. *Fortschritte Gebeit Röntgenstrahlen* 1987;146:548–550.
26. Holm CL. Primary synovial chondromatosis of the ankle. *J Bone Joint Surg [Am]* 1970;58:878–880.
27. Dunn WA, Whisler JH. Synovial chondromatosis of the knee with associated extracapsular chondromas. *J Bone Joint Surg [Am]* 1973;55:1747–1748.
28. Akhtar M, et al. Synovial chondromatosis of the temporomandibular joint: report of a case. *J Bone Joint Surg [Am]* 1977; 59:266–267.
29. Silver CM, Simon SD, Litchman HM, et al. Synovial chondromatosis of the temporomandibular joint: a case report. *J Bone Joint Surg [Am]* 1971;53:777–780.
30. Nokes ST, King PS, et al. Temporomandibular joint chondromatosis with intracranial extension: MR and CT contributions. *AJR* 1987;148:1173–1174.
31. Norman A, Steiner GC. Bone erosion in synovial chondromatosis. *Radiology* 1986;161:749–752.
32. Hermann G, Abdelwahab IF, Klein M, et al. Synovial chondromatosis. *Skeletal Radiol* 1995;24:298–300.
33. Szypryt P, Twining P, et al. Synovial chondromatosis of the hip joint presenting as a pathological fracture. *Br J Radiol* 1986; 59: 399–401.
34. Eisenberg KS, Johnston JO. Synovial chondromatosis of the hip joint presenting as an intrapelvic mass: a case report. *J Bone Joint Surg [Am]* 1972;54:176–178.
35. Claudon M, Aymard B, et al. Scanographie et chondrometaplasie synoviale. *J Radiol* 1986;67:871–880.
36. Hamilton A, Davis RI, et al. Chondrosarcoma developing in synovial chondromatosis. *J Bone Joint Surg* 1987;69:137–140.
37. Kaiser TE, Ivins JC, Unni KK. Malignant transformation of extra-articular synovial chondromatosis. *Skeletal Radiol* 1980; 5:223–226.

AVN

38. Mitchell DG, Rao VM, et al. Femoral head avascular necrosis: correlation of MR imaging, radiographic staging, radionuclide imaging, and clinical findings. *Radiology* 1987;162:709–715.

Trevor's Disease

39. Connor JM, Horan FT, Beighton P. Dysplasia epiphysealis hemimelica. *J Bone Joint Surg [Br]* 1983;65:350–354.

Capsular Constriction of the Hip

40. Lequesne M, Becker J, Bard M, et al. Capsular constriction of the hip: arthrographic and clinical considerations. *Skeletal Radiol* 1981;6:1–10.
41. Griffiths HJ, Utz R, et al. Adhesive capsulitis of the hip and ankle. *AJR* 1988;144:101–105.
42. Maloney MD, Sauser DD, et al. Adhesive capsulitis of the wrist: arthrographic diagnosis. *Radiology* 1988;167:187–190.

Myositis Ossificans Circumscripta

43. Kegal VW. Kausistischer beitrag zum krankheitsbild der myositis ossificans localisata. *Fortschritte Gebeit Röntgenstrahlen* 1981; 135:613–614.

44. Paterson DC. Myositis ossificans circumscripta. *J Bone Joint Surg [Br]* 1970;52:296–301.
45. Chung BS. Drug-induced myositis ossificans circumscripta. *JAMA* 1973;226:469.
46. Vas W, Cockshott WP, Martin RF, et al. Myositis ossificans in hemophilia. *Skeletal Radiol* 1981;7:2–31.
47. Yaghmai I. Myositis ossificans: diagnostic value of arteriography. *AJR* 1977;128:811–816.
48. Amendola MA, Glazer GM, Agha FP, et al. Myositis ossificans circumscripta: computed tomographic diagnosis. *Radiology* 1983;149:775–779.
49. Kramer KL, Kurtz AB, Rubin C, et al. Ultrasound appearance of myositis ossificans. *Skeletal Radiol* 1979;4:1–20.
50. Drane WE. Myositis ossificans and the three phase bone scan. *AJR* 1984;142:179–180a.
51. Kransdorf MJ, Meis JM, Jelinek JS. Myositis ossificans: MR appearance with radiology-pathologic correlation. *AJR* 1991;157:1243–1248.
52. De Smet AA, Norris MA, Fisher DR. Magnetic resonance imaging of myositis ossificans: analysis of seven cases. *Skeletal Radiol* 1992;21:503–507.
53. Voss H. Uber die parostalen und para-artikularen knochen-neubildugen bie organischen nervenkrankheiten. *Fortschritte Gebeit Röntgenstrahlen* 1937;55:423–441.

Tumors Involving Joints

Synovial Sarcoma
54. Genest P, Kim TH, Katsarkas A, et al. Calcified synovial sarcoma of the oropharynx. *Br J Radiol* 1983;56:580–582.
55. Enzinger FM, Weiss SW. *Soft-tissue tumors,* 2nd ed. St. Louis: CV Mosby, 1988.
56. Azouz EM, Vicker DB, Brown KLB. Computed tomography of synovial sarcoma of the foot. *J Can Assoc Radiol* 1984;35:85–87.
57. Morton MJ, Berquist TH, McLeon RA, et al. MR imaging of synovial sarcoma. *AJR* 1991; 56:337–340.

Chordoma
58. Firooznia H, et al. Chordoma: radiologic evaluation of 20 cases. *AJR* 1976;127:797–805.
59. Yuh WTC, Flickinger FW, et al. MR imaging of unusual chordomas. *J Comput Assist Tomogr* 1988;12:30–35.
60. Stratt B, Steiner RM. The radiologic findings in posterior mediastinal chordoma. *Skeletal Radiol* 1980;5:171–173.
61. deBruine FT, Kroon HM. Spinal chordoma: radiologic features in 14 cases. *AJR* 1988;150:861–863.
62. Wang AM, Joachim CL, Shillito J, et al. Cervical chordoma presenting with intervertebral foramen enlargement mimicking neurofibroma: CT findings. *J Comput Assist Tomogr* 1984;8:529–535.
63. Smith J, Ludwig RL, et al. Sacrococcygeal chordoma. *Skeletal Radiol* 1987;16:37–44.
64. Rosenthal DI, Scott JA, et al. Sacrococcygeal chordoma: magnetic resonance imaging and computed tomography. *AJR* 1985;145:143–147.
65. Sze G, Uichanco LE III, et al. Chordomas: MR imaging. *Radiology* 1988;166:187–191.

Bone Tumors That May Affect Joints

Aneurysmal Bone Cyst
66. Bonakdarpour A, Levy WM, Aegerter E. Primary and secondary aneurysmal bone cyst: a radiological study of 75 cases. *Radiology* 1978;126:75–83.
67. Slowick FA, Campbell CJ, Kettlekamp DB. Aneurysmal bone cyst: an analysis of 13 cases. *J Bone Joint Surg [Am]* 1968;50:1142–1151.
68. Diercks RL, Sauter AJM, et al. Aneurysmal bone cyst in association with fibrous dysplasia: a case report. *J Bone Joint Surg [Br]* 1986;68:144–146.
69. Dabezies EJ, D'Ambrosia RD, Chuinard RG, et al. Aneurysmal bone cyst after fracture. *J Bone Joint Surg [Am]* 1982;64:617.
70. Buirski G, Watt I. The radiological features of "solid" aneurysmal bone cysts. *Br J Radiol* 1984;57:1057–1065.
71. Chateil JR, Coindre JM, et al. Localisation rachidienne d'un kyste aneurysmal solide: Aspects cliniques, radiographiques et histopathologiques. *J Radiol* 1987;68:805–808.
72. Hay MC, Paterson D, Taylor TKF. Aneurysmal bone cysts of the spine. *J Bone Joint Surg [Br]* 1978;60:406.
73. Burns-Cox CJ, Higgins AT. Aneurysmal bone cyst of the frontal bone. *J Bone Joint Surg [Br]* 1969;51:344–345.
74. O'Gorman, Kirkham TH. Aneurysmal bone cyst of the orbit with unusual angiographic features. *AJR* 1976;126:896–899.
75. Huettig G, Rittmeyer K. Multiple aneurysmatische knochenzysten bei 3 monate altem saeugling. *Fortschritte Gebeit Röntgenstrahlen* 1978;129:796.
76. Dyer R, Stelling CB, Fechner RE. Epiphyseal extension of an aneurysmal bone cyst. *AJR* 1981;173:172–173.
77. Henley FT, Richetts GL. Aneurysmal bone cyst presenting as a chest mass: a case report. *Radiology* 1969;92:1103–1104.
78. Capanna R, Van Horn JR, Biagini R, et al. Aneurysmal bone cyst of the sacrum. *Skeletal Radiol* 1989;18:109–113.
79. Hertzanu Y, Mendelsohn DB, Gottschalk F. Aneurysmal bone cyst of the calcaneus. *Radiology* 1984;151:51–52.
80. Hudson TM. Fluid levels in aneurysmal bone cysts. *AJR* 1984;142:1001–1004.
81. Hudson TM. Scintigraphy of aneurysmal bone cysts. *AJR* 1984;142:761–765.
82. Yaghmai I. *Angiography of bone and soft-tissue lesions.* New York: Springer-Verlag, 1979.
83. Beltran J, Simon DC, et al. Aneurysmal bone cysts: MR imaging at 1.5T. *Radiology* 1986;158:689–690.

Chondroblastoma
85. Nolan DJ, Middlemiss H. Chondroblastoma of bone. *Clin Radiol* 1975;26:343–350.
86. Plum GE, Pugh DG. Roentgenologic aspects of benign chondroblastoma of bone. *AJR* 1958;79:584–591.
87. Schajowicz F, Gallardo H. Epiphyseal chondroblastoma of bone. *J Bone Joint Surg [Br]* 1970;52:205–226.
88. Sundaram TKS. Benign chondroblastoma. *J Bone Joint Surg [Br]* 1966;48:92–104.
89. Hudson TM, Hawkings IF. Radiological evaluation of chondroblastoma. *Radiology* 1981;139:1–10.
90. Fechner RE, Wilde HD. Chondroblastoma in the metaphysis of the femoral neck. *J Bone Joint Surg [Am]* 1974;56:413–415.
91. Kricun ME, Kricun R, Haskin ME. Chondroblastoma of the calcaneus: radiographic features with emphasis on location. *AJR* 1977;128:613–616.
92. Cohen J, Cohen I. Benign chondroblastoma of the patella: a case report. *J Bone Joint Surg [Am]* 1963;45:824–826.
93. Moser RP Jr, Brockmole DM, et al. Chondroblastoma of the patella. *Skeletal Radiol* 1988;17:413–419.
94. Neviaser RJ, Wilson JRN. Benign chondroblastoma of the finger. *J Bone Joint surg [Am]* 1972;54:389–392.
95. Matsuno T, Hasegawa I, et al. Chondroblastoma arising in the triradiate cartilage. *Skeletal Radiol* 1987;16:216–222.
96. Braunstein E, Martel W, Weatherbee L. Periosteal bone apposition in chondroblastoma. *Skeletal Radiol* 1979;4:34–36.

97. Brower AC, Moser RP, Kransdorf MJ. The frequency and diagnostic significance of periostitis in chondroblastoma. *AJR* 1990; 154:309–314.

98. Hayes CW, Conway WF, Sundaram M. Misleading aggressive MR imaging appearance of some benign musculoskeletal lesions. *Radiographics* 1992;12:111–134.

99. Gohel VK, Dalinka MK, Edeiken J. Ischemic necrosis of the femoral head simulating chondroblastoma. *Radiology* 1973; 107:545–546.

100. Bloem JL, Mulder JD. Chondroblastoma: a clinical and radiological study of 104 cases. *Skeletal Radiol* 1985;14:1–9.

101. McLaughlin RE, Sweet DE, Webster T, et al. Chondroblastoma of the pelvis suggestive of malignancy: report of an unusual case treated by wide pelvic excision. *J Bone Joint Surg [Am]* 1975;57: 549–550.

102. Dahlin DC, Unni KK. *Bone tumors*, 4th ed. Springfield, IL: Charles C Thomas, 1986.

Osteoid Osteoma

103. Lechner G, Knahr K, Riedl P. Das osteoid-osteom (osteoid osteoma). *Fortschr Geb Rontgenstr* 1978;128:511–520.

104. Swee RG, McLeod RA, Beabout JW. Osteoid osteoma. *Radiology* 1979;130:117–123.

105. Bilchik T, Heyman S, Siegel A, et al. Osteoid osteoma: the role of radionuclide bone imaging, conventional radiography and computed tomography in its management. *J Nucl Med* 1992; 33:269–271.

106. Pettine KA, Klassen RA. Osteoid-osteoma and osteoblastoma of the spine. *J Bone Joint Surg [Am]* 1986;68:354–361.

107. Kehl DK, Alonson JE, Lovell WW. Scoliosis secondary to an osteoid-osteoma of the rib. *J Bone Joint Surg [Am]* 1983;65: 701–703.

108. Scott M, Lignelli GJ, Shea FJ. Cervical radicular pain secondary to osteoid osteoma of spine. *JAMA* 1971;217:964–965.

109. Lawrie TR, Aterman K, Path FC, et al. Painless osteoid osteoma: a report of 2 cases. *J Bone Joint Surg [Am]* 1970;52:1357–1363.

110. Herndon JH, Eaton RG, Littler JW. Carpal-tunnel syndrome: an unusual presentation of osteoid-osteoma of the capitate. *J Bone Joint Surg [Am]* 1974;56:1715–1718.

111. Moser RP, Kransdorf MJ, Brower AC, et al. Osteoid osteoma of the elbow. *Skeletal Radiol* 1990;19:181–186.

112. Greenfield GB. *Radiology of bone diseases*, 5th ed. Philadelphia: JB Lippincott, 1990.

113. Brabants K, Greens S, et al. Subperiosteal juxta-articular osteoid osteoma. *J Bone Joint Surg* 1986;68:320–324.

114. Kattapuram SV, Kushner DC, Phillips WC, et al. Osteoid osteoma: an unusual cause of articular pain. *Radiology* 1983;147: 383–387.

115. Norman A, Abdelwhab IF, et al. Osteoid osteoma of the hip stimulating an early onset of osteoarthritis. *Radiology* 1986; 158:417–420.

116. Habermann ET, Stern RE. Osteoid osteoma of the tibia in an 8-month-old boy: a case report. *J Bone Joint Surg [Am]* 1974; 56: 633–636.

117. Shereff MJ, Cullivan WT, Johnson KA. Osteoid osteoma of the foot. *J Bone Joint Surg [Am]* 1983;65:638–641.

118. Daly JG. Case report: osteoid osteoma of the skull. *Br J Radiol* 1973;46:392–393.

119. Prabhakar B, Reddy DR, Dayananda B, et al. Osteoid osteoma of the skull. *J Bone Joint Surg [Br]* 1972;54:146–148.

120. Alcalay M, Clarac JP, Bontoux D. Double osteoid-osteoma in adjacent carpal bones. *J Bone Joint Surg [Am]* 1982;64: 779–780.

121. Glynn JL, Lichtestine L. Osteoid osteoma with multicentric nidus. *J Bone Joint Surg [Am]* 1973;55:855–858.

122. Rand JA, Sim FH, Unni KK. Two osteoid-osteomas in one patient. *J Bone Joint Surg [Am]* 1982;64:1243–1245.

123. O'Dell CW, et al. Osteoid osteomas arising in adjacent bones: report of a case. *J Can Assoc Radiol* 1976;27:298–300.

124. Sherman FS. Osteoid osteoma associated with changes in the adjacent joint: report of 2 cases. *J Bone Joint Surg* 1947;29: 483–490.

125. Sharr JW, Abell MR, Martel W. Lymphofollicular synovitis with osteoid osteoma. *Radiology* 1973;106:557–560.

126. Cronemeyer RL, Kirchmer NA, DeSmet AA, et al. Intra-articular osteoid-osteoma of the humerus simulating synovitis of the elbow. *J Bone Joint Surg [Am]* 1981;63:1172–1174.

127. Gamba JL, Martinez S, Apple J, et al. Computed tomography of axial skeletal osteoid osteomas. *AJR* 1984;142:769–772.

128. Schlesinger AE, Hernandez RJ. Intracapsular osteoid osteoma of the proximal femur: Findings on plain film and CT. *AJR* 1990154:1241–1244.

129. Bassett LWH, Webber MM. Radionuclide bone imaging. *Radiol Clin North Am* 1981;19:675–702.

130. Helms CA, Hattner RS, Vogler JB. Osteoid osteoma: radionuclide diagnosis. *Radiology* 1984;151:779–784.

131. Ghelman B, Vigorita VJ. Postoperative radionuclide evaluation of osteoid osteomas. *Radiology* 1983;146:509–512.

132. Goldman AB, Schneider R, Pavlov H. Osteoid osteomas of the femoral neck: report of four cases evaluated with isotopic bone scanning, CT, and MR imaging. *Radiology* 1993;186:227–232.

133. Woods ER, Martel W, Mandel SH, et al. Reactive soft-tissue mass associated with osteoid osteoma: correlation of MR imaging features with pathologic findings. *Radiology* 1993;186: 221–225.

134. Biebuyck JC, Katz LD, McCauley T. Soft-tissue edema in osteoid osteoma. *Skeletal Radiol* 1993;22:37–41.

135. Bettelli G, Tigani D, Picci P. Recurring osteoblastoma initially presenting as a typical osteoid osteoma. Report of two cases. *Skeletal Radiol* 1991;20:1–4.

Giant Cell Tumor

136. Jaffe HL. *Tumors and tumorous conditions of the bones and joints*. Philadelphia: Lea & Febiger, 1958.

137. Campanacci M, Baldini N, et al. Giant-cell tumor of bone. *J Bone Joint Surg* 1987;69:106–114.

138. Dahlin DC. Giant cell tumor of bone: highlights of 407 cases. *AJR* 1985;144:955–960.

139. Jacobs P. The diagnosis of osteoclastoma (giant-cell tumour): a radiological and pathological correlation. *Br J Radiol* 1972; 45:121–136.

140. McInerney DP, Middlemiss JH. Giant-cell tumor of bone. *Skeletal Radiol* 1978;2:195–204.

141. Mnaymneh WA, Dudley HR, Mnaymneh LG. Giant-cell tumor of bone: an analysis and follow-up study of the 41 cases observed at the Massachusetts General Hospital between 1925 and 1960. *J Bone Joint Surg [Am]* 1964;46:63–75.

142. Murray JA, Schlafly B. Giant-cell tumors in the distal end of the radius. *J Bone Joint Surg* 1986;68:687–694.

143. Wilkerson JA, Cracchiolo A. Giant-cell tumor of the tibial diaphysis. *J Bone Joint Surg [Am]* 1969;51:1205–1209.

144. Tubbs WS, Brown LR, et al. Benign giant-cell tumor of bone with pulmonary metastases: clinical findings and radiologic appearance of metastases in 13 cases. *AJR* 1992;158:331–334.

145. Gould ES, Cooper JM, et al. Case report 740. *Skeletal Radiol* 1992;21:335–338.

146. Hanna RM, Kyriakos M, Quinn SF. Case report 757. *Skeletal Radiol* 1992;21:482–488.

147. Mechlin MB, Krikun ME, Stead J, et al. Giant cell tumor of tarsal bones. *Skeletal Radiol* 1984;11:266–270.

148. Shankman S, Greenspan A, et al. Giant cell tumor of the is-chium: a report of two cases and review of the literature. *Skeletal Radiol* 1988;17:46–51.
149. Peison B, Feigenbaum J. Metaphyseal giant-cell tumor in a girl of 14 years. *Radiology* 1976;118:145–146.
150. Sherman M, Fabricus R. Giant-cell tumor in the metaphysis of a child: report of an unusual case. *J Bone Joint Surg [Am]* 1961;43:1225–1229.
151. Kransdorf MJ, Sweet DE, et al. Giant cell tumor in skeletally immature patients. *Radiology* 1992;184:233–237.
152. Schutte HE, Taconis WK. Giant cell tumor in children and adolescents. *Skeletal Radiol* 1993;22:173–176.
153. Yao L, Mirra JM, et al. Case report 715. *Skeletal Radiol* 1992;21:124–127.
154. Shaw JA, Mosher JF. A giant-cell tumor in the hand presenting as an expansile diaphyseal lesion. *J Bone Joint Surg [Am]* 1983;65:692–695.
155. deSantos LA, Murray JA. Evaluation of giant-cell tumor by computerized tomography. *Skeletal Radiol* 1978;2:205–212.
156. Brady TJ, Gebhardt MC, Pykett IL, et al. NMR imaging of forearms in healthy volunteers and patients with giant-cell tumor of bone. *Radiology* 1982;144:549–552.
157. Herman SD, Mesgarzadeh M, et al. The role of magnetic resonance imaging in giant cell tumor of bone. *Skeletal Radiol* 1987;16:635–643.
158. Hudson TM, Shiebler M, Springfield I, et al. Radiology of giant cell tumors of bone: computed tomography, arthrotomography, and scintigraphy. *Skeletal Radiol* 1984;11:85–95.
159. Levin E, DeSmet AA, Neff JR, et al. Scintigraphic evaluation of giant cell tumor of bone. *AJR* 1984;143:343–348.

Osteosarcoma
160. Unni KK, Dahlin DC. Osteosarcoma: pathology and classification. *Semin Roentgenol* 1989;24:143–152.
161. Edeiken-Monroe B, Edeiken J, Jacobson HG. Osteosarcoma. *Semin Roentgenol* 1989;24:153–173.
162. deSantos LA, et al. Osteogenic sarcoma after the age of 50: a radiographic evaluation. *AJR* 1978;131:481–484.
163. Lee ES. Osteosarcoma: a reconnaissance. *Clin Radiol* 1975;26:5–25.
164. Miller CW, McLaughlin RE. Osteosarcoma in siblings: report of 2 cases. *J Bone Joint Surg [Am]* 1977;59:261–262.
165. Miller TT, Abdelwahab IF, et al. Case report 735. *Skeletal Radiol* 1992;21:277–279.
166. Coffre C, Vanel D, et al. Problems and pitfalls in the use of computed tomography for the local evaluation of long bone osteosarcoma: report on 30 cases. *Skeletal Radiol* 1985;13:147–153.
167. Schreiman JS, Crass JR, et al. Osteosarcoma: role of CT in limb-sparing treatment. *Radiology* 1986;161:485–488.
168. Azouz ME, Esseltine DW, Chevalier L. Radiologic evaluation of osteosarcoma. *J Can Assoc Radiol* 1982;33:167–171.
169. Gillespy T III, Manfrini M, et al. Staging of intraosseous extent of osteosarcoma: correlation of preoperative CT and MR imaging with pathologic macroslides. *Radiology* 1988;167:765–767.

Ewing's Sarcoma
170. Dahlin DC, Coventry MB, Scanlon PW. Ewing's sarcoma: a critical analysis of 165 cases. *J Bone Joint Surg [Am]* 1961;43:185–192.
171. Whitehouse GH, Griffiths GJ. Roentgenologic aspects of spinal involvement by primary and metastatic Ewing's tumor. *J Can Assoc Radiol* 1976;27:290–297.
172. Lacey SH, Danish EH, et al. Ewing's sarcoma of the proximal phalanx of a finger. *J Bone Joint Surg* 1987;69:931–934.
173. Dick HM, Francis KC, Johnston AD. Ewing's sarcoma of the hand. *J Bone Joint Surg [Am]* 1971;53:345–348.
174. Reinus WR, Gilula LA, et al. Radiographic appearance of Ewing's sarcoma of the hands and feet. *AJR* 1985;144:331–336.
175. Escobedo EM, Bjorkengren AG, Moore SG. Case report. Ewing's sarcoma of the hand. *AJR* 1992;159:101–102.
176. Vacher H, Lavenu MCV, Sauvegrain J. Etude anatomo-radio-clinique des sarcomes d'Ewing's du rachis lombaire. *J Radiol* 1981;62:425–428.
177. Weinstein JB, Siegel MJ, Griffith RC. Spinal Ewing's sarcoma: misleading appearances. *Skeletal Radiol* 1984;11:262–265.
178. Klaassen MA, Hoffman G. Ewing's sarcoma presenting as spondylolisthesis: report of a case. *J Bone Joint Surg* 1987;69:1089–1092.
179. Levine E, Levine C. Ewing's tumor of rib: radiologic findings and computed tomography contribution. *Skeletal Radiol* 1983;9:227–233.
180. Azouz ME. Massee intrathoracique dans le sarcome d'Ewing des cotes. *J Radiol* 1983;64:391–395.

Chondrosarcoma
181. Patel MR, Pearlman HS, Engler J, et al. Chondrosarcoma of the proximal phalanx of the finger: review of the literature and report of a case. *J Bone Joint Surg [Am]* 1977;59:401–403.
182. Dahlin DC, Unni KK. *Bone tumors,* 4th ed. Springfield, IL: Charles C Thomas, 1986.
183. Jaffe H. *Tumors and tumorous conditions of the bones and joints.* Philadelphia: Lea & Febiger, 1958.
184. Hermann G, Sacher M, et al. Chondrosarcoma of the spine: an unusual radiographic presentation. *Skeletal Radiol* 1985;14:178–183.
185. Pinstein ML, Sebes JI, Scott RL. Transarticular extension of chondrosarcoma. *AJR* 1984;142:779–780.
186. Norman A, Sissons HA. Radiographic hallmarks of peripheral chondrosarcoma. *Radiology* 1984;151:589–596.

Non-Hodgkin's Lymphoma
187. Griffiths HJ. Marrow tumors. In *Bone tumors,* vol 5. Berlin: Springer-Verlag, 1977.
188. Ivins JC, Dahlin DC. Reticulum-cell sarcoma of bone. *J Bone Joint Surg [Am]* 1953;35:835–842.
189. Parker F, Jackson H. Primary reticulum-cell sarcoma of bone. *Surg Gynecol Obstet* 1939;68:45–51.

Multiple Myeloma
190. Gompels BM, Vataw ML, Martel W. Correlation of radiological manifestations of multiple myeloma with immunoglobulin abnormalities and prognosis. *Radiology* 1972;104:509–514.

MRI OF RHEUMATOID ARTHRITIS AND COMMON ARTHRITIDES

JOHN A. ARRINGTON

The text and images of this chapter highlight the current applications of magnetic resonance imaging (MRI) in rheumatoid arthritis and the common arthritides. MRI of the inflammatory or degenerative nature of the common arthritides as well as the sequelae of spine and joint involvement are reviewed. MRI does not currently have a defined or established role in the evaluation of the early manifestations, effectiveness of treatment, or staging of the common arthritides, even though MRI has the capability to image cartilage and subtle osseous erosion that cannot be imaged with radiographs or computed tomography (CT).

Radiographs have a well-established role in assessing the severity of arthritic involvement in the spine and joints, but this assessment is limited to osseous changes, and narrowing of disc and joint spaces. MRI does not currently have an established role in assessing the severity of spine and joint involvement in rheumatoid arthritis (RA) or most of the common arthritides. MRI does have a well-established role in evaluating joints for internal derangement, and for evaluating spinal pathology in arthritis patients as well as nonarthritis patients.

MRI provides excellent soft-tissue contrast (multiplanar and tomographic capability), which allows for effective evaluation of cartilage, subchondral bone, and the soft-tissue structures of joints. MRI is more sensitive than radiographs in detecting the early manifestations of inflammatory and degenerative arthritis. MRI can detect cartilaginous and small osseous erosions that cannot be detected on radiographs. MR imaging effectively evaluates the soft-tissue structures of joints (fibrocartilage, ligaments, tendons) and spine (spinal cord, nerve roots). MRI defines the soft tissues and osseous anatomy of the joints and spine delineating any internal derangement or pathology. MRI is better suited than radiographs to monitor response to therapy and evaluate for either improvement or deterioration. This should

significantly impact treatment plans. Even with the superior imaging capabilities of MRI, there is currently not a defined role for MRI in the assessment of disease severity or evaluation of treatment.

MRI is currently being utilized to image the long-term manifestations and complications (e.g., chronic rotator cuff tear, degenerative meniscal tear, tendon rupture, and severe C1-C2 instability) of the joints and spine. There is great potential for MRI in RA patients; therefore, there is great hope for a better way to evaluate early disease, response to therapy, and improved treatment plans for RA. As the treatment for RA patients and MRI technology continue to evolve and improve, the role of MRI will become better defined and MRI utilization will expand. It is expected that MRI utilization in patients with arthritis will significantly increase. MRI can successfully image the early manifestations and progression of disease, as well as the response to therapy. In the near future, the focus of MRI will shift to the routine imaging of early or mild synovitis and cartilage erosion as treatment plans begin to depend on the MR staging of the severity of the synovitis and cartilage erosion. There will be a reduced need to image complications of disease such as chronic rotator cuff tears with earlier and more effective treatment intervention. Prerequisite for expanded MRI utilization are treatment regimens that are effective interventions for early disease, and treatment plans that incorporate varied responses to therapy. If treatment regimens depend on or change with specific imaging findings, MRI will have a significant role in the overall care of the patient with arthritis.

COMPARISON OF IMAGING MODALITIES

MRI provides superior soft-tissue contrast with multiplanar and multislice capability. With current MRI technology, detailed noninvasive imaging of the spine and joints is routinely obtained. Soft-tissue structures including the spinal cord, nerve roots, cartilage, synovial tissue, ligaments, and tendons are all exquisitely imaged with MRI using standard techniques and currently available equipment. Images can be obtained in any plane with multiple or contiguous slices, giving MRI a tomographic capability. This gives MRI a critical advantage over radiographs and CT in evaluating the osseous joints and spine, especially for subtle bony pathology, including osseous erosion, intraarticular extension of osseous cysts, and stress fractures.

MRI provides a more detailed evaluation of the soft-tissue and osseous anatomy of the spine and joints than any other imaging modality or the clinical examination. In the cervical spine, MRI provides adequate bone detail of odontoid erosion with superior soft-tissue contrast and the ability to image in the sagittal plane, and MRI gives exquisite detail regarding the amount of periodontotic pannus and spinal cord compression. The combination of superior soft-tissue contrast and multiplane/multislice imaging gives MRI a unique ability in evaluating the cervical spine manifestations of rheumatoid arthritis. In joints, MRI effectively images synovium, cartilage, subchondral bone, ligaments, and tendons. MRI adequately evaluates synovial hypertrophy, as well as cartilaginous and osseous erosion. MRI exquisitely details intraosseous cysts, meniscal tears, as well as tendon and ligament pathology.

CT has superior bone detail and resolution in comparison to MRI and plain films, but is limited to the axial plane for most anatomic structures. CT is more sensitive to subtle osseous erosion, but cannot image the spine and larger joints in the sagittal or coronal planes. The soft-tissue contrast obtained with CT is superior to radiographs, but is far inferior to MRI. In the cervical spine, CT imaging provides superior bone resolution and detail of odontoid erosion, and adequate images of periodontotic pannus. Noncontrast CT cannot image the spinal cord or evaluate for cord compression. In joints, noninvasive CT scanning does not adequately define the anatomy or delineate pathology of soft-tissue structures.

CT arthrography can adequately evaluate some soft-tissue structures of some joints. A shoulder CT arthrogram effectively evaluates the articular cartilage and the fibrocartilage (labrum) of the glenohumeral joint, but does not adequately image the rotator cuff. CT arthrography of the wrist can effectively evaluate the triangular fibrocartilage complex (TFC) but not the tendons. CT imaging of the knee is limited to the axial plane, and even with arthrography, cannot effectively image the menisci, ligaments, or tendons. For CT imaging to effectively evaluate the soft-tissue structures of the spine and joints, direct coronal and sagittal scanning is required. This is not currently possible in the spine and larger joints. It is possible but cumbersome for the smaller joints of most patients.

Radiographs of joints are a better positive than negative imaging test in arthritis patients. A normal hand radiograph does not exclude synovitis or cartilaginous erosion. Radiographs are insensitive to the early manifestations of RA, including detection of subtle osseous erosion or soft-tissue involvement. Plain films are also limited in evaluating the effects of treatment. Radiographs accurately measure the atlantodens distance and evaluate the stability of the cervical spine, but are insensitive to subtle odontoid erosion and cannot evaluate periodontotic pannus or the spinal cord.

ARTHRITIDES

Normal articular cartilage is critical to the functioning of joints. Cartilage failure is basic to the development of degenerative arthritis and cartilage erosion is an integral component of inflammatory arthritis. Noninvasive imaging of cartilage is a key component in the advancement of our understanding of the arthritis. Effective noninvasive imaging of cartilage allows for the evaluation of early manifestations of the arthritides. MRI provides a reliable, noninvasive way to image articular cartilage. Imaging of articular cartilage or any of the soft-tissue and osseous structures of the joints and spine needs to be noninvasive for several reasons. To evaluate response to therapy, repeat imaging is required. Multiple joints may need to be imaged because many of the arthritides are polyarticular.

Rheumatoid Arthritis

RA is characterized by an inflammatory synovitis that leads to marked thickening and hyperplasia of the synovium, and results in cartilaginous and bone erosion. Joint involvement tends to be symmetrical and polyarticular. The cervical spine is one of the most commonly involved sites. The hands, wrist, and knee joints are among the most commonly affected joints followed by the shoulder, elbow, hips, ankle, and foot.

MRI OF JOINT INVOLVEMENT

The early erosion of cartilage and subchondral bone by the inflammatory synovitis typically begins at the margins of the joints. MRI now provides high-resolution imaging of articular cartilage and subtle osseous erosion can be imaged (Figs. 9.1–9.3). The ability to image cartilage and bone erosion with MRI is in part owing to the multiplanar imaging and tomographic capability of MRI, as well as to the superior soft-tissue contrast. Multiplanar imaging capability allows for imaging a joint in any plane to optimally demonstrate the cartilage and subchondral cortex. The ability to obtain multiple slices in any plane gives MRI a tomographic capability. High-resolution imaging with volume acquisition is now possible with both fast spin echo (FSE) and gradient echo (GRE) technique. Higher spatial resolution and

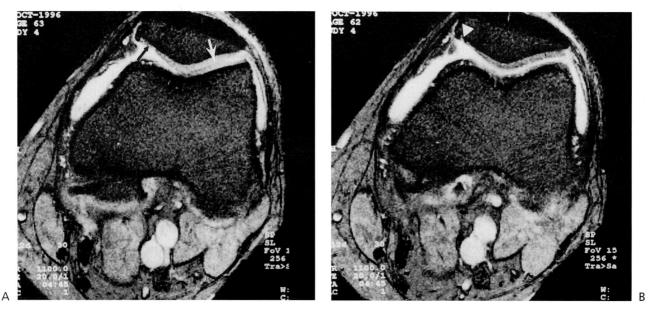

FIGURE 9.1. Rheumatoid arthritis involvement of the knee. Two-dimensional gradient echo axial images **(A,B)** through the femoropatellar joint. Note erosion of the articular cartilage of the medial patellar facet (*black arrow*). This is compared to the normal cartilage of the lateral patellar facet (*white arrow*). Also demonstrated is subtle osseous erosion (*white arrowhead*) of the medial patellar facet.

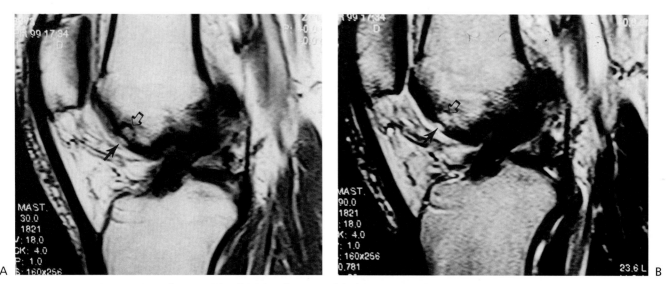

FIGURE 9.2. Rheumatoid arthritis involvement of the knee. Proton density weight (PDW) and T2-weighted sagittal FSE images of the knee **(A,B)** demonstrate erosion of the articular cartilage of the femur (*black arrows*), and osseous erosion of the underlying cortex (*open black arrows*). Note the high contrast between the joint fluid and articular cartilage, as well as the contrast between normal and abnormal cartilage on the T2-weighted FSE image. Also noted is osseous erosion of the posterior lateral tibial plateau (*black arrowheads*) on the T1-weighted coronal SE image **(C)**, and coronal STIR images **(D)**.

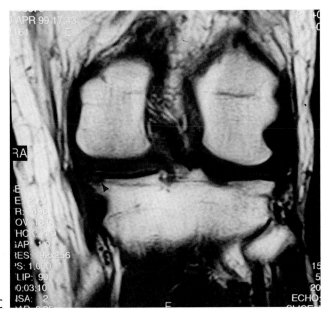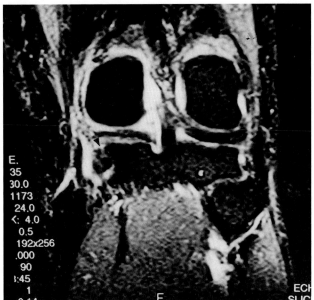

FIGURE 9.2. *(continued)*

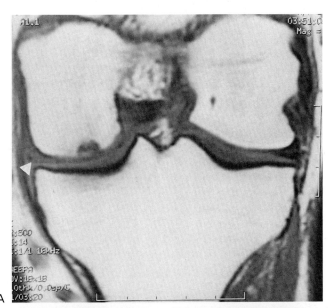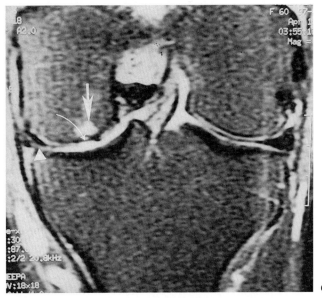

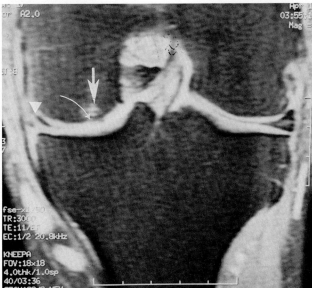

FIGURE 9.3. Erosive changes of the knee. T1-weighted coronal SE **(A)**, and fat suppressed PD- and T2-weighted SE images **(B,C)** demonstrate subchondral erosion of the medial femoral condyle (*white arrows*). The T2-weighted FSE image also demonstrates erosion of the cartilage (*small white arrows*). The cartilage erosion is seen as an area of high signal intensity contrasted with the low signal intensity of normal cartilage on this image. There is also a degenerative tear of the posterior horn medial meniscus (*white arrowheads*).

thinner slice thickness are achieved with three-dimensional technique. The ability to obtain serial thin section images in any plane allows for detection of very subtle cartilaginous or subchondral bony erosion or damage.

Successful MRI of articular cartilage depends on the contrast between articular cartilage and joint fluid, signal to noise ratio, and spatial resolution. T2-weighted spin echo (SE) imaging has historically offered the best contrast. Superior cartilage contrast has been achieved with a much greater signal to noise ratio with the advancement and development of the FSE technique (Figs. 9.3 and 9.4). Normal articular cartilage has much lower signal intensity than joint fluid on heavily T2-weighted FSE images. The FSE technique is superior to the GRE technique, even though higher resolution can be achieved with three-dimensional GRE

imaging. The additional capabilities of fat-suppressed SE imaging has also added to our ability to evaluate articular cartilage both noninvasively, as well as with MR arthrography. Continued evolution of MRI technology will provide further advances in our ability to image and evaluate articular cartilage.

Bone erosion is best seen on T1-weighted SE and T2-weighted FSE images (Figs. 9.1, 9.3, and 9.5–9.15). The erosion typically is seen as an area of low signal intensity in the subchondral bone on the T1-weighted SE and the high signal intensity on T2-weighted FSE images. Fat suppression (FS) is an exceptionally helpful technique to enhance conspicuity of osseous pathology in the spine and joints. Suppression of the signal intensity from normal marrow increases the contrast or signal difference between normal and

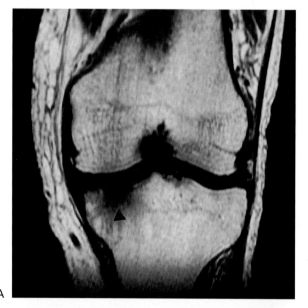

A

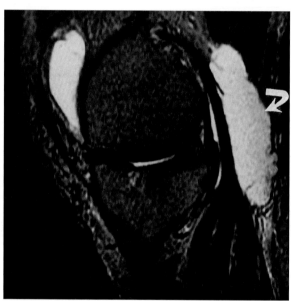

C

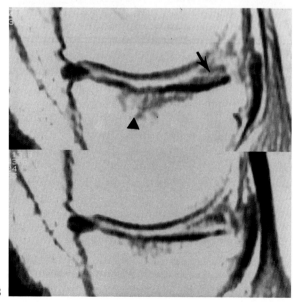

B

FIGURE 9.4. Rheumatoid arthritis involvement of the knee. T1-weighted coronal **(A)**, and sagittal PD- and T2-weighted **(B,C)** SE images of the knee. Note a subchondral cyst of the medial tibial plateau (*black arrowheads*). The PD meniscal windows show degeneration and thinning of the medial meniscus with a degenerative tear (*black arrow*). A large Baker's cyst is noted posteromedially (*curved white arrow*).

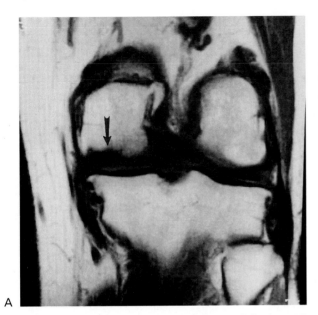
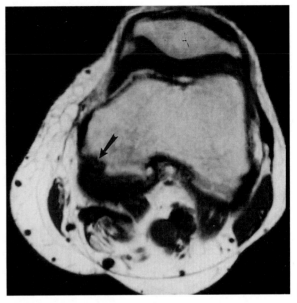

FIGURE 9.5. Osseous erosion of the knee. T1-weighted coronal **(A)** and axial **(B)** SE images demonstrate erosion of the posterior medial femoral condyle (*black arrows*).

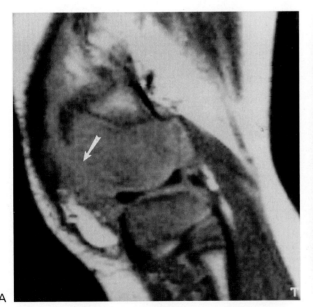
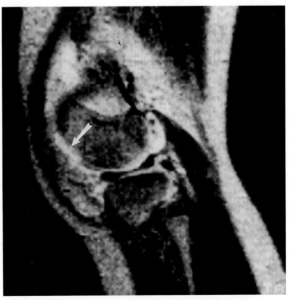

FIGURE 9.6. Juvenile rheumatoid arthritis (JRA) involvement of the knee. PD- **(A)** and T2-weighted **(B)** SE images of the knee demonstrate erosive changes of the lateral femoral epiphysis (*white arrows*). This is best seen on the T2-weighted SE images.

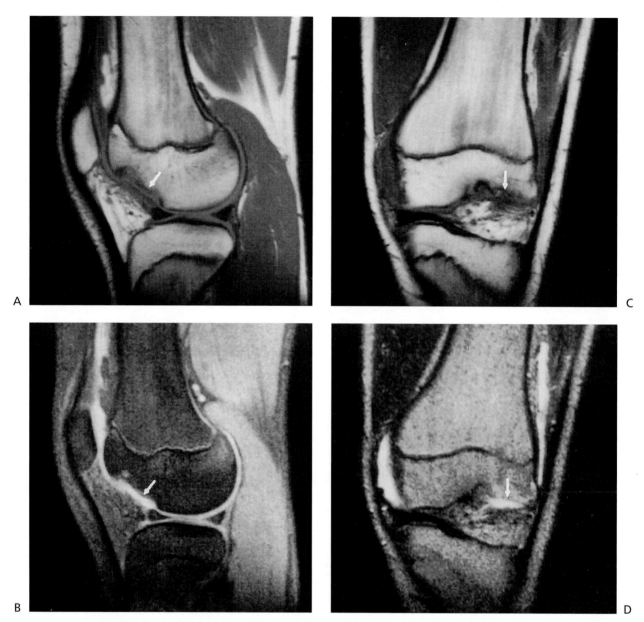

FIGURE 9.7. JRA involvement of the knee. Sagittal T1-weighted SE and two-dimensional T2-weighted GRE **(A,B)**, and coronal T1- and T2-weighted SE **(C,D)**, and PD- and T2-weighted sagittal SE images **(E-H)**. The sagittal and coronal images demonstrate erosion of the femoral epiphysis (*white arrows*), as well as synovial hypertrophy and an infiltrative appearance to the infrapatellar fat pad (*black arrows*).

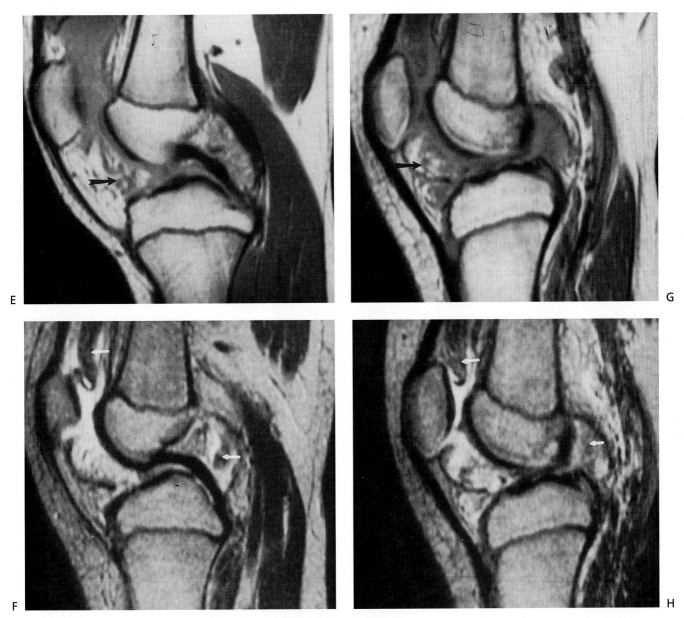

FIGURE 9.7. *(continued)*

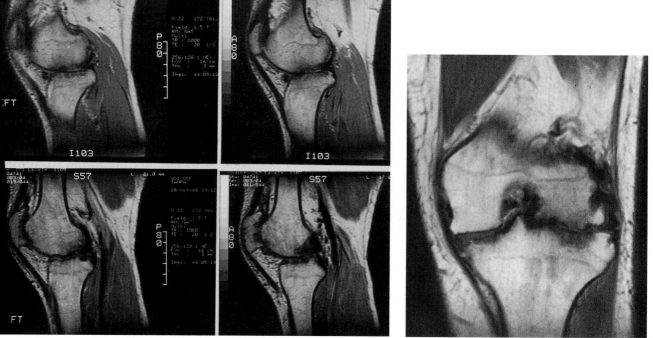

FIGURE 9.8. Hemophilic arthropathy of the knee. T1-weighted sagittal SE **(A)**, and coronal **(B)** images demonstrate degenerative changes of the femoropatellar and femorotibial joint spaces with osseous erosion in a 22-year-old hemophiliac patient.

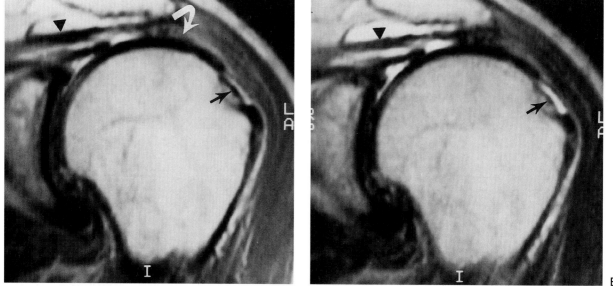

FIGURE 9.9. Osseous erosion of the humeral head. Oblique coronal PD- **(A)** and T2-weighted **(B)** demonstrate erosion of the lateral humeral head (*black arrows*). The erosion fills with joint fluid on the T2-weighted image. A retracted supraspinatus muscle (*black arrowheads*) and a full-thickness tear of the supraspinatus tendon (*curved white arrow*) are also present.

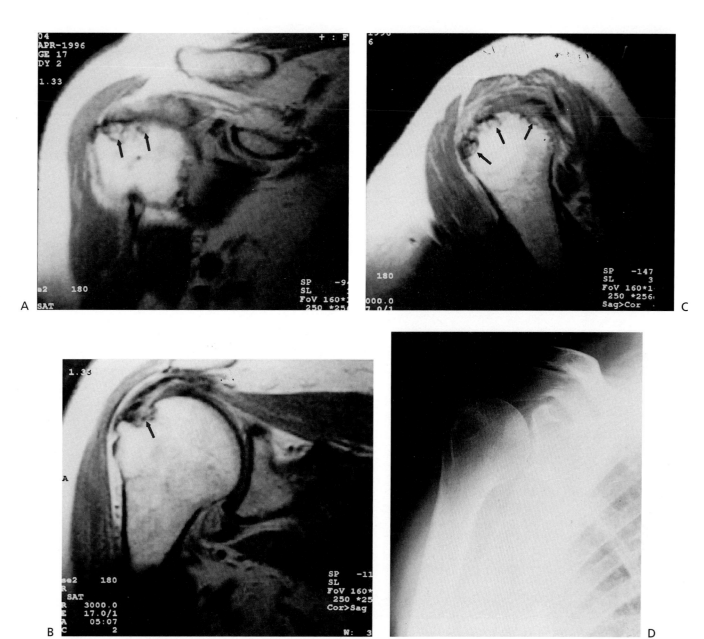

FIGURE 9.10. Osseous erosion of the shoulder. Oblique coronal PD-weighted **(A,B)**, and oblique sagittal PD-weighted SE images **(C)**, and AP radiograph **(D)**. The oblique coronal and sagittal images demonstrate subchondral erosion of the lateral humeral head (*black arrows*). The eroded areas are not clearly identified on the radiograph.

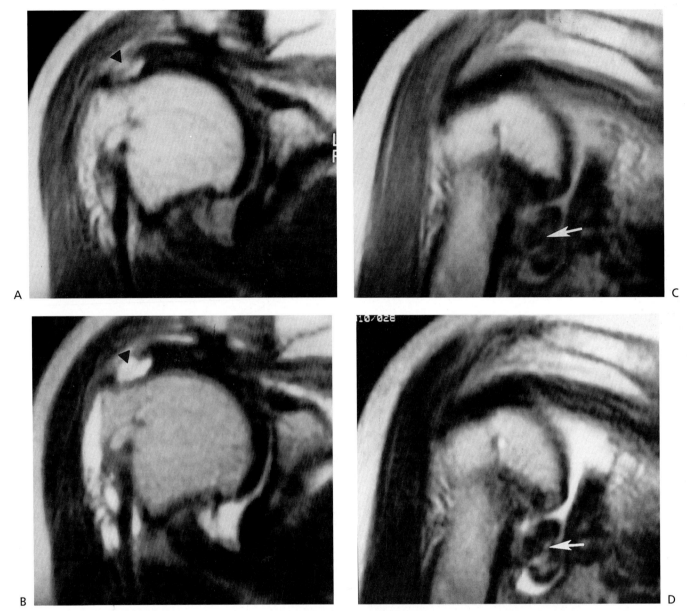

A

B

C

D

FIGURE 9.11. Large humeral head spur with multiple loose bodies. Oblique coronal PD- and T2-weighted images at the level of the AC joint **(A,B)**, and through the posterior joint **(C,D)**. Oblique sagittal PD- and T2-weighted images at the level of the medial humeral head and axillary recess **(E,F)**, and more laterally through the subdeltoid bursa and lateral humeral head **(G,H)**. Axial T2-weighted GRE images through the inferior glenohumeral joint space **(I,J)**. Internal and external rotation plain films **(K,L)**. The multiplanar images show multiple rounded and oval intraarticular masses *(white arrows)*. These are clearly lower signal intensity than the joint effusion and bursal fluid. The intraarticular loose bodies are more numerous in the axillary recess and posterior joint. A large spur originates from the posterior medial humeral head *(black arrows)*. A small rotator cuff tear *(black arrowheads)* and marked subdeltoid bursitis are present.

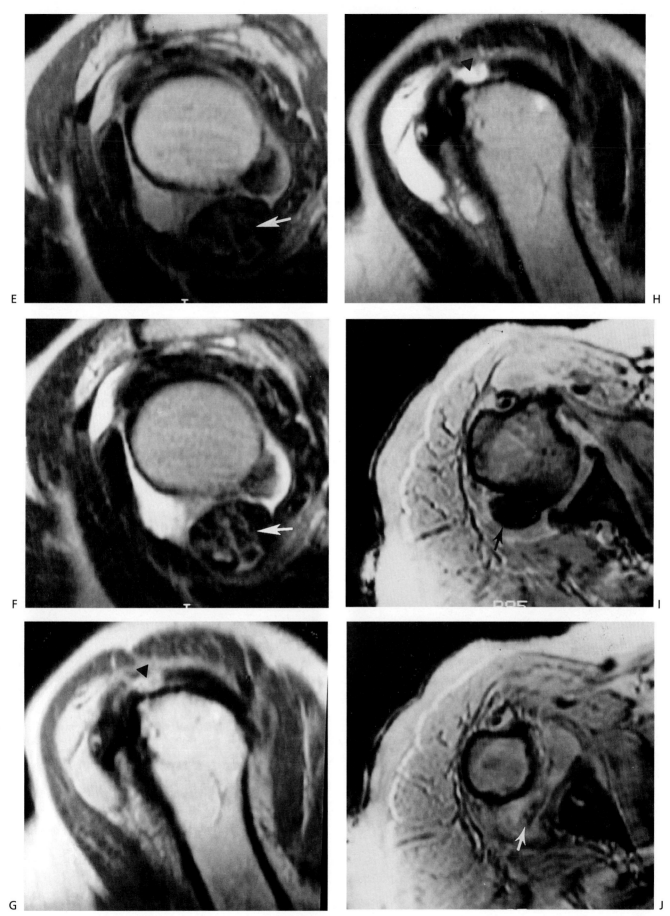

FIGURE 9.11. *(continued)*

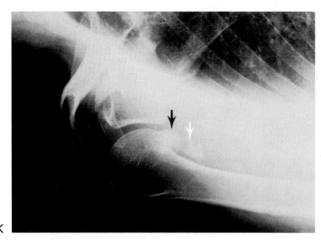

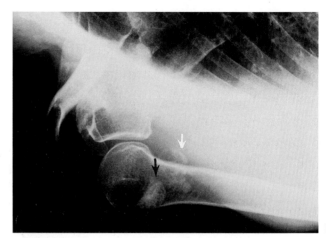

K

L

FIGURE 9.11. *(continued)*

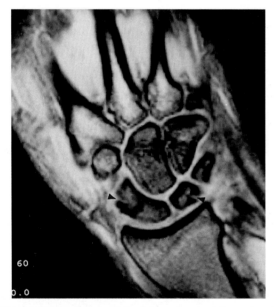

FIGURE 9.12. Osseous erosion of the wrist. Two-dimensional T2-weighted coronal GRE images demonstrate subtle erosion (*black arrowheads*) of the scaphoid and lunate carpal bones.

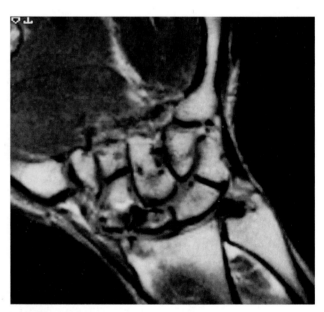

FIGURE 9.13. Osseous erosion of the wrist. T1-weighted coronal SE image demonstrates osseous erosion of the lunate and scaphoid, as well as of the lateral radius, and to a lesser degree the capitate.

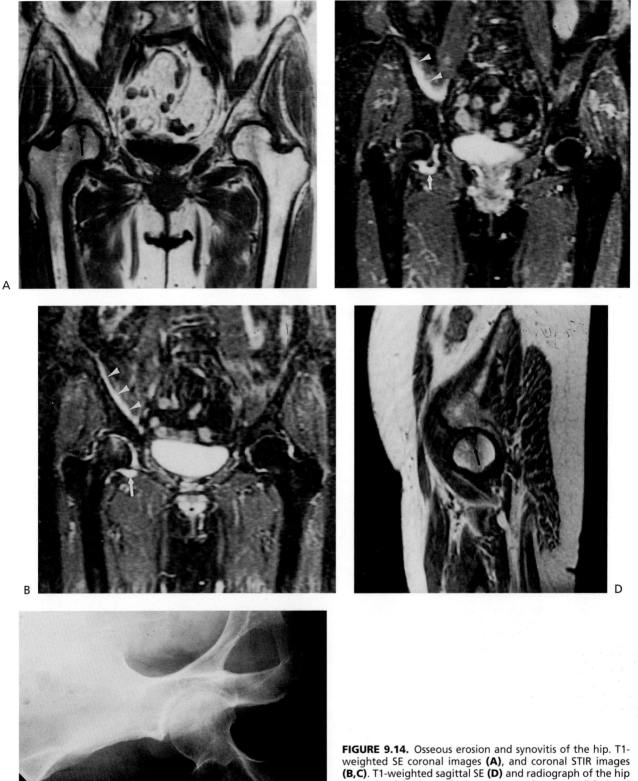

FIGURE 9.14. Osseous erosion and synovitis of the hip. T1-weighted SE coronal images **(A)**, and coronal STIR images **(B,C)**. T1-weighted sagittal SE **(D)** and radiograph of the hip and pelvis **(E)**. The multiplanar images show a small femoral erosion of the femoral head (*black arrows*), and a moderate joint effusion (*white arrows*). The STIR images demonstrate fluid located between the ilium and the iliacus muscle (*white arrowheads*). The erosion is not seen on the radiograph.

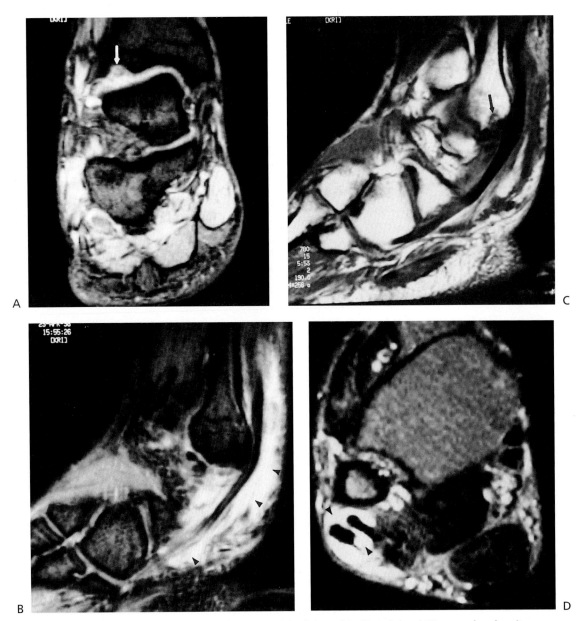

FIGURE 9.15. Osseous erosion and tenosynovitis of the ankle. T2-weighted GE coronal and sagittal **(A,B)**, T1-weighted sagittal SE **(C)**, and T2-weighted axial SE images **(D)**. The coronal T2-weighted images demonstrate erosion of the tibial plafond (*white arrow*). There is marked acute tenosynovitis with some synovial hypertrophy of the peroneus longus and brevis tendons, seen as fluid distending the tendon sheaths (*white arrowheads*). There is also erosion of the distal fibular (*black arrowheads*).

abnormal marrow. When fat suppression imaging is utilized, either with short T1 inversion time (STIR) or the fat-suppressed T2-weighted FSE technique, the contrast between erosion and normal bone are maximized. The erosion is seen as an area of high signal intensity within very low signal intensity normal bone (Figs. 9.3, 9.4, and 9.16). The bone erosion typically will enhance if intravenous gadolinium is administered, and the cartilaginous and osseous erosion will fill with contrast on MR arthrography.

Intraosseous cysts are commonly seen with rheumatoid arthritis in addition to erosion of bone. Although larger in-

traosseous cysts can be identified with radiographs, intraosseous cysts are better evaluated with MRI. MRI has been shown to be more sensitive than radiographs in evaluating these cysts and detecting smaller cysts. An intraosseous cyst can arise primarily within bone or as an extension from a joint (Figs. 9.4, 9.16, and 9.17). Intraosseous cysts that originate from the joint communicate with the joint throughout their development. Intraosseous cysts that arise within the bone may not initially communicate with the joint, but only communicate intraarticularly as the cyst expands into the joint.

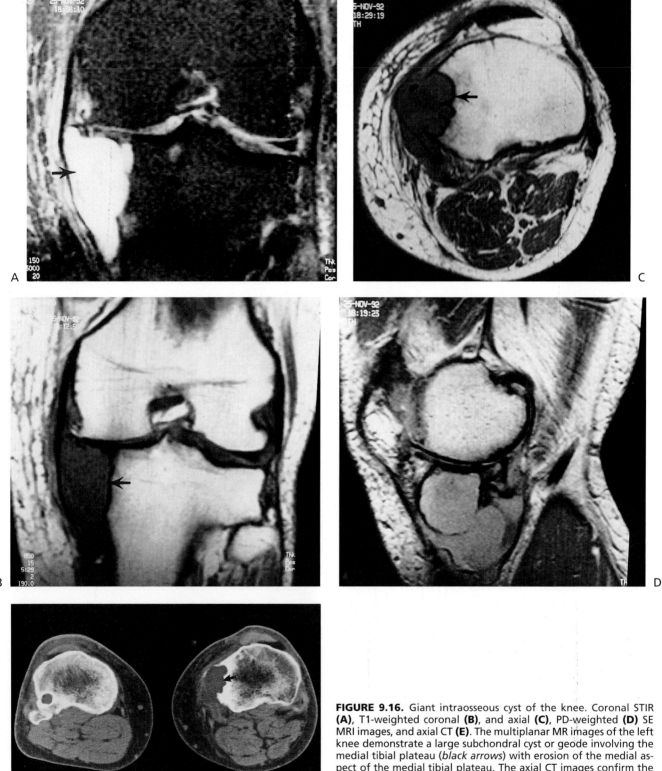

FIGURE 9.16. Giant intraosseous cyst of the knee. Coronal STIR **(A)**, T1-weighted coronal **(B)**, and axial **(C)**, PD-weighted **(D)** SE MRI images, and axial CT **(E)**. The multiplanar MR images of the left knee demonstrate a large subchondral cyst or geode involving the medial tibial plateau (*black arrows*) with erosion of the medial aspect of the medial tibial plateau. The axial CT images confirm the osseous erosion and also demonstrate a smaller of the lateral tibial plateau of the knee.

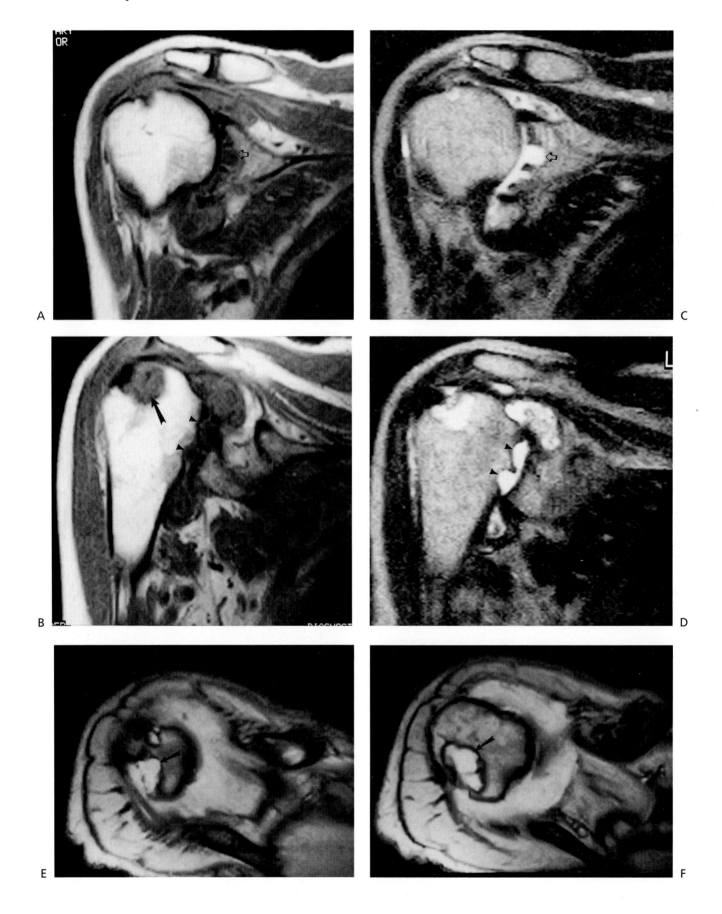

Joint effusion or fluid is easily demonstrated by MRI. A joint effusion is seen as decreased signal or low signal intensity on T1-weighted images and increased signal or bright signal intensity on T2-weighted images. The intraarticular or bursal location of fluid is easily demonstrated on MRI. A joint effusion greatly enhances MRI's ability to image and evaluate synovium. In the absence of a joint effusion, MR arthrography or intravenous contrast is necessary to adequately evaluate changes in the synovium. On SE MRI, both normal and abnormal synovial tissue is low or intermediate signal intensity on T1- and PD-weighted images, and remains low signal intensity on T2-weighted images. Although the contrast between synovium and joint fluid can be affected by technical factors such as echo time, echo train, and fat suppression, hypertrophied synovium is easily separated from joint fluid on any reasonably T2-weighted image. FSE imaging allows for heavily T2-weighted image acquisition with excellent signal to noise ratio and a decreased acquisition time. Hyperplastic synovium has similar signal intensity similar to joint effusion on T1- and PD-weighted images, and is usually difficult to distinguish from joint fluid. Hyperplastic synovium resulting from inflammatory arthritis is easily separated from joint fluid on T2-weighted images (Figs. 9.7 and 9.18–9.21). Hyperplastic synovium is intermediate in signal intensity, which is in contrast to the high signal intensity of fluid on T2-weighted images. It has also been shown that active pannus demonstrates enhancement after intravenous (IV) administration of gadolinium. Synovial involvement is typically diffuse but may be focal or nodular in certain inflammatory arthritides. Hyperplastic synovium can appear masslike in the nodular form or pigmented villonodular synovitis (Fig. 9.20). A larger field of view must be utilized to ensure that the entire extent of the inflammatory involvement is imaged in the diffuse form of PNS (Figs. 9.19 and 9.21). Care must be taken to cover the superior extent of the suprapatellar bursa and the inferior extent of the popliteus bursa in the knee. If areas of very low signal intensity are identified within hypertrophied synovium on MRI, this may represent areas of fibrosis or hemosiderin deposition from prior hemorrhage.

Rheumatoid synovitis can invade ligaments, tendons, and fibrocartilage. These structures normally have low signal intensity or appear black on all MRI images (T1-weighted, PD-weighted, T2-weighted), as well as with all MRI pulse sequences (SE, GRE, and IR). Any increased signal intensity within a ligament, tendon, or fibrocartilage is abnormal; it may indicate involvement by the synovitis in patients with RA. The involvement from erosion or invasion may result in degeneration or tear. Bone erosion may result in the fraying of a tendon or ligament insertion and lead to avulsion or tear of these structures. Invasion of tendons leads to structural weakening, thinning, and eventual rupture of the tendon. It is critical to evaluate both the morphology and signal intensity of ligaments, tendons, and fibrocartilage on MRI. The earliest MRI changes are typically increased signal within an otherwise normal appearing ligament, tendon, or fibrocartilage. The morphology becomes abnormal with progression of disease, with the structure appearing thinned or frayed. Eventually this may lead to a complete tear, which is demonstrated on MRI as complete disruption of the fibers of the ligament or tendon, and as signal extending to an articular surfaces of fibrocartilage such as a knee meniscus (Figs. 9.3 and 9.4). Acute tenosynovitis is seen as high signal intensity fluid on T2-weighted MRI (Fig. 9.15) distending the tendon sheath. Hyperplastic synovium may also thin the tendon sheath, but is typically intermediate in signal intensity on T2-weighted images.

Synovial cysts associated with joint pathology are a common finding in patients with arthritis. These fluid-filled cysts are lined with synovial cells and may or may not communicate with the joint. Synovial cysts are associated with pathology of the adjacent joint. In the knee, meniscal cysts are seen with meniscal tears, and popliteal (Baker's) cysts are associated with internal derangement. Popliteal cysts are the most common synovial cyst in the body, and their incidence increases with age. MRI of synovial cysts of the knee demonstrates well-demarcated fluid signal intensity collections either in the gastrocnemio-semimembranous bursa (popliteal cyst) extending from a meniscal tear (meniscal cyst). The role of imaging is not only to anatomically define the cyst, but also to evaluate associated intraarticular pathology (Fig. 9.4).

Intraspinal synovial cysts are uncommon but may mimic disc disease when they result in nerve root compression. They are more common in the lower lumbar spine, usually at the L4-5 level. Synovial cysts are more common on the posterior (or dorsal) aspect of the facet joints and are usually asymptomatic. Cysts that originate from the anterior or ventral surface of a facet joint may extend into the spinal canal and cause thecal sac compression and nerve root impingement. Patients with degeneration of apophyseal or facet

FIGURE 9.17. Intraosseous cyst and osseous erosion of the shoulder. Oblique coronal T1-weighted SE **(A,B)**, and oblique coronal T2-weighted SE **(C,D)**, and axial two-dimensional T2-weighted GRE **(E,F)** images demonstrate severe degenerative changes with narrowing of the glenohumeral joint space and prominent intraosseous cyst of the posterolateral humeral head (*black arrows*), and erosion of the medial humeral head (*black arrowhead*) and glenoid (*open black arrows*). The intraarticular communication of the posterolateral humeral cyst is seen on the axial and T1-weighted coronal images.

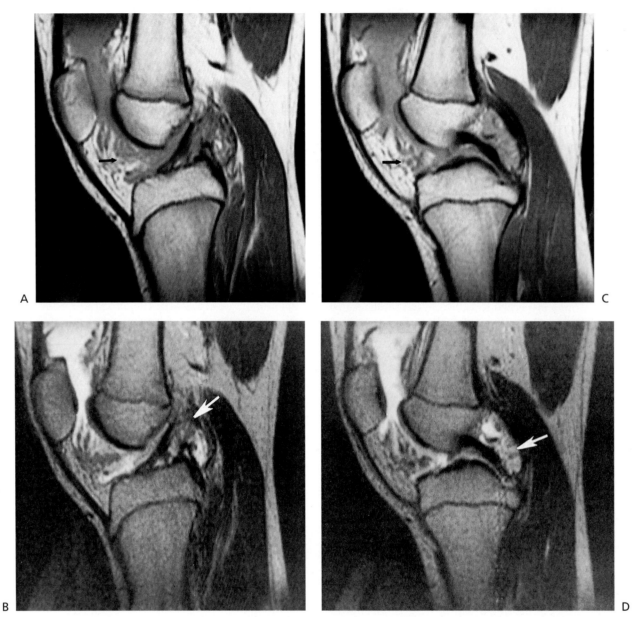

FIGURE 9.18. JRA involvement of the knee. PD- **(A,C)** and T2-weighted **(C,D)** sagittal SE images demonstrate synovial hypertrophy *(white arrows)* as well as infiltration of the infrapatellar fat pad *(black arrows)*.

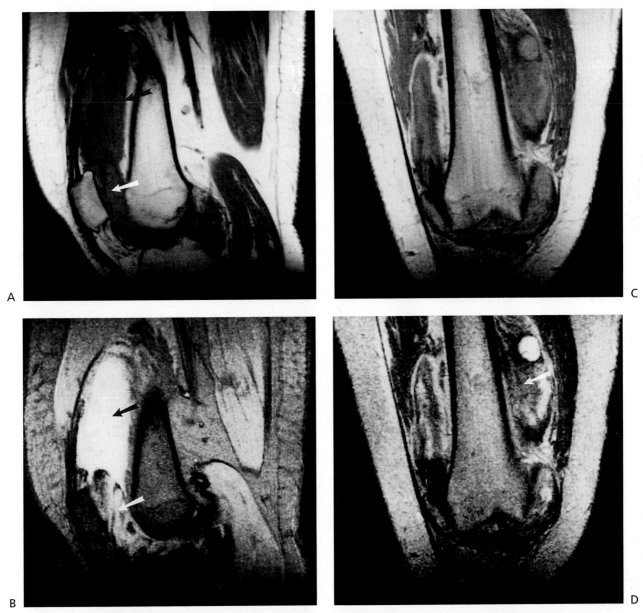

FIGURE 9.19. Pigmented villonodular synovitis involvement of the knee. T1-weighted sagittal SE **(A)**, and T2-weighted sagittal two-dimensional GRE **(B)** images, and coronal PD- **(C)** and T2-weighted **(D)** SE images. The multiplanar images demonstrate a synovial process/mass in the suprapatellar bursa with abnormal intermediate signal intensity on the T2-weighted images within the femoropatellar joint space and suprapatellar bursa with synovial hypertrophy (*white arrows*). A large joint effusion is also present (*black arrows*).

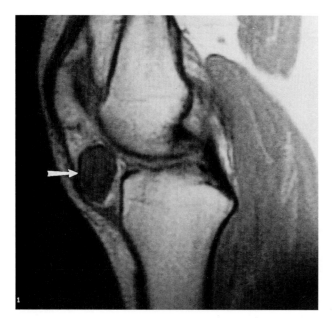

FIGURE 9.20. Focal involvement of PNS of the knee. PD-weighted SE sagittal image demonstrates a well-demarcated intermediate signal intensity mass in the infrapatellar fat of the knee (*white arrow*). This represents an organized inflammatory mass of hyperplastic synovium.

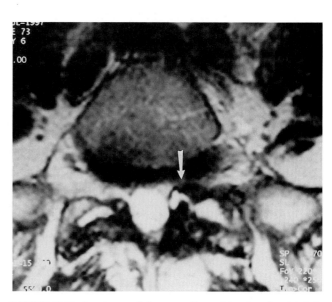

FIGURE 9.22. Erosion and degeneration of lumbar facet joint. Axial T2-weighted SE image of the lumbar spine demonstrate severe erosive and arthritic changes of the L5-S1 facet joints bilaterally with greater left lateral recessed stenosis (*white arrow*). This results in impingement on the left S1 nerve root.

joints of the lumbar spine (Fig. 9.22) may have associated synovial cysts (Figs. 9.23 and 9.24).

The complications of inflammatory or degenerative arthritis are not limited to the disease process itself, but also to the sequelae of treatment. Steroids are commonly administered and can result in osteoporosis, which in turn can lead to stress fractures (Fig. 9.25). Long-term corticosteroid

treatment can also result in avascular necrosis (AVN) of joints (Fig. 9.26).

RA commonly affects the knee, and less frequently involves the shoulder, hip, and ankle. MRI is rarely utilized to detect and evaluate synovitis or early cartilage erosion in the larger joints. MRI is used to evaluate painful joints for internal derangement, including the knee (Figs. 9.3, 9.4, 9.8,

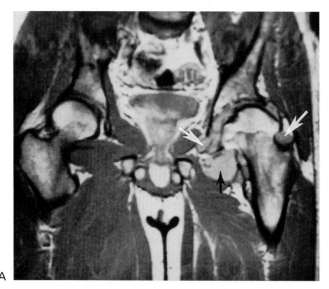

A

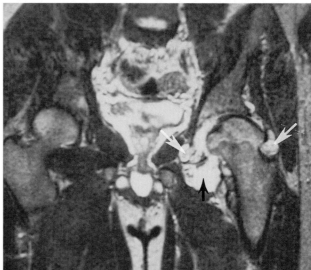

B

FIGURE 9.21. Pigmented villonodular synovitis of the hip. PD-weighted and T2-weighted coronal SE **(A,B)** demonstrate an extremely large left joint effusion (*black arrows*) with abnormal synovial process with synovial hypertrophy (*white arrows*). There are erosive changes of the acetabula.

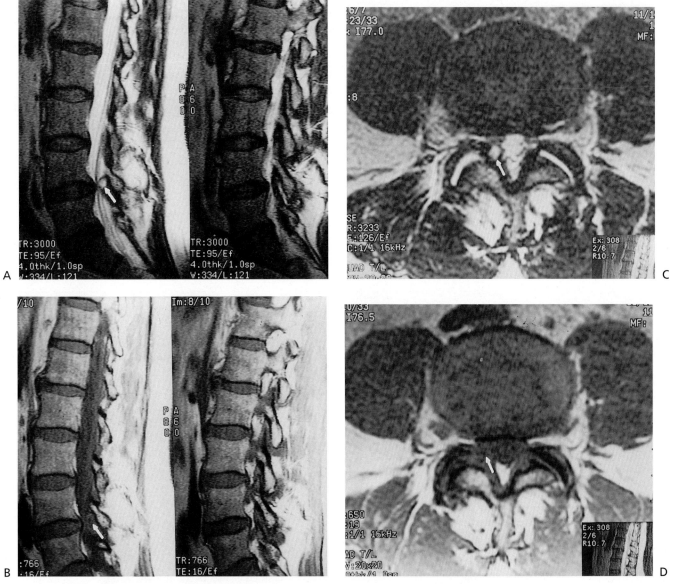

FIGURE 9.23. Synovial cyst of facet joint. Sagittal T2- and T1-weighted **(A,B)**, and axial T2- and T1-weighted **(C,D)** SE images demonstrate erosive and degenerative changes of the L4-5 facet joints and a small synovial cyst (*white arrows*) projecting from the right L4-5 facet joint extending into the right lateral recess and impinging upon the right L-5 nerve root.

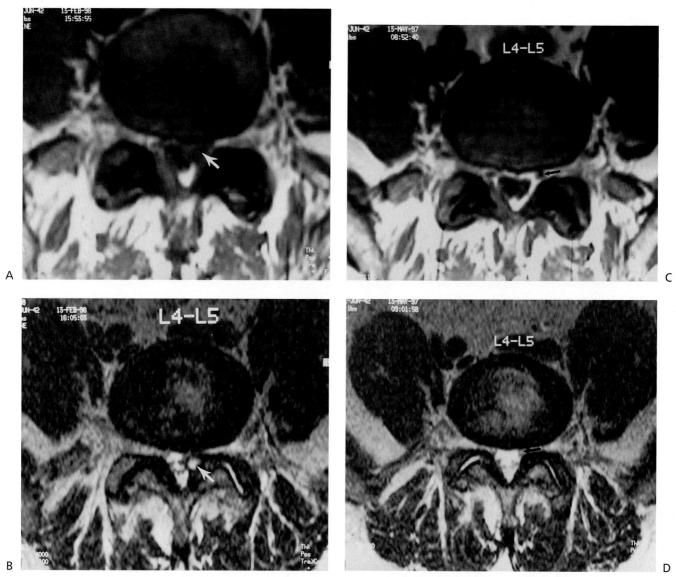

FIGURE 9.24. Synovial cyst of facet joint. Axial T1- and T2-weighted images **(A,B)**, and follow-up axial T1- and T2-weighted images **(C,D)** on a follow up scan. The patient had acute left L-5 radicular symptoms at the time images **(A)** and **(B)** were obtained. They demonstrate a synovial cyst (*white arrows*) projecting from the left L4-5 facet joint into the left lateral recess with compression of the left L-5 nerve root. The follow-up images **(C,D)** were obtained when the patient was asymptomatic; they demonstrate resolution of the synovial cyst with no compression of the left L-5 nerve root. The nerve root is seen surrounded by normal epidural fat (*black arrows*).

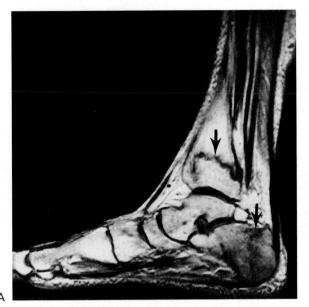
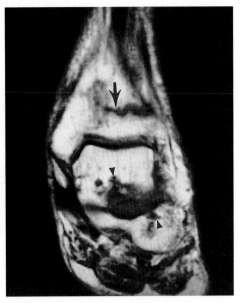

FIGURE 9.25. Stress fracture of the ankle. T1-weighted sagittal and coronal **(A,B)** SE images of the ankle. The examination demonstrates a stress fracture of the distal tibia and of the calcaneus (*black arrows*). There is greater bone marrow edema associated with the calcaneal fracture that is comminuted. The coronal images also demonstrate erosion of the talus and calcaneus (*black arrowheads*).

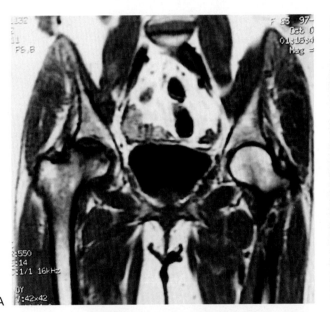
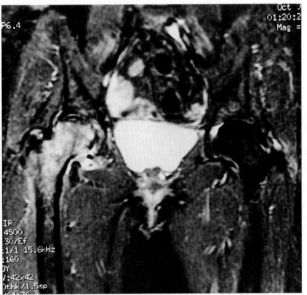

FIGURE 9.26. AVN of the hip. T1-weighted coronal SE **(A)**, and STIR coronal **(B)** images through the hips demonstrate typical signal changes of AVN of the right hip. Curvilinear decreased signal is noted on the T1-weighted images. The STIR images demonstrate marked edematous changes of the femoral head and neck.

and 9.16), ankle (Fig 9.15), and hip joint (Figs. 9.14 and 9.26) in both arthritis and nonarthritis patients. Tendon and ligament involvement by rheumatoid arthritis is frequently not considered clinically in larger joints early in the disease, and may go undiagnosed, resulting in extensive degeneration and possible tear.

MRI allows for early detection and treatment with surgical intervention. This is of particular importance in the eval-

uation of rotator cuff pathology. Early diagnosis and repair is critical to the surgical outcome of rotator cuff repair and significantly impacts shoulder function in the postoperative patient. MRI provides far greater information about the shoulder than any other imaging modality (Figs. 9.11, 9.17, and 9.27). The articular cartilage of the glenohumeral joint is usually destroyed evenly across the entire joint and erosion of the glenoid occurs medially in inflammatory arthritis.

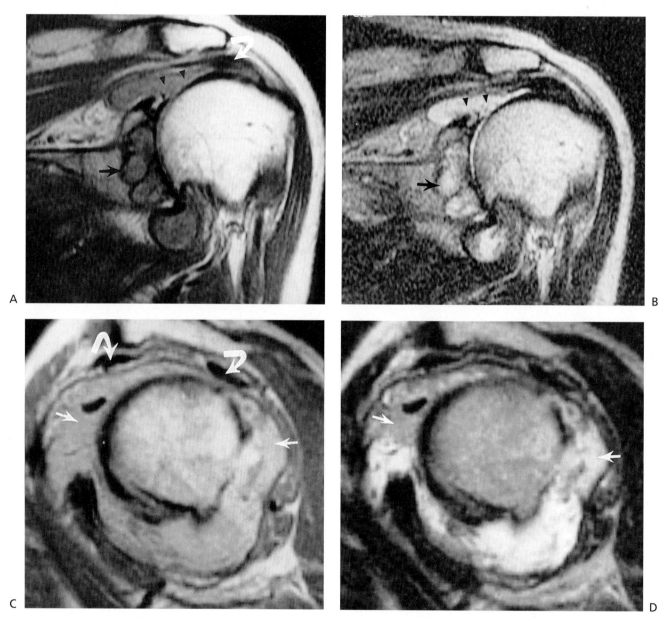

FIGURE 9.27. Rheumatoid arthritis of the shoulder. Oblique coronal PD- and T2-weighted SE images **(A,B)**. Oblique sagittal PD- and T2-weighted SE images at the level of the humeral head **(C,D)**, and at the level of the glenoid **(E,F)**, and axial T2-weighted GRE images through the glenohumeral joint **(G,H)**. AP **(I)**, and lateral **(J)** radiographs. The images demonstrate narrowing of the glenohumeral joint, subchondral cysts of the glenoid, and lateral humeral head (*black arrows*). The joint effusion (*black arrowheads*) and synovial hypertrophy (*white arrows*) have similar signal intensity on the PDW image **(C)**, but can be distinguished on the T2-weighted image **(D)**. The long head of the biceps tendon and the supraspinatus and infraspinatus tendons are seen as very low signal intensity black structures (*curved white arrows*).

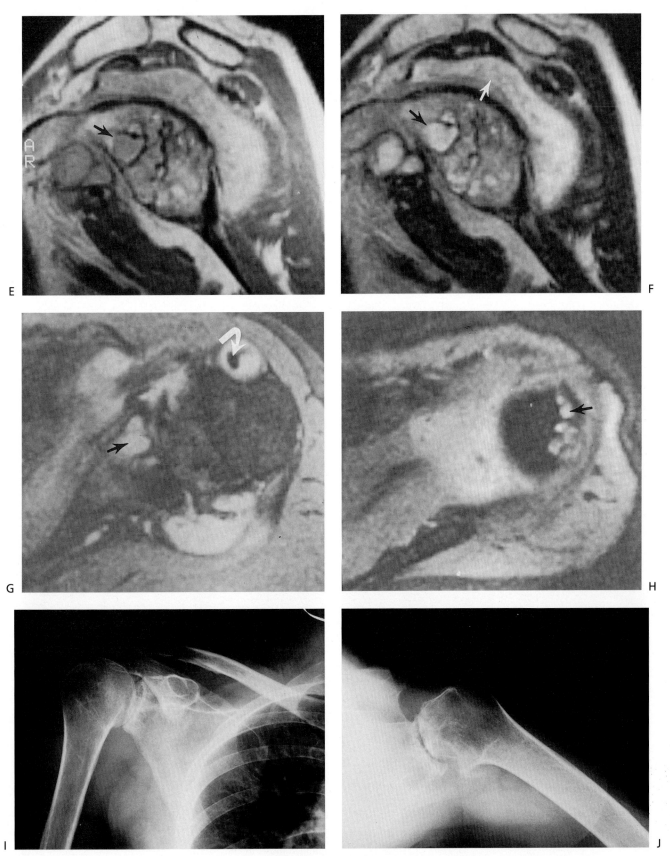

FIGURE 9.27. *(continued)*

Long-term involvement leads to osteopenia and more severe erosion. The osteopenia can be hastened by steroid administration. MRI demonstrates early erosion as well as small and large intraosseous cysts (Figs. 9.9, 9.10, 9.17, and 9.27). MRI is sensitive to mild synovitis as well as to the detection of hypertrophied synovium (Fig. 9.27). MRI also demonstrates the quality of the rotator cuff (degree of degeneration or tear), and is sensitive to early degeneration or involvement from RA. Between 25% and 45% of patients with RA develop rotator cuff tears. Early or small tears, as well as partial thickness tears, are routinely demonstrated by MRI (Fig. 9.11). MR arthrography of the shoulder is more sensitive to partial tears and small full-thickness tears of the rotator cuff.

MRI OF THE SPINE

MRI is the preferred imaging modality for evaluation of the spine, both for disc disease and spinal cord pathology. Spinal stenosis resulting from combined degeneration of the inter-

vertebral disc and facet joints is more common in the lower lumbar spine (Fig. 9.28). The end-stage manifestations of ankylosing spondylitis (AS) are also most severe in the cervical spine (Fig. 9.29). MRI is ideally suited in evaluating RA involvement of the cervical spine (Figs. 9.30–9.32). Spinal involvement by RA is mainly limited to the cervical spine. Thoracic and lumbar spine involvement by RA is infrequent and usually insignificant. Approximately 50% of patients with RA have involvement of the cervical spine. The severity of rheumatoid involvement of the cervical spine frequently does not correlate with the clinical symptoms, including neurologic findings. Also, significant pannus formation and cord compression may be present with relatively little or minimal C1-2 instability on radiographs. Even though there is frequent involvement of the cervical spine, surgery is necessary in only a small percentage of patients with RA. The goals of surgery are to relieve spinal cord or brainstem compression (Fig. 9.31), and stabilize the cervical spine.

Radiographs with flexion lateral views are the gold standard in the evaluation of the stability of the cervical spine,

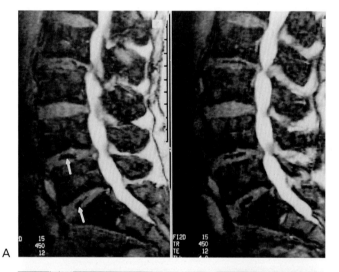

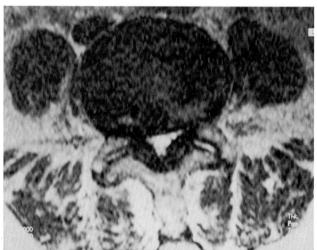

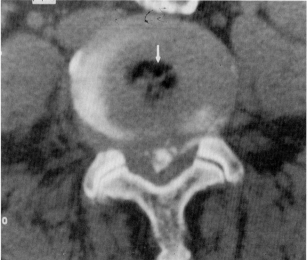

FIGURE 9.28. Degenerative disc disease of the lumbar spine. Two-dimensional T2-weighted GRE sagittal and T2-weighted axial spin echo **(A,B)**, and axial CT myelogram **(C)** demonstrate severe spinal stenosis at the L4-5 level owing to a combination of diffusely bulging annulus and marked ligamentous and facet hypertrophy. The sagittal image shows the multilevel stenosis as well as the multilevel degenerative changes with vacuum cleft involvement of multiple disc spaces (*white arrows*).

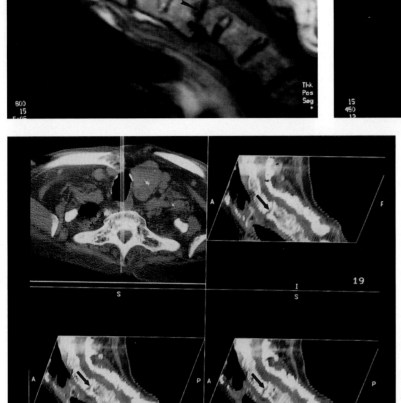

FIGURE 9.29. Ankylosing spondylitis involvement of the cervical spine. T1-weighted sagittal SE **(A)**, and T2-weighted sagittal GRE images **(B)**, and sagittally reconstructed CT images **(E,F)** demonstrate near complete fusion of the cervical intervertebral disc spaces with a resultant flexion deformity. There is a fracture through the C6-7 disc space (*black arrows*) with mild offset with impingement on the ventral cord (*white arrow*).

including the C1-2 level. Radiographs also clearly document degenerative disc disease and erosion of the odontoid from pannus, but they are limited to the osseous findings and narrowing of the disc spaces. The ability to image the osseous and soft-tissue structures of the spine in the sagittal plane is of critical importance in patients with RA. The common and significant sequelae of rheumatoid involvement of the cervical spine is best demonstrated in the lateral view or sagittal plane. Compression of the cervical spinal cord typically occurs between the odontoid process or periodontotic pannus and the posterior arch of C-1 in patients with RA who have C1-2 laxity (Fig. 9.32). MRI in the sagittal plane is ideally suited for the detection and evaluation of spinal cord compression, and is commonly used in presurgical planning. MRI scans can be obtained in the sagittal plane with the patient's spine in neutral and hyperextension/flexion positions (Fig. 9.30) to evaluate and visualize the degree of cord compression with positional change. MRI also allows for evaluation of the cervical spinal cord for myelopathy or signal changes associated with cord compression. Additionally, MRI is helpful in

evaluating the postoperative patient following decompressive stabilizing surgery to ensure there has been adequate surgical decompression and relief of spinal cord compression (Fig. 9.32).

Rheumatoid synovitis can involve multiple joints and synovial-lined spaces of the cervical spine. The inflammatory synovitis can involve the facet and uncovertebral joints of Luschka, the articulations of the occipital condyles and the atlas, as well as the synovial lined space between the odontoid and the transverse ligament. The most frequent imaging findings are seen in the upper cervical spine at the C1-2 level and occiput. Three common cervical spine abnormalities can result from rheumatoid involvement: C1-2 subluxation, subaxial subluxation (subluxation below the level of C-2), and superior migration of the odontoid. C1-2 subluxation and subaxial subluxation may lead to compression of the cervical spinal cord, whereas basilar invagination may result in compression of the brainstem (medulla). Subluxations in the cervical spine in patients with RA are most common at C1-2. Subaxial subluxations occur more commonly at C2-3 and C3-4.

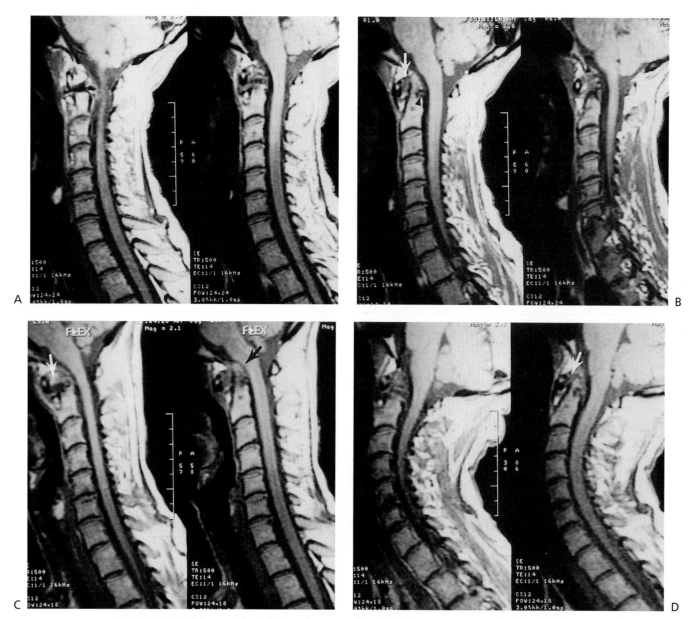

FIGURE 9.30. Rheumatoid arthritis involvement of the cervical spine. T1-weighted sagittal SE images and neutral **(A,B)**, flexion **(C)**, and extension **(D)**. T2-weighted sagittal SE images **(E,F)**, axial T2-weighted GRE **(G)**, T1-weighted axial SE **(H)**, axial CT **(I)**, coronal **(J)**, and sagittal **(K)** plane CT reconstructions. The sagittal MR images demonstrate abnormal widening of the atlantodens distance (*white arrows*). This increases with flexion and decreases with extension. There is also impingement on the cervicomedullary junction with flexion (*black arrow*). Also noted is degenerative change with hypertrophic spurring of the left C1-2 articulation. The spurring extends into the left lateral canal and recess (*open black arrows*). There is also erosion of the odontoid tip (*black arrowheads*).

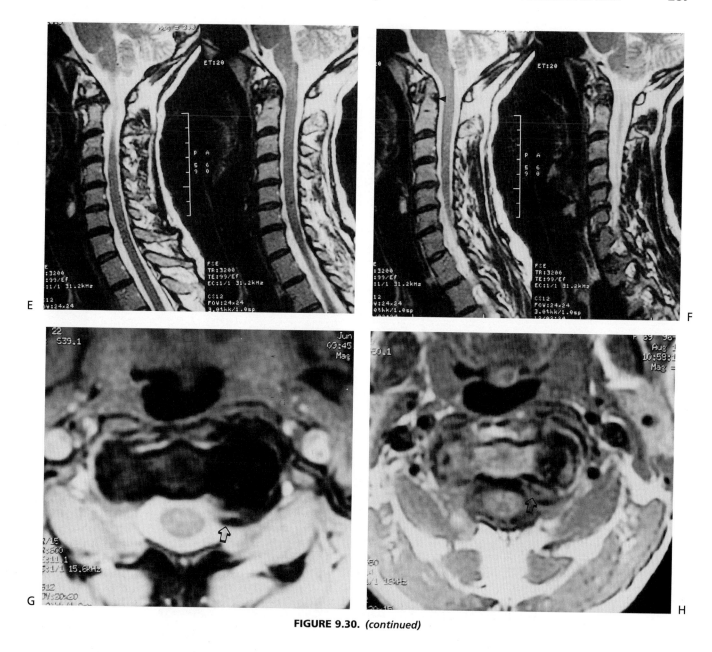

FIGURE 9.30. *(continued)*

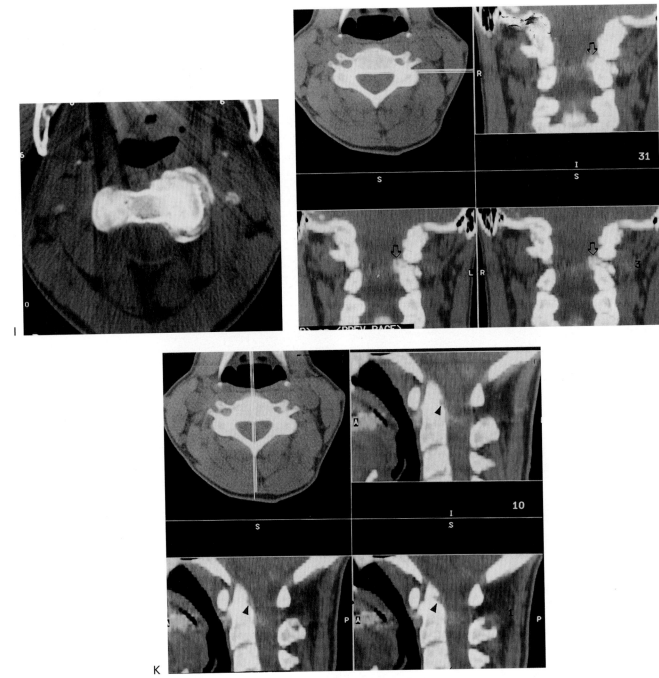

FIGURE 9.30. *(continued)*

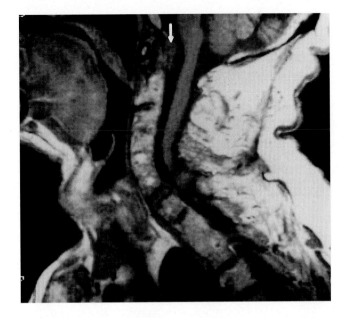

FIGURE 9.31. Rheumatoid arthritis involvement of the cervical spine. T1-weighted sagittal SE image demonstrates abnormal soft tissue representing pannus (*white arrow*) posterior to the odontoid process and erosive changes of the odontoid. Also note the near complete fusion of the cervical disc spaces.

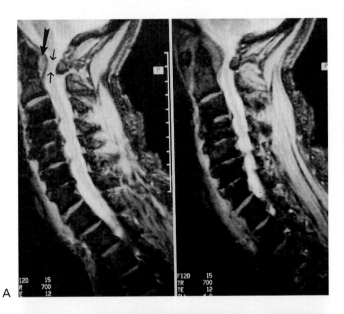

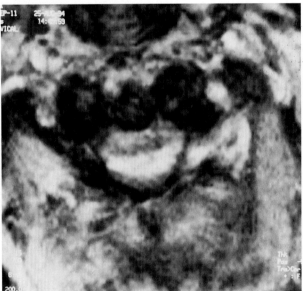

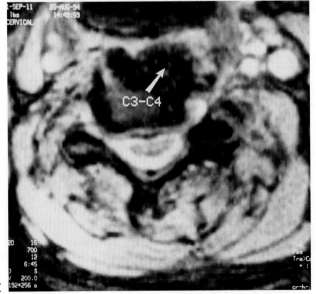

FIGURE 9.32. Rheumatoid arthritis involvement of the cervical spine. Two-dimensional T2-weighted GRE sagittal **(A)** and axial **(B-D)** and T1-weighted sagittal and axial **(E,F)**, and postsurgical T1-weighted sagittal spin echo images **(G)**. The multiplanar images demonstrate abnormal soft-tissue mass posterior to the odontoid process representing pannus (*black arrows*). There is compression of the cervical spinal cord between the pannus and posterior arch of C-1 (*small black arrows*). The spinal cord compression is relieved by the posterior decompression (white arrowhead). Also noted are the marked degenerative changes of the cervical disc spaces and uncovertebral joints (*white arrows*).

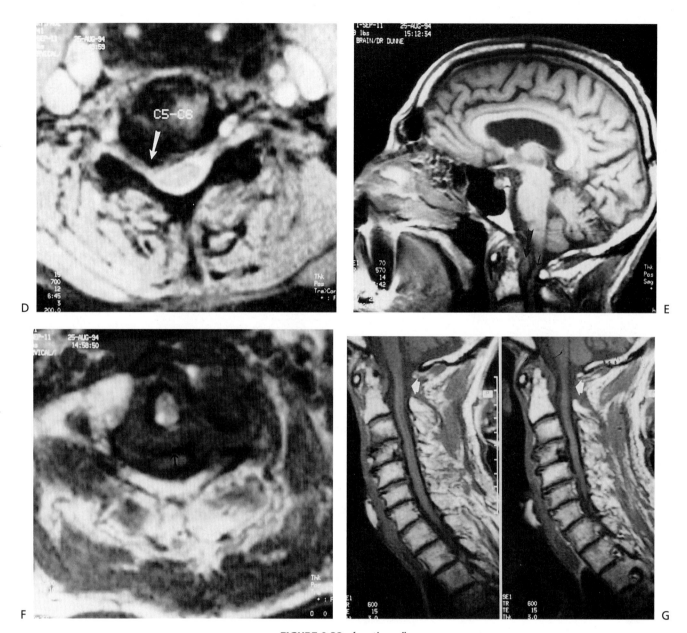

FIGURE 9.32. *(continued)*

Atlantoaxial instability is the most common instability seen with RA and results from rheumatoid involvement of the C1-2 articulation and the invasion of the alar and transverse ligaments, which hold and stabilize the anterior arch of C-1 to the odontoid process. When involved by rheumatoid synovitis the C1-2 joint becomes lax and allows abnormal motion or movement of C-1 on C-2 (Fig. 9.30). A synovial-lined space separates the transverse ligament and the odontoid. Rheumatoid synovitis involvement of this space leads to laxity of the transverse ligament and allows for widening of the atlantodens distance and atlantoaxial subluxation. Invasion or destruction of the transverse and alar ligaments leads to greater C1-2 instability. With progression of the inflamma-

tory process, granulation tissue or pannus may extensively invade the periodontotic soft tissues and erode the odontoid. The periodontotic pannus may compress the cervical spinal cord or cervicomedullary junction (Figs. 9.30 and 9.31).

Anterior subluxation of C-1 leads to widening of the atlantodens distance on lateral radiographs and MRI. The normal atlantodens distance is 3 mm or less in adults. This distance can measure greater than 10 mm in patients with RA. This is most accurately measured with lateral radiographs, but can also be detected with MRI. The distance between the posterior margin of the odontoid and the anterior arch of C-1 is the space available for the cervical spinal cord. As the atlantodens instability worsens, the distance between the odontoid and the posterior arch of C1 decreases. If peri-odontotic pannus is present, this further decreases the distance between the odontoid and posterior arch of C1 and decreases the space available for the cervical spinal cord and can result in spinal cord compression. The periodontotic pannus progression of disease may erode the dens (Fig. 9.30). Bone erosion of the dens is best evaluated on CT, but is also demonstrated with MRI and radiographs.

Rheumatoid synovitis may involve the apophyseal or facet joints and invade the anterior and posterior longitudinal ligaments. This can result in laxity of the facet joints and ligaments that eventually leads to instability. The discovertebral junction can become involved in patients with RA (spondylodiscitis) either by invasion of pannus from the uncovertebral joints or the biomechanical instability caused by laxity of the facet and uncovertebral joints and anterior/posterior longitudinal ligament laxity. This can also result in fusion of the disc spaces (Fig. 9.31). The instability can lead to subluxation or vertebral body offset and may result in cord compression. When the instability and subluxation is combined with disc disease (either disc bulge, protrusions, or spondylosis), significant cord compression and myelopathy may occur in the cervical spine below the C-2 level, usually centered at the disc spaces.

Involvement of the C1-2 facet joints and the articulation of the occipital condyles and atlas can result in erosion and collapse of the structures. This allows the odontoid to migrate superiorly or vertically. The odontoid can extend into the foramen magnum and compress the brainstem.

SUMMARY

MRI is more sensitive than radiographs in detecting the early or subtle cartilaginous and osseous erosion of RA. Radiographs are limited to the bony changes. Radiographs document bone erosion and osseous sequelae, but cannot image cartilage. Articular cartilage thinning or erosion is implied by narrowing of a joint space. MRI permits direct visualization, and therefore, assessment of both the soft-tissue and osseous sequelae of RA. MRI demonstrates not only subtle and significant bone erosion, but also allows visualization of synovitis, hyperplastic synovium, pannus, and the involvement of ligaments, tendons, and fibrocartilage.

MRI provides soft-tissue and osseous information that cannot be obtained from the clinical examination or any other imaging modality. Even with these advantages, MRI does not currently have a clear-cut or defined role in the staging or evaluation of RA or the common arthritides. With the continued evolution and refinement of treatment and MRI, MRI is expected to have a more clearly defined role in the evaluation, assessment, and staging of patients with RA in the future.

REFERENCES

1. Abu-Shakra M, Toker R, Flusser D. Clinical and radiographic outcomes of rheumatoid arthritis patients not treated with disease-modifying drugs. *Radiology* 1998;209:591.
2. Adam G, Dammer M, Bohndorf K, et al. Rheumatoid arthritis of the knee: value of gadopentetate dimeglumine-enhanced MR imaging. *AJR* 1991;156:125.
3. Aisen AM, Martel W, Ellis JH, et al. Cervical spine involvement in rheumatoid arthritis: MR imaging. *Radiology* 1987;165:159.
4. Albert K, Michel S, Gunther U, et al. 13C NMR investigation of synovial fluids. *MRI Med* 1993;30:236.
5. Babyn PS, Kim HKW, Lemaire C. High-resolution magnetic resonance imaging of normal porcine cartilaginous epiphyseal maturation. *JMRI* 1996;6:172.
6. Bacic G, Liu KJ, Goda F, et al. MRI contrast enhanced study of cartilage proteoglycan degradation in the rabbit knee. *MRI Med* 1997;37:764.
7. Bashir A, Gray MI, Burstein D. Gd-DTPA^2 as a measure of cartilage degradation. *MRI Med* 1996;36:665.
8. Bell GR, Stearns KL. Flexion-extension MRI of the upper rheumatoid cervical spine. *Orthopedics* 1991;14:973.
9. Beltran J, Campanini DS, Knight C, et al. The diabetic foot: magnetic resonance imaging evaluation. *Skeletal Radiol* 1990; 19:37–41.
10. Beltran J, Caudill JL, Herman LA, et al. Rheumatoid arthritis: MR imaging manifestations. *Radiology* 1987;165:153.
11. Bjorkengren AG, Geborek P, Rydholm U, et al. MR imaging of the knee in acute rheumatoid arthritis: synovial uptake of Gadolinium-DOTA. *AJR* 1990;155:329.
12. Bjorkengren AG, et al. Spontaneous osteonecrosis of the knee: value of MR imaging in determining prognosis. *AJR* 1990; 154:331.
13. Blandino A, Salvi L, Chirico G, et al. Synovial osteochondromatosis of the ankle: MR findings. *Clin Imag* 1992;16:34.
14. Boden SD, Dodge LD, Bohlman HH, et al. Rheumatoid arthritis of the cervical spine: long-term analysis with predicators of paralysis and recovery. *Radiology* 1994;191:882.
15. Braun J, Bollow M, Eggens U, et al. Use of dynamic magnetic resonance imaging with fast imaging in the detection of early and advanced sacroiliitis in spondyloarthropathy patients. *Arthritis Rheumatol* 1994;37:1039.
16. Britton CA, Wasko MC. Rheumatoid arthritis. *Roentgenology* 1996;31:198.
17. Broderick LS, Turner DA, Renfrew DL, et al. Severity of articular cartilage abnormality in patients with osteoarthritis: evaluation with fast spin-echo MR vs arthroscopy. *AJR* 1994; 162:99–103.
18. Brown DG, Edwards NL, Greer JM, et al. Magnetic resonance imaging in patients with inflammatory arthritis of the knee. *Clin Rheumatol* 1990;9:73.
19. Bundschuh C, Modic MT, Kearney F, et al. Rheumatoid arthritis of the cervical spine: surface-coil MR imaging. *AJR* 1988; 151:181.
20. Castelijns JA, van den Brekel MWM, Tobi H, et al. Laryngeal carcinoma after radiation therapy: correlation of abnormal MR imaging signal patterns in laryngeal cartilage with the risk of recurrence. *Radiology* 1996;198:151.
21. Chan WP, Lang P, Chieng PU, et al. Three-dimensional imaging of the musculoskeletal system: an overview. *J Formos Med Assoc* 1991;90:713–722.
22. Chan WP, Lang P, Stevens MP, et al. Osteoarthritis of the knee: comparison of radiography, CT, and MR imaging to assess extent and severity. *AJR* 1991;157:799–806.

23. Cole PR, Jasani MK, Wood B, et al. High resolution, high field magnetic resonance imaging of joints: unexpected features in proton images of cartilage. *Br J Radiol* 1990;63:907–909.

24. Corvetta A, Giovagnoni A, Baldelli S, et al. MR imaging of rheumatoid hand lesions: comparison with conventional radiology in 31 patients. *Clin Exp Rheumatol* 1992;10:217.

25. Dardzinski BJ, Mosher TJ, Li S, et al. Spatial variation of T2 in human articular cartilage. *Radiology* 1997;205:456.

26. Disler DG. Fat-suppressed three-dimensional spoiled gradient-recalled MR imaging: assessment of articular and physeal hyaline cartilage. *AJR* 1997;169:1117.

27. Disler DG, McCauley TR, Kelman CG, et al. Fat-suppressed three-dimensional spoiled gradient-echo MR imaging of hyaline cartilage defects in the knee: comparison with standard MR imaging and arthroscopy. *AJR* 1996;167:127.

28. Drapé JL, Thelen P, Gay-Depassier P, et al. Intraarticular diffusion of Gd-DOTA after intravenous injection of the knee: MR imaging evaluation. *Radiology* 1993;188:227.

29. Drapé JL, Pessis E, Auleley GR, et al. Quantitative MR imaging evaluation of chondropathy in osteoarthritic knees. *Radiology* 1998;208:49.

30. Duyvuri U, Reddy R, Patel SD, et al. T_{1P}-relaxation in articular cartilage: effects of enzymatic degradation. *MRI Med* 1997;38:863.

31. Eckstein F, Sittek H, Gavazzeni A, et al. Magnetic resonance chondro-crassometry (MR CCM): method for accurate determination of articular cartilage thickness? *MRI Med* 1996;35:89.

32. Eckstein F, Tieschky M, Faber SC, et al. Effect of physical exercise on cartilage volume and thickness in vivo: MR imaging study. *Radiology* 1998;207:243.

33. Eckstein F, Westhoff J, Sittek H, et al. In vivo reproducibility of three-dimensional cartilage volume and thickness measurements with MR imaging. *AJR* 1998;170:593.

34. Einig M, Higer HP, Meairs S, et al. Magnetic resonance imaging of the craniocervical junction in rheumatoid arthritis: value, limitations, indications. *Skeletal Radiol* 1990;19:341.

35. Ensign MF. Magnetic resonance imaging of hip disorders. *Semin Ultrasound CT MRI* 1990;11:288.

36. Erickson SJ, Cox IH, Hyde JS, et al. Effect of tendon orientation on MR imaging signal intensity: a manifestation of the "magic angle" phenomenon. *Radiology* 1991;181:389.

37. Erickson SJ, Prost RW. Laminar structures on MR imaging of articular cartilage. *Radiology* 1997;204:16.

38. Erickson SJ, Waldschmidt JG, Czervionke LF, et al. Hyaline cartilage: truncation artifact as a cause of trilaminar appearance with fat-suppressed three-dimensional spoiled gradient-recalled sequences. *Radiology* 1996;201:260.

39. Fagerlund M, Björnebrink J, Ekelund L, et al. Ultra low field MR imaging of cervical spine involvement in rheumatoid arthritis. *Acta Radiol* 1992;33:89.

40. Fezoulidis I, Neuhold A, Wicke L, et al. Diagnostic imaging of the occipito-cervical junction in patients with rheumatoid arthritis: plain films, computed tomography, magnetic resonance imaging. *Eur J Radiol* 1989;9:5.

41. Flandry F, Hughston JC, McCann SB, et al. Diagnostic features of diffuse pigmented villonodular synovitis of the knee. *Clin Orthop Rel Res* 1994;298:212.

42. Frank LR, Brossmann J, Buxton RB. MR imaging truncation artifacts can create a false laminar appearance in cartilage. *AJR* 1997;168:547.

43. Freeman DM, Bergman G, Glover G. Short TE MR microscopy: accurate measurement and zonal differentiation of normal hyaline cartilage. *MRI Med* 1997;38:72.

44. Fry ME, Jacoby RK, Hutton CW, et al. High-resolution magnetic resonance imaging of the interphalangeal joints of the hand. *Skeletal Radiol* 1991;20:273–277.

45. Gilkeson G, Polisson R, Sinclair H, et al. Early detection of carpal erosions in patients with rheumatoid arthritis: a pilot study of magnetic resonance imaging. *J Rheumatol* 1988;15:1361.

46. Goodwin DW, Wadghiri YZ, Dunn JF. Micro-imaging of articular cartilage: T2, proton density, and the magic angle effect. *Acad Radiol* 1998;5:790.

47. Graudal NA, Jurik AG, de Carvalho A, et al. Radiographic progression in rheumatoid arthritis: long-term prospective study of 109 patients. *Radiology* 1998;209:887.

48. Gründer W, Biesold M, Wagner M, et al. Improved nuclear magnetic resonance microscopic visualization of joint cartilage using liposome entrapped contrast agents. *Invest Radiol* 1998;33:193.

49. Gründer W, Wagner M, Werner A. MR-microscopic visualization of anisotropic internal cartilage structures using the magic angle technique. *MRI Med* 1998;39:376.

50. Gubler FM, Algra PR, Maas M, et al. Gadolinium-DTPA enhanced magnetic resonance imaging of bone cysts in patients with rheumatoid arthritis. *Ann Rheum Dis* 1993;62:716.

51. Hajnal JV, Saeed N, Saor EJ, et al. A registration and interpolation procedure for subvoxel matching of serially acquired MR images. *J Comput Assist Tomogr* 1995;19:289–296.

52. Hardy PA, Recht MP, Piraino D, et al. Optimization of a dual echo in the steady state (DES) free-precession sequence for imaging cartilage. *JMRI* 1996;6:329.

53. Harris EDJ. Rheumatoid arthritis: pathophysiology and implications for therapy. *N Engl J Med* 1990;322:1277.

54. Havdrup T, Hulth A, Telhag H. The subchondral bone in osteoarthritis and rheumatoid arthritis of the knee: a histologic and microradiographical study. *Acta Orthop Scand* 1976;47:345.

55. Herberhoid C, Stammberger T, Faber S, et al. MR-based technique for quantifying the deformation of articular cartilage during mechanical loading in an intact cadaver joint. *MRI Med* 1998;39:843.

56. Hervé-Somma CMP, Sebah GH, Prieur AM, et al. Juvenile rheumatoid arthritis of the knee: MR evaluation with Gd-DOTA. *Radiology* 1992;182:92.

57. Herzog S, Mafee M. Synovial chondromatosis of the TMJ: MR and CT findings. *AJNR* 1990;11:742.

58. Hodler J, Resnick D. Current status of imaging of articular cartilage. *Skeletal Radiol* 1996;25:703.

59. Iannauzzi L, Dawson N, Zein N, et al. Does any therapy slow radiographic progression in rheumatoid arthritis? *N Engl J Med* 1983;309:1023.

60. Insko EK, Reddy R, Leigh JS. High resolution, short echo time sodium imaging of articular cartilage. *JMRI* 1997;7:1056.

61. Jaffe IA. New approaches to the management of rheumatoid arthritis. *J Rheumatol* 1992;19(Suppl 36):2.

62. Jaramillo D, Connolly SA, Mulkern R, et al. Developing epiphysis: MR imaging characteristics and histologic correlation in the newborn lamb. *Radiology* 1998;207:49.

63. Jelinek JS, Kransdorf MJ, Utz JA, et al. Imaging of pigmented villonodular synovitis with emphasis on MR imaging. *AJR* 1989;152:337.

64. Jevtic V, Watt I, Rozman B, et al. Distinctive radiological features of small hand joints in rheumatoid arthritis and seronegative spondyloarthritis demonstrated by contrast-enhanced (Gd-DTPA) magnetic resonance imaging. *Skeletal Radiol* 1995;24:351.

65. Jevtic V, Watt I, Rozman B, et al. Precontrast and postcontrast (Gd-DTPA) magnetic resonance imaging of hand joints in patients with rheumatoid arthritis. *Clin Radiol* 1993;48:176.

66. Karasick D, Schweitzer ME. Tear of the posterior tibial tendon causing asymmetric flatfoot: radiologic findings. *AJR* 1993;161:1237.

67. Kawaida H, Sakou T, Moprizono Y, et al. Magnetic resonance imaging of upper cervical disorders in rheumatoid arthritis. *Spine* 1989;14:1144.
68. Kaye JJ. Radiographic methods of assessment (scoring) of rheumatoid disease. *Rheumatol Dis Clin North Am* 1991; 17:457.
69. Kieft GH, Dijkmans BAC, Bloem JL, et al. Magnetic resonance imaging of the shoulder in patient with rheumatoid arthritis. *Ann Rheumatic Dis* 1990;49:7.
70. Kim DK, Ceckler TL, Hascall VC, et al. Analysis of water-macromolecule proton magnetization transfer in articular cartilage. *MRI Med* 1993;29:211–215.
71. Konig H, Sieper J, Wolf KJ. Rheumatoid arthritis: evaluation of hypervascular and fibrous pannus with dynamic MR imaging enhanced with Gd-DTPA. *Radiology* 1990;176:473.
72. Kottal RA, Vogler JBI, Matamoros A, et al. Pigmented villonodular synovitis: a report of MR imaging in two cases. *Radiology* 1987;163:551.
73. Kramer J, Jolesz F, Kleefield J. Rheumatoid arthritis of the cervical spine. *Rheumatic Dis Clin North Am* 1991;17:757.
74. Kramer J, Recht M, Deely DM, et al. MR appearance of idiopathic synovial osteochondromatosis. *J Comput Assist Tomogr* 1993;17:772.
75. Kramer J, Recht MP, Imhof H, et al. Postcontrast MR arthrography in assessment of cartilage lesions. *J Comput Assist Tomogr* 1994;18:218–224.
76. Krodel A, Refior HJ, Westermann S. The importance of functional magnetic resonance imaging (MRI) in the planning of stabilizing operations on the cervical spine in rheumatoid patients. *Arch Orthop Trauma Surg* 1989;109:30.
77. Kuksaka Y, Grunder W, Rumpel H, et al. MR microimaging of articular cartilage and contrast enhancement by manganese ions. *MRI Med* 1992;24:137–148.
78. Kursunoglu-Brahme S, Riccio T, Wiesman MH, et al. Rheumatoid knee: role of gadopentetate-enhanced MR imaging. *Radiology* 1990;176:831.
79. Lang P, Genant HK, Jergesen HE, et al. Imaging of the hip joint. Computed tomography versus magnetic resonance imaging. *Clin Orthop Rel Res* 1992;274:135.
80. Larsson EM, Holtas S, Zygmunt S. Pre- and postoperative MR imaging of the craniocervical junction in rheumatoid arthritis. *AJR* 1989;152:561.
81. Lavid NE, DePaolis DC, Pope TW, et al. Analysis of three-dimensional computerized representations of articular cartilage lesions. *Invest Radiol* 1996;31:577.
82. Law TC, Chong SF, Iu PP, et al. Bilateral subacromial bursitis with macroscopic rice bodies: ultrasound, CT and MR appearance. *Australas Radiol* 1998;42:161.
83. Lehtinen A, Paimela I, Kreula J, et al. Painful ankle region in rheumatoid arthritis: analysis of soft-tissue changes with ultrasonography and MR imaging. *Acta Radiol* 1996;37: 572.
84. Lesperance LM, Gray ML, Burstein D. Determination of fixed charge density in cartilage using nuclear magnetic resonance. *J Orthop Res* 1992;10:1–13.
85. Li KC, Higgs J, Aisen AM, et al. MRI in osteoarthritis of the hip: gradation of severity. *MRI Imaging* 1988;6:229.
86. Lupetin AR, Daffner RH. Rheumatoid iliopsoas bursitis: MR findings. *J Comput Assist Tomog* 1990;14:1035.
87. Matsuda Y, Miyazaki K, Tada K, et al. Increased MR signal intensity due to cervical myelopathy: analysis of 29 surgical cases. *J Neurosurg* 1991;74:887.
88. Maurice H, Crone M, Watt I. Synovial chondromatosis. *J Bone Joint Surg [Br]* 1988;70:807.
89. McCauley TR, Disler DG. MR imaging of articular cartilage. *Radiology* 1998;209:629.
90. McGibbon CA, Dupuy DE, Palmer WE, et al. Cartilage and subchondral bone thickness distribution with MR imaging. *Acad Radiol* 1998;5:20.
91. Milbrink J, Nyman R. Posterior stabilization of the cervical spine in rheumatoid arthritis: clinical results and magnetic resonance imaging correlation. *J Spinal Disord* 1990;3:308.
92. Mitchell M, Howard B, Haller J, et al. Septic arthritis. *Radiol Clin North Am* 1988;26:1295–1313.
93. Modl JM, Sether LA, Haughton VM, et al. Articular cartilage: correlation of histologic zones with signal intensity at MR imaging. *Radiology* 1991;181:853–855.
94. Moore EA, Jacoby RK, Ellis RE, et al. Demonstration of a geode by magnetic resonance imaging: a new light on the cause of juxta-articular bone cysts in rheumatoid arthritis. *Ann Rheum Dis* 1990;49:785.
95. Moore TE, Yuh WTC, Kathol MH, et al. Abnormalities of the foot in patients with diabetes mellitus: findings on MR imaging. *AJR* 1991;157:813–816.
96. Morishita Y, Rubin SJ, Hicks DG, et al. MR imaging of rabbit hip cartilage with a clinical imager and specifically designed surface coils. *Acad Radiol* 1998;5:365.
97. Munk PL, Vellet AD, Levin MF, et al. Intravenous administration of gadolinium in the evaluation of rheumatoid arthritis of the shoulder. *Can Assoc Radiol J* 1993;44:99.
98. Murphy FP, Dahlin DC, Sullivan CR. Articular synovial chondromatosis. *J Bone Joint Surg [Am]* 1962;44:77.
99. Nakahura N, Uetani M, Hayashi K, et al. Gadolinium-enhanced MR imaging of the wrist in rheumatoid arthritis: value of fat suppression pulse sequences. *Skeletal Radiol* 1996; 25:639.
100. Nokes SR, King PS, Garcia R Jr, et al. Temporomandibular joint chondromatosis with intracranial extension: MR and CT contributions. *AJR* 1987;148:1173.
101. Ogilvie-Harris DJ, McLean J, Zarnett ME. Pigmented villonodular synovitis of the knee. *J Bone Joint Surg [Am]* 1992; 74:119.
102. Oneson SR, Timins ME, Scales LM, et al. MR imaging diagnosis of triangular fibrocartilage pathology with arthroscopic correlation. *AJR* 1997;168:1513.
103. Ostergaard M, Gideon P, Henrikson O, et al. Synovial volume: a marker of disease severity in rheumatoid arthritis? Quantification by MRI. *Scand J Rheumatol* 1994;23:197.
104. Papadopoulos SM, Dickman CA, Sonntag VKH. Atlantoaxial stabilization in rheumatoid arthritis. *J Neurosurg* 1991;74:1.
105. Paul PK, Jasani MK, Sebok D, et al. Variation in MR signal intensity across normal human knee cartilage. *JMRI* 1993; 3:569–574.
106. Peterfy CG, Genant HK. Emerging applications of magnetic resonance imaging in the evaluation of articular cartilage. *Radiol Clin North Am* 1996;34:195.
107. Peterfy CG, Majumdar S, Lang P, et al. MR imaging of the arthritic knee: improved discrimination of cartilage, synovium and effusion with pulsed saturation transfer and fat-suppressed T1-weighted sequences. *Radiology* 1994;191:413–419.
108. Peterfy CG, van Dijke CF, Janzen DL, et al. Quantification of articular cartilage in the knee by pulsed saturation transfer and fat-suppressed MRI: optimization and validation. *Radiology* 1994;192:485–491.
109. Peterfy CG, van Dijke CF, Lu Y, et al. Quantification of articular cartilage in the metacarpophalangeal joints of the hand: accuracy and precision of 3D MR imaging. *AJR* 1995; 165:371–375.
110. Pettersson H, Larsson EM, Holtas S, et al. MR imaging of the cervical spine in rheumatoid arthritis. *AJNR* 1988;9:573.
111. Pilch L, Stewart C, Gordon D, et al. Assessment of cartilage volume in the femorotibial joint with magnetic resonance imaging

and 3D computer reconstruction. *J Rheumatol* 1994;21: 2307–2321.

112. Poleksic L, Zdravkovic D, Jablanovic D, et al. Magnetic resonance imaging of bone destruction in rheumatoid arthritis: comparison with radiography. *Skeletal Radiol* 1993;22:577.

113. Poletti SC, Gates HS, Martinez SM, et al. The use of magnetic resonance imaging in the diagnosis of pigmented villonodular synovitis. *Orthopedics* 1990;13:185.

114. Polisson RP, Schoenberg OI, Fischman A, et al. Use of magnetic resonance imaging and positron emission tomography in the assessment of synovial volume and glucose metabolism in patients with rheumatoid arthritis. *Arthritis Rheumatol* 1995;38:819.

115. Quinn SF, Rose PM, Brown TR, et al. MR imaging of the patellofemoral compartment. *MRI Clin North Am* 1994;2: 425–439.

116. Rau R, Herborn G. Healing phenomena of erosive changes in rheumatoid arthritis patients undergoing disease-modifying antirheumatic drug therapy. *Radiology* 1996;199:886.

117. Recht MP, Kramer J, Marcelis S, et al. Abnormalities of articular cartilage in the knee: analysis of available MR techniques. *Radiology* 1993;187:473–478.

118. Reddy R, Insko EK, Leigh JS. Triple quantum sodium imaging of articular cartilage. *MRI Med* 1997;38:279.

119. Reddy R, Insko EK, Noyszewski EA, et al. Sodium MRI of human articular cartilage in vivo. *MRI Med* 1998;39:697.

120. Reddy R, Li S, Noyszewski EA, et al. In vivo sodium multiple quantum spectroscopy of human articular cartilage. *MRI Med* 1997;38:207.

121. Regan-Smith MG, O'Connor GT, Kwoh CK. Lack of correlation between the Steinbrocker staging of hand radiographs and the functional health status of individuals with rheumatoid arthritis. *Arthritis Rheum* 1989;32:128.

122. Reijnierse M, Bloem JL, Dijkmans BAC, et al. Cervical spine in rheumatoid arthritis: relationship between neurologic signs and morphology on MR imaging and radiographs. *Skeletal Radiol* 1996;25:113.

123. Reiser MF, Bongarts GPM, Erlemann R, et al. Gadolinium-DTPA in rheumatoid arthritis and related diseases: first results with dynamic magnetic resonance imaging. *Skeletal Radiol* 1989;18:591.

124. Roca A, Bernreuter WK, Alarcon GS. Functional magnetic resonance imaging should be included in the evaluation of the cervical spine in patients with rheumatoid arthritis. *J Rheumatol* 1993;20:1485.

125. Rominger MG, Bernreuter WK, Kenney PJ, et al. MR imaging of the hands in early rheumatoid arthritis: preliminary results. *Radiographics* 1993;13:37.

126. Rose PM, Demlow TA, Szumowski J, et al. Chondromalacia patellae: fat-suppressed MR imaging. *Radiology* 1994;193: 437–440.

127. Rubens DJ, Blebea JS, Totterman S, et al. Rheumatoid arthritis: evaluation of wrist extensor tendons with clinical examination versus MR imaging: a preliminary report. *Radiology* 1993; 187:831.

128. Rubenstein JD, Kim JK, Henkelman RM. Effects of compression and recovery on bovine articular cartilage appearance on MR imagings. *Radiology* 1996;201:843.

129. Rubenstein JD, Li JG, Majumdar S, et al. Image resolution and signal-to-noise ratio requirements for MR imaging of degenerative cartilage. *AJR* 1997;169:1089.

130. Rubenstein JD, Kim JK, Morava-Protzner I, et al. Effects of collagen orientation on MR imaging characteristics of bovine cartilage. *Radiology* 1993;188:219–226.

131. Rubenstein J, Recht M, Disler DG, et al. Laminar structures on MR imaging of articular cartilage. *Radiology* 1997;204:15.

132. Schiller J, Arnhold J, Sonntag K, et al. NMR studies on human, pathologically changed synovial fluids: role of hypochlorous acid. *MRI Med* 1996;35:848.

133. Seo GS, Aoki J, Moriya H, et al. Hyaline cartilage: in vivo and in vitro assessment with magnetization transfer imaging. *Radiology* 1996;201:525.

134. Shanley DJ, Auber AE, Watabe JT, et al. Pigmented villonodular synovitis of the knee demonstrated on bone scan. Correlation with US, CT, and MRI. *Clin Nucl Med* 1992;17:9801.

135. Shanley DJ, Evans EM, Buckner AB, et al. Synovial osteochondromatosis demonstrated on bone scan: correlation with CT and MRI. *Clin Nucl Med* 1992;17:338.

136. Sharp JT. Radiologic assessment as an outcome measure in rheumatoid arthritis. *Arthritis Rheum* 1989;32:221.

137. Singson RD, Zalduondo FM. Value of unenhanced spin-echo MR imaging in distinguishing between synovitis and effusion of the knee. *AJR* 1992;159:569.

138. Smith JH, Pugh DG. Roentgenographic aspects of articular pigmented villonodular synovitis. *AJR* 1962;87:1146.

139. Solloway S, Hutchinson CE, Waterton JC, et al. Use of active shape models for making thickness measurements of articular cartilage from MR images. *MRI Med* 1997;37:943.

140. Spitzer CE, Dalinka MK, Kressel HY. Magnetic resonance imaging of pigmented villonodular synovitis: report of two cases. *Skeletal Radiol* 1987;16:316.

141. Starok M, Eilenberg SS, Resnick D. Rheumatoid nodules: MRI characteristics. *Clin Imag* 1998;22:216.

142. Stiskal M, Szolar DH, Stenzel I, et al. Magnetic resonance imaging of Achilles tendon in patients with rheumatoid arthritis. *Invest Radiol* 1997;32:602.

143. Sugimoto H, Takeda A, Masuyama J-I, et al. Early-stage rheumatoid arthritis: diagnostic accuracy of MR imaging. *Radiology* 1996;198:185.

144. Sundaram M, McGuire MH, Fletcher J, et al. Magnetic resonance imaging of lesions of synovial origin. *Skeletal Radiol* 1986; 15:110.

145. Takahashi M, Yamashita Y, Sakamoto U, et al. Chronic cervical cord compression: clinical significance of increased signal intensity on MR images. *Radiology* 1989;173:219.

146. Tan TCF, Wilcox DM, Frank L, et al. MR imaging of articular cartilage in the ankle: comparison of available imaging sequences and methods of measurement in cadavers. *Skeletal Radiol* 1996;25:749.

147. Tebben PJ, Pope TW, Hinson G, et al. Three-dimensional computerized reconstruction: illustration of incremental articular cartilage thinning. *Invest Radiol* 1997;32:475.

148. Tervenen O, Dietz MJ, Carmichael SW, et al. MR imaging of knee hyaline cartilage: evaluation of two- and three-dimensional sequences. *JMRI* 1993;3:663–668.

149. Totterman SMS, Miller RJ, McCance SE, et al. Lesions of the triangular fibrocartilage complex: MR findings with a three-dimensional gradient recalled-echo sequence. *Radiology* 1996; 199:227.

150. Trattnig S, Huber M, Breitenseher MJ, et al. Imaging articular cartilage defects with 3D fat-suppressed echo planar imaging: comparison with conventional 3D fat-suppressed gradient echo sequence and correlation with histology. *JCAT* 1998;22:8.

151. Tuckman G, Wirth CZ. Synovial osteochondromatosis of the shoulder: MR findings. *J Comput Assist Tomogr* 1989;13:360.

152. van Dijke CF, Kirk BA, Peterfy CG, et al. Arthritic temporomandibular joint: correlation of macromolecular contrast-enhanced MR imaging parameters and histopathologic findings. *Radiology* 1997;204:823.

153. van der Linden E, Kroon HM, Doornbos J, et al. MR imaging of hyaline cartilage at 0.5T: quantitative and qualitative in vitro

evaluation of three types of sequences. *Skeletal Radiol* 1998; 27:297.

154. van der Heide A, Remme CA, Hofman DM, et al. Prediction of progression of radiologic damage in newly diagnosed rheumatoid arthritis. *Radiology* 1996;198:916.

155. Vellet AD, Marks P, Fowler P, et al. Occult posttraumatic lesions of the knee, prevalence, classification, and short-term sequelae evaluated with MR imaging. *Radiology* 1991;178:271–276.

156. Wacker FK, Bolze X, Felsenberg D, et al. Orientation-dependent changes in MR signal intensity of articular cartilage: manifestation of the "magic angle" effect. *Skeletal Radiol* 1998; 27:306.

157. Waldschmidt JG, Rilling RJ, Kajdacsy-Balla AA, et al. In vitro and in vivo MR imaging of hyaline cartilage: zonal anatomy, imaging pitfalls, and pathologic conditions. *Radiographics* 1977; 17:1387.

158. Weissman BN. Use of radiographs to measure outcome of rheumatoid arthritis. *Am J Med* 1987;83(Suppl 4B): 96.

159. Weissman BN, Winalski CS, Hussan S, et al. Following patients with rheumatoid arthritis: observation on assessment of effusion and synovium by MR and clinical methods. *Radiology* 1991; 181:303.

160. Wilson AJ, Murphy WA, Hardy DC, et al. Transient osteoporosis: transient bone marrow edema? *Radiology* 1988;167: 757.

161. Winalski CS, Aliabadi P, Wright JR, et al. Enhancement of joint fluid with intravenously administered gadopentetate dimeglumine: technique, rationale, and implications. *Radiology* 1993; 187:179.

162. Winalski CS, Mulkern RV, Utz PJ, et al. In vivo T2 relaxation times of synovium and joint fluid in rheumatoid arthritis: optimization of nonenhanced MR imaging. *Radiology* 1994; 193:206.

163. Winalski CS, Palmer WE, Rosenthal DI, et al. Magnetic resonance imaging of rheumatoid arthritis. *Radiol Clin North Am* 1996;34:243.

164. Xia Y. Relaxation anisotropy in cartilage by NMR microscopy (FMRI) at 14 Fm resolution. *MRI Med* 1998;39:941.

165. Xia Y, Farquhar T, Burton-Wurster N, et al. Origin of cartilage laminae in MRI. *JMRI* 1997;7:887.

166. Yamashita Y, Takahashi M, Sakamoto Y, et al. Atlantoaxial subluxation: radiography and magnetic resonance imaging correlated to myelopathy. *Acta Radiology (Sweden)* 1989;30:135.

167. Yanagawa A, Takano K, Nishioka K, et al. Clinical staging and gadolinium-DTPA enhanced images of the wrist in rheumatoid arthritis. *J Rheumatol* 1993;20:781.

168. Yao I, Gentili A, Thomas A. Incidental magnetization transfer contrast in fast spin-echo imaging of cartilage. *JMRI* 1996;6: 108.

169. Yulish BS, Montanez J, Goodfellow DB, et al. Chondromalacia patellae: assessment with MR imaging. *Radiology* 1987;164: 763–766.

170. Zygmunt S, Saveland H, Brattstrom H, et al. Reduction of rheumatoid periodontotic pannus following posterior occipitocervical fusion visualised by magnetic resonance imaging. *Br J Neurosurg* 1988;2:315.

PATHOLOGIC ASPECTS OF DISEASES OF THE JOINT AND JUXTAARTICULAR TISSUES

CARLOS A. MURO-CACHO

The human body has 327 joints of various sizes, complexities, and motion capabilities.[1] *Syndesmoses* (e.g., cranial sutures) allow almost no movement, *synchondroses* (e.g., vertebral bodies) allow limited movement, and *diarthrodial joints* allow free movement along several axes and have synovial fluid in a space lined by a synovial membrane. Joints are supported by a capsule that is continuous with the periosteum and by ligaments that attach one bone to another. Blood flows from feeder arteries through fenestrated capillaries in the synovium. Diffusion of nutrients across synovial intima, synovial fluid, and cartilage matrix is facilitated by joint motion. A rich network of arterial, venous, and lymphatic anastomoses ensures the removal of products of catabolism and is responsible for the physiological and pathological interdependence of the various anatomic compartments.[2]

COMPONENTS OF THE JOINT

Bone

Bone is organized as either a structurally important, dense compact bone or as a metabolically active, spongy cancellous bone. Compact bone accounts for 70% of the skeleton and is found in cortex, diaphysis of long bones, walls of vertebral bodies, and subchondral plate of concave joints (acetabulum, glenoid fossa). Cancellous bone is found in epiphyses beneath articular surfaces and within vertebral bodies and forms a network of bony *trabeculae* oriented along lines of stress and continuous with the inner cortex.[3] Bone is formed by deposition of inorganic calcium hydroxyapatite crystals (77% of bone's dry weight) that are responsible for resistance to high compressive forces into a complex organic matrix that has evolved to resist high tension forces.[4,5] *Osteoblasts* differentiate from pluripotential bone marrow stem cells and become embedded in the matrix that they produce, adopting a cuboidal morphology with the nucleus polarized to the side of the cell away from the bone surface. They have receptors for parathyroid hormone (PTH) and $1,25(OH)_2$ vitamin D, and secrete alkaline phosphatase.[6] Osteoblasts are not capable of division and at the end of their metabolic life (approximately 6 months) the majority flattens out and outline the bone surface (*lining cells*). They remain, however, responsive to PTH and vitamin D.[4,6] Approximately 10% to 15% of osteoblasts become *osteocytes*, the most abundant cell in the bone. Osteocytes reside inside the organic matrix within 15 μm *lacunae* and send cytoplasmic extensions via *canaliculi* to neighboring osteocytes and lining cells forming the *osteocytic membrane system*.[6-8] This system regulates calcium metabolism and the transmission of small piezoelectrical currents in response to stress and strain. Bone resorption is the responsibility of the *osteoclast*, a multinucleated giant cell measuring 20 to 100 μm and found within the superficial *Howship's lacunae* and

the deep *cutting cones*. Osteoclasts result from the fusion of mononuclear precursors and although related to macrophages they are the end result of an independent line of differentiation. The surface of the osteoclast is notably increased by long cytoplasmic extensions and their cytoplasm contains proteases and tartrate-resistant acid phosphatase.[6-10] Osteoclasts respond to vitamin D, interleukins, and prostaglandins but they lack PTH receptors; therefore, osteoblast mediation is necessary for bone resorption. The lacunae where osteocytes reside are evenly distributed along the organic matrix known as *osteoid*. Osteoid is composed of type I collagen (90%) and a mixture of proteoglycans and noncollagenous proteins such as osteocalcin (involved in the initiation of bone turnover in response to vitamin D), osteonectin (it binds to collagen and apatite crystals and may function as initiator or moderator of mineralization), osteopontin, sialoproteins, serum proteins, and growth factors (e.g., TGFβ, insulinlike growth factor, fibroblast growth factor, bone morphogenetic proteins).[6-12] In mature bone, collagen fibers are located within 3 to 7 μm *lamellae* oriented perpendicular to the fibers of adjacent lamellae. In the inner and outer cortex, however, lamellae are concentrically arranged around the bone shaft in *outer* and *inner circumferential layers* respectively.[12,13] Compact bone is made up of *osteons* or *haversian systems*, 50 μm in diameter and 1 cm in length, oriented parallel to the long axis of the bone. Osteons have a central *haversian canal* that contains one or two capillaries and a nerve fiber and is surrounded by 8 to 15 concentric lamellae. The osteons in mature bone are outlined by *cement lines* (evidence of previous remodeling) within surrounding *interstitial systems*.[8-10] This tissue architecture allows all osteocytes to be only within 0.1 to 0.2 mm from the closest blood vessel. Another system of blood vessels is located within *Volkmann's canals* that run perpendicular to the osteons and connect the haversian canals with marrow cavity and periosteum. Compact bone is covered outside by *periosteum* and inside by *endosteum*, both capable of haversian remodeling. In cancellous bone, osteons are incomplete and trabeculae are subjected to continuous osteoclastic resorption and osteoblastic formation.[12,13]

Bone Remodeling

Bone remodeling is a continuous process in which bone is removed in tiny increments and replaced by new bone (in childhood and healing fractures the newly formed bone is known as "*woven*" bone).[13-15] Remodeling occurs at different rates in compact (2% per year) and cancellous (25% per year) bone, resulting in 18% of the skeleton being replaced every year and the entire skeleton being renewed every 5 years.[16-18] In the *activation* phase, a layer of osteoid 10 μm in thickness is deposited by osteoblasts. During the next 20 days (*mineralization lag time*) small matrix vesicles detach from the cytoplasm and ionic calcium and phosphate begins to precipitate inside the vesicles helped by alkaline-phosphatase hydrolysis of the mineralization inhibitor pyrophosphate. Eventually, crystals leak into the extracellular fluid and mineralization of the matrix proceeds for approximately 1 year. In lamellar bone, however, mineralization begins within the collagen fibrils independently from matrix vesicles.[19,20] The *resorption* phase lasts one month and occurs within 50 μm cavities in cancellous bone and in the 2.5 mm cutting zones in compact bone. In response to a resorption signal (via local factors or PTH-osteoblast mediated), lining cells secrete proteases that digest the unmineralized matrix layer exposing the mineralized surface.[16–19] Osteoclasts attach themselves to the surface and secrete proteases that digest proteins and protons that acidify the environment and dissolve the minerals. Osteoclasts also produce a matrix rich in proteoglycans and poor in collagen that glues the bone to the newly formed cavity. This substance forms the remodeling blue lines that accumulate with age as a result of previous remodeling events. The *reversal* phase lasts 1 or 2 weeks. Coupling signals attract osteoblasts to the cavity and fill it with new bone, completely in cancellous bone and only partially in compact bone where the central region is left nonossified to become the haversian canal.[13–19]

Cartilage

Contact surfaces of adjacent bones are covered by a smooth and slippery hyaline articular cartilage composed of chondrocytes embedded in lacunae and surrounded by extracellular matrix. The matrix is composed of water (60% to 80%) trapped in a framework of negatively charged proteoglycan aggregates (chondroitin and keratan sulfates) and type II collagen fibers.[21–24] Minor amounts of other collagen types (V, VI, IX, X, and XI) are also found in specific areas. The articular cartilage can be divided into four zones, depending on the relative proportions of proteoglycans and collagen fibers.[21] The *superficial zone* is poor in proteoglycans and rich in collagen fibers, which are oriented parallel to the surface (*lamina splendens*). In the *transitional zone* below, the number of proteoglycans increases and collagen fibers are curved. In the third zone, immediately underneath, proteoglycans are abundant and water content is low. In the deepest region, the *zone of calcified cartilage*, collagen fibers are perpendicular to the bone and separated from the other layers by the *tidemark*. Also, proteoglycans are abundant around chondrocytes, in the *pericellular region*, whereas collagen fibers are more numerous away from the chondrocytes, in the *territorial zone*. Between these two regions, in the *interterritorial area*, collagen fibers and proteoglycans are maximally concentrated.[24,25] Renewal and breakdown of this extracellular matrix is the responsibility of chondrocytes. Owing to the absence of blood vessels and nerves, chondrocytes receive nutrients from adjacent tissues via the synovial fluid. The synovial fluid also removes matrix fragments and carries them to the blood via lymphatics. The overall structure functions as a turbid gel and provides a

unique system of pressurization that makes hyaline cartilage firm and resilient and allows it to act as a coiled spring sustaining pressures of three or more atmospheres. Joints in areas of tensile stress (e.g., crescentic menisci over tibial plateau, roof of acetabulum, costosternal joints, pubic symphysis) have another type of cartilage known as *fibrocartilage*. In fibrocartilage, chondrocytes are surrounded by larger fibrils of type I collagen and its characteristics are intermediate between cartilage and ligaments/tendons.[22–24]

Synovium

The synovium is a loose fibrovascular structure with various amounts of fat that can be described as *areolar, adipose,* or *fibrous* depending of its tissue composition. The synovium represents only 1/10,000th of the total body mass but when inflamed it causes serious disability.[25–28] The specialized form (areolar synovium) is composed of type A (macrophagelike) and type B (fibroblastlike) cells in a well-organized microfibrillary matrix of chondroitin-6-sulfate rich proteoglycans containing hyaluronic acid, laminin, fibronectin, and small amounts of collagen types I, III, IV, V, and VI.[29–32] The so-called "synovial membrane" is only 25 to 35 μm in thickness but its surface is increased by numerous villous fronds containing one or two layers of cells that secrete some of the components of the synovial fluid. This synovial membrane covers all intraarticular surfaces with subtle histological variations depending on location. A rich network of capillaries is found beneath the surface and veins and lymphatics are found in deeper layers.[32–39]

Synovial Fluid

Normal synovial fluid production is the result of a regulated balance between transudation from plasma and removal from lymphatics. The fluid is in direct continuity with the matrix of the synovium and cartilage without any separating boundaries, contains molecules produced by type B synoviocyte (fibroblastlike) and is kept free of debris by the action of type A synoviocytes (macrophagelike). This special arrangement allows all joint components to work as a single functional unit. As a result, cellular and biochemical changes in the fluid are a reflection of abnormalities in the joint and represent an optimal target for diagnostic analysis. The fluid should be anticoagulated and submitted to the laboratory within 24 hours.[40–50]

Gross examination of normal fluid reveals a clear, yellow, and viscous appearance. In bleeding processes it can be red or orange, in inflammatory processes white, and in septic processes it may adopt different colors depending on the etiologic agent. The fluid becomes turbid with increase in cellularity or debris. In inflammatory conditions viscosity can be reduced by enzymatic digestion. Normal fluid contains less than 200 cells/mm^3. In inflammatory conditions it is not unusual to find 1,000 cells/mm^3, and in rheumatoid and septic arthritis the cell count can reach 25,000 cells/mm^3. A quick wet preparation allows the identification of crystalline (monosodium urate monohydrate and calcium pyrophosphate crystals) and noncrystalline (fragments of fibrocartilage, ligaments, plastic and metal debris, foreign bodies) particles by microscopic analysis. The number of ragocytes (cells of various lineages with granules in the cytoplasm) is increased in inflammatory conditions and in large numbers is strongly associated with either rheumatoid arthritis (>70%) or septic arthritis (>95%). Dilution of the fluid, cytocentrifugation, and staining of cytospins with Giemsa followed by microscopic analysis allow the identification of microorganisms and cells of special significance. Quantitation of inflammatory mediators (cytokines, enzymes), proteins of the complement system, antibodies (rheumatoid factor), and byproducts of the degradation of cartilage proteoglycans and noncollagenous proteins can be correlated with disease activity. Finally, culture methods for bacteria, fungi, and viruses should be requested as needed according to clinical considerations.

Ligaments, Tendons, Tendon Sheaths, and Bursae

Ligaments are strong bundles of parallel type I collagen fibers that insert on the entheses of bones where they link with Sharpey's fibers to prevent inappropriate motions. Tendons are histologically similar to ligaments but they function as active drivers of joint motion. Tendons often run within tendon sheaths that isolate them from surrounding tissues and are protected by bursae in areas of friction (i.e., next to bony prominences, under the skin). Tendon sheaths and bursae are lubricated by a fluid similar to synovial fluid.[51–53]

DISEASES INVOLVING THE JOINT AND JUXTAARTICULAR TISSUES

The inflammation of joints and juxtaarticular tissues is generally known as arthritis. There are more than 100 clinical types of arthritis that can be placed in several broad categories on the basis of clinical and pathologic features and pathogenetic mechanisms.[54]

GENETIC

Neurofibromatosis

Neurofibromatosis 1 (von Recklinghausen's disease) is the most common single gene disorder in humans, with over 100,000 Americans affected.[55] It is mostly transmitted as an autosomal dominant disorder with 100% penetrance and several degrees of severity; it affects the skeleton in 30% to

60% of cases. Neurofibromatosis 2 is very rare and does not involve the skeleton. Half of the patients present with scoliosis owing to vertebral abnormalities with vertebral body wedging and scalloping and approximately 13% of patients present with pseudoarthrosis.[55–57]

Lysosomal Storage Diseases

Lysosomal storage diseases are caused by a defect in synthesis of lysosomal enzymes necessary for digestion of cellular breakdown products. Some of the three dozen known diseases in this category affect the bone and the joints secondarily.

Gaucher's Disease

Inherited as an autosomal recessive disorder, Gaucher's disease is characterized by the accumulation of glucosylceramide in macrophages (Gaucher's cells) that have a wrinkled tissue paper appearance in the cytoplasm. Skeletal manifestations are osteonecrosis (55% of patients) usually of the femoral head resulting from intraosseous vascular compression.[56–64]

Mucopolysaccharidoses

Deficiencies in the enzymes that catabolize glycosaminoglycans affect hyaline cartilage, resulting in vertebral and hip abnormalities known as *dysostosis multiplex* and characterized by frequent joint dislocations. Metachromatic inclusions are present within vacuoles in lymphocytes (Gasser cells).[65–70]

Alkaptonuria (Ochronosis)

A deficiency in homogentisic acid oxidase results in an inability to catabolize homogentisic acid that accumulates in tissues leading to black pigmentation. The spine is usually the first region to be affected with pigment deposition in discs, paravertebral and paraarticular soft tissues, and intraarticularly (intraarticular vacuum radiographically). Large joints (hips and knees) are affected later in the disease. The articular cartilage is severely pigmented and becomes brittle, with fragments detaching into the joint and becoming embedded into the synovial membrane, resulting in severe synovitis and secondary osteoarthritis with calcified loose bodies. The synovial fluid is typically noninflammatory and contains 100 to 700 cells/mm^3, mostly mononuclear cells.[66–76]

Skeletal Dysplasias

Skeletal dysplasias are owing to abnormalities in osteogenesis, chondrogenesis, fibrogenesis, or other mechanisms and may or may not involve the joints.[77–80]

Osteogenesis Imperfecta

This is the most common genetic disease of the skeleton affecting 15,000 to 20,000 people in the United States. Abnormalities in collagen type I lead to bone and joint deformities. Cortical thickness and trabecular volume are diminished, bone turnover is reduced, and woven bone persists. The growth plate is thin and islands of hyaline cartilage persist in metaphysis and epiphysis.[81]

Spondyloepiphyseal Dysplasia

This is a heterogeneous group of disorders in which abnormal spine and dysplastic epiphyses result in joint deformities and premature osteoarthritis. The articular cartilage shows chondrocyte inclusions owing to dilated endoplasmic reticulum.[82]

Metaphyseal Chondrodysplasia

Metaphyseal changes caused by growth plate abnormalities lead to lordosis and various knee deformities with widened and irregular growth plates that are often mistaken for rickets. Microscopically, there are irregular cartilaginous masses without column orientation composed by chondrocytes with granular precipitates in the endoplasmic reticulum.[83]

Enchondromatosis (Ollier's Disease)

In Ollier's disease, excess hypertrophic cartilage that is not resorbed and ossified in the growing ends of the bones migrates progressively during longitudinal growth into the metaphyses and diaphyses, producing chondromas that undergo sarcomatous changes in 20% of the cases, usually into a chondrosarcoma.[84]

Multiple Epiphyseal Dysplasia

A delay in ossification centers retard skeletal growth with malformed epiphyses and symmetric joint involvement and secondary coxa vara, genu valgum, severe osteoarthritis, and osteonecrosis.[78-80]

Pseudoachondroplasia

Defective proteoglycan synthesis results in accumulation of laminated cytoplasmic inclusions within chondrocytes, joint deformities, and premature osteoarthritis.[83,84]

METABOLIC

Crystal Arthropathies

The term "crystal deposition disease" refers to the presence of crystals in healthy tissues where they elicit pathologic changes. The term "crystal arthropathy" assumes no etiopathogenic role for the crystal. Intrinsic or endogenous crystals are associated with acute, self-limited inflammation, chronic joint disease, or asymptomatic (lanthanic) deposition. Several types of crystals, and mixtures of them, can be identified in the joints: monosodium urate, calcium phosphates (pyrophosphate, hydroxyapatite, octacalcium phosphate, dicalcium phosphate dihydrate), oxalate, cholesterol, proteins (immunoglobulins, paraproteins, Charcot-Leyden crystals), corticosteroid depots, and prosthetic fragments.

Gout

Gout is the clinical manifestation of a disorder of purine metabolism characterized by chronic hyperuricemia and recurrent episodes of inflammatory arthritis (*gouty arthritis*). It is caused by precipitation of monosodium urate crystals and can lead to the formation of large urate deposits (*tophi*) in joints, periarticular tissues, ear lobes, nasal cartilages, kidney, and skin (Fig. 10.1).[85-88] Uric acid is the final breakdown product of purine, one of the building blocks of nucleic acids. Urate is the ionized form of uric acid and normally exists in a monosodium form in plasma, extracellular fluid, and synovial fluid. Hyperuricemia is a serum or plasma urate level above 6.8 mg/dL.[89] Higher concentrations exceed the solubility limit for urate in plasma at normal pH and body temperature. Hyperuricemia, however, is not the sole determining factor for gout because it is found in approximately 10% of the population and gout affects only 0.1% to 0.4% of individuals.[90-92] Gout typically affects men (95% of all cases) in the fifth decade. It is the most common inflammatory arthritis in men over 40 and occurs infrequently in women after menopause. A family history of gout is obtained in 25% of cases.[90-93] The natural history of gout progresses along four phases:

1. Asymptomatic hyperuricemia
2. Acute gouty arthritis
3. Intercritical gout
4. Chronic tophaceous gout

Gouty nephropathy and uric acid renal stones also occur in 10% to 25% of patients with gout.[93] Hyperuricemia and gout are classified as *primary* and *secondary* types. There is also an idiopathic form characterized by elevated serum urate without gout.[90] Patients with *primary hyperuricemia* may have familial or nonfamilial gout caused by either an overproduction of uric acid (10% of cases) or renal underexcretion of uric acid (90% of cases). In cases owing to overproduction of uric acid, two heritable (X-linked) enzyme defects have been identified: hyperactivity of PRPP (5-phosphoribosyl-1-pyrophosphate) synthase and partial deficiency of HGPRT (hypoxanthine-guanine phosphoribosyltransferase).[90-93] These enzymes are involved in the de novo and salvage pathways of purine synthesis, respectively. Men with either of these genetic defects usually develop gouty

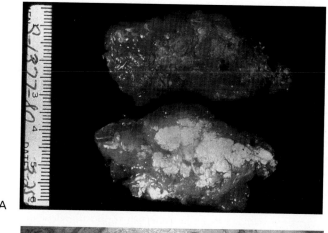

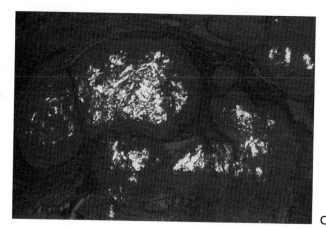

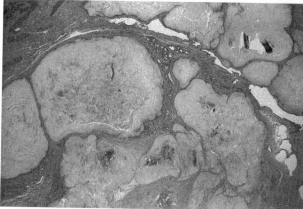

FIGURE 10.1. Chronic gout. **A:** Gross appearance of tophi within synovial tissue. **B:** Granulation tissue and multinucleated giant cells surrounding tophi. **C:** Crystals under polarized light.(See Color Figure 10.1.)

arthritis at a young age and also have a high incidence of uric acid renal stones. The basic renal defect leading to underexcretion of uric acid is not well established. The following mechanisms may be involved: reduced glomerular filtration of uric acid, decreased tubular secretion of uric acid, and increased tubular resorption of uric acid. Patients with *secondary hyperuricemia* may have familial or nonfamilial gout caused by either overproduction of uric acid or renal underexcretion of uric acid. In patients with overproduction of uric acid, the uric acid surplus is usually owing to excessive breakdown of cells and increased turnover of nucleic acids (myeloproliferative disorders, leukemias, multiple myeloma, some carcinomas, hemolytic anemias, or after massive cell lysis produced by cytotoxic drug therapy). Another cause of overproduction is the Lesch-Nyhan syndrome, characterized by self-mutilation and neurologic abnormalities inherited in an X-linked manner.[90] In this syndrome, a complete deficiency of HGPRT results in accumulation of PRPP and increased purine synthesis de novo. Secondary hyperuricemia caused by renal underexcretion of uric acid may result from chronic renal disease, diuretic drug treatment (which interferes with the renal secretion of uric acid and causes blood volume contraction),

salicylates, and ethanol. Patients with glucose-6-phosphatase deficiency (von Gierke's disease/glycogen storage disease) have both an overproduction of uric acid and renal underexcretion of uric acid.

Acute Gouty Arthritis

Acute gouty arthritis is usually monarticular in onset (50% of cases) and typically (75% or cases) involves the metatarsophalangeal joint of the big toe (*acute podagra*), tarsal joint, ankle, or knee. The inflammation resembles a septic joint with sudden onset of joint pain, exquisite tenderness, swelling, and redness. Prominent neutrophilic inflammatory infiltrate and fibrin deposition are present in the synovial membrane. The synovial effusion shows an increased white cell count with numerous urate crystals. These 5 to 25 μm crystals are identified under polarized light as needle-shaped and show strong negative birefringence (Fig. 10.1C).[92–95] In the synovial fluid, the crystals are coated with proteins that mediate ingestion by neutrophils, macrophages, and synovial lining cells. After phagocytosis, the protein coat is enzymatically degraded. The crystals along with enzymes and inflammatory mediators (interleukin-1, prostaglandins, leukotrienes, oxygen radicals, and chemotactic factors), are released from the phagocytic cells into the extracellular environment. The cycle of crystal-induced inflammatory arthritis is repeated over again until the process of crystal formation subsides. Urate deposits are water soluble and are dissolved by routine histologic procedures. They are best preserved by alcohol fixation and visualized by polarized light microscopy or special silver stains.[92–95]

Chronic Gouty Arthritis

In untreated or poorly controlled patients, crystal deposition continues and, following multiple recurrences or polyarticular involvement (usually over a period of about 10 years after the first attack), gross deposits of urates (*tophi*) form in joints, bursae, tendons, and subcutaneous tissue (chronic tophaceous gout) (Fig. 10.1A).[96] The synovial fluid is a poorer solvent than plasma and crystallization is favored in peripheral joints (feet, hand) because of lower temperatures. The initial microtophi appear as acellular amorphous material surrounded by macrophages, fibroblasts, and multinucleate foreign body–type giant cells that can be confused with microorganisms. With time, tophi become chalky masses that may reach several centimeters in diameter. As urates precipitate in the synovial lining and encrust the articular surfaces, the phagocytic (type A) synovial lining cells proliferate, resulting in a diffuse synovitis with fibrosis and a *pannus* that eventually erodes the underlying cartilage and subchondral bone, resulting in permanent joint changes.[96]

Calcium Pyrophosphate Dihydrate Deposition Disease

Calcium pyrophosphate dihydrate deposits (calcium pyrophosphate dihydrate deposition disease [CPPD]) typically appear as punctate and linear densities in the cartilage and menisci of the knees of 3% of asymptomatic individuals less than 70 years of age and 30% to 60% of adults older than 85.[97] The disease has a female predominance and is recognized radiologically as *calcinosis*.[98] A tendency to form deposits can be inherited in an autosomal dominant pattern or can be seen in patients who suffered a previous injury to the joint, myocardial infarction, stroke, hyperparathyroidism, hypercalcemia, gout, or hemochromatosis.[99] The disease presents as an acute synovitis involving one (most commonly the knee) or rarely more joints (*pseudogout*) in 25% of patients. Alternatively, it may present as a *chronic pyrophosphate arthropathy* involving knees, hips, wrists, and metacarpophalangeal joints of the hand. Occasionally, deposits are found in the soft tissues (*tophaceous pseudogout*) mimicking a neoplasm. CPPD is probably caused by a failure of chondrocytes to maintain the homeostasis of the extracellular matrix, resulting in

shedding of calcium pyrophosphate dihydrate deposits from the hyaline cartilage or fibrocartilage into the adjacent synovial cavity, ligaments, and joint capsule. The synovial fluid is usually turbid or stained with blood and contains numerous neutrophils. The intracellular crystals, best visualized by polarized light microscopy, appear as rhomboids 2 to 10 μm long with weak birefringence. These features distinguish them from urate crystals (needle-shaped and negatively birefringent) and hydroxyapatite deposits (nonbirefringent clumps). The crystals are primarily deposited in cartilage and secondarily affect the synovium, tenosynovioma, and bursae. There is usually minimal or no inflammatory reaction except in synovial membranes. The earliest damage is perilacunar, but tophuslike deposits can be widespread. The chondrocytes are hyperplastic, the cartilage loses basophilia and undergoes mucoid degeneration, and the subchondral bone may undergo cystic changes. The crystals are known to activate complement, stimulate production of TNFα and IL-6, and induce oxygen radical damage.[100–103]

Calcium Hydroxyapatite Deposition Disease

Apatite is a form of calcium phosphate that can be found in periarticular tissues (*calcific periarthritis*) or intraarticularly.[104] In calcific periarthritis, the presence of crystals is often asymptomatic and can be observed in childhood in the shoulders of approximately 3% of the general population and also in the knees, elbow, wrist, and ankle joints.[105] However, the crystals can elicit an acute inflammatory reaction or chronic pain syndrome. Intraarticular calcifications are found in the synovial fluid of 30% to 60% patients with knee osteoarthropathy. In the acute form, the synovial fluid is hypocellular and may contain calcium deposits mixed with inflamed tissue that appear as toothpaste. The crystals are needle-shaped, measuring less than 0.1 μm in length and form aggregates that are not birefringent. Calcifications are located in tendons, peritendinous areas, bursae, or ligaments.[105–108]

Amyloid Deposition

In amyloidosis, proteins become insoluble and form fibrillar deposits that are Congo red positive and show apple green birefringence under polarized light. Most amyloid precursors have a β-pleated sheet secondary structure in soluble state, whereas deposited fibrils have an antiparallel β-sheet structure.[109–111] Amyloid deposition may be localized or systemic and can be classified according to the chemical nature of the fibrils. In joints, it is usually the manifestation of primary amyloidosis (AL) and myeloma or secondary to renal dialysis caused by poor filtering of β_2-microglobulin.[112,113] Synovial amyloidosis is usually bilateral and symmetrical, affecting shoulders, hips, wrists, and knees. In tenosynovial tissues, amyloid can produce carpal tunnel syndrome. Amyloid deposits may lead to subchondral cysts and erosive arthropathy, mostly in humeral and femoral heads, hand, and spine. Secondary fractures may occur.

DEGENERATIVE

Chondromalacia Patellae

The articular cartilage of the patella can be affected either by: "surface degeneration," which occurs in young individuals and deteriorates with increasing age predisposing to degenerative arthritis, or "basal degeneration," in which there is a fasciculation of collagen in the middle and deep zones of cartilage without initially affecting the surface. The pathogenesis of basal degeneration may be influenced by the subchondral space, and metaplasia of the tidemark may play a significant part. Many cases are clinically silent but cartilage damage usually is present.[114–116]

Internal Knee Derangement

The mediopatellar plica is a fold of synovial tissue attaching medially at the undersurface of the quadriceps tendon that extends distally around the patella and over the medial femoral condyle to insert into the fat pad. An extensor mechanism of derangement may be produced by a mediopatellar plica that has lost its pliability because of fibrosis or hyalinization. Lesions usually are found in the triangular area of the medial condyle and on a small strip of the lateral condyle. Similar lesions have been described in association with flexion deformities in rheumatoid and osteoarthritic knees.[117–122]

Osteoarthritis

Osteoarthritis (OA; degenerative joint disease, hypertrophic arthritis, osteoarthrosis) is the most common joint disease and affects elderly men, and especially women, of all ethnic groups. OA is rare in individuals younger than 40 (10% to 20%) but is found in 100% of individuals older than 65 years of age at autopsy.[123–125] It is characterized by a progressive deterioration of the articular cartilage accompanied by the formation of bony outgrowths (*osteophytes*) at the margins of the joints and thickening and sclerosis of the subchondral bone. It can be *primary* or *secondary* to osteonecrosis, crystal arthropathy, trauma, congenital dysplasia, or inflammatory arthritis. It is often asymptomatic, but joint pain, motion limitation, crepitus (a crackling sensation when the joint is moved), and joint deformity are common.[124] Clinical symptoms do not correlate with radiographic severity, but in secondary OA they appear 10 years earlier than in primary OA. OA can involve any joint, although hips, knees, spine, wrist, and particularly the small joints of the hand are more commonly affected. Only the hip is involved in approximately 5% of individuals older than 55 years. This presentation may correspond to a different disease because only one joint is involved and the distribution is equal in men and women. Conventional OA typically presents in one of three major distribution patterns: (a) in White men, affecting primarily the hip with little involvement of other joints; (b) in obese hypertensive women, affecting primarily the knee; and (c) in a familial form (associated with HLA-A1, B8), affecting middle-aged women and typically involving hands, knee, and occasionally hips. This is known as *generalized* or *disseminated OA of Kellgren*; patients frequently develop *Heberden's nodes* and subcutaneous nodules in the fingers secondary to osteophyte formation.[123–125]

The pathogenesis of OA is not completely understood. Heredity, ligament laxity, gait, disuse, and body habitus determine joint shape. A long prevailing hypothesis is that OA is caused by daily biomechanical stresses accompanied by abnormal cartilage renewal associated with aging. Although trauma caused by overuse may result in OA, many older people have no OA symptoms, and the ankle, a joint subject to constant pressures, is rarely involved. Also, patients with osteoporosis rarely have the disease, whereas patients with osteopetrosis or Paget's disease of the bone are almost always affected. Thus, the etiology of OA is most likely the result of a combination of genetic, biomechanical, biochemical, hormonal, and immunologic factors. Central to the pathogenesis of OA, however, is an abnormal cartilaginous extracellular matrix. Mutations in the collagen type II gene lead to OA before 40 years of age. Also, there is an increased synthesis of structurally abnormal proteoglycans in OA that aggregate less efficiently with hyaluronic acid and are easily degraded by chondrocyte metalloproteinase under the control of interleukin-1.[125] This results in decreased amounts of proteoglycans, collagen damage (fibrillation), and compensatory increase in water content with marked alterations in the quality and function of the extracellular matrix. Continued use and injury splits and fragments the articular cartilage. Cartilage initially responds with clonal proliferation of chondrocytes that synthesize proteoglycans and collagen II. In later stages, however, cartilage renewal and repair decreases and injured or dead chondrocytes, synoviocytes, and inflammatory cells release lytic enzymes (proteases, collagenases) that further degrade the cartilage matrix. This process of degradation exceeds repair and finally the cartilage is eroded irreversibly.[123]

The main pathologic feature of OA is progressive damage of the articular cartilage followed by alterations in the shape of the articular surfaces (Fig. 10.2). The earliest pathologic change is a disruption of the *lamina splendens*, the most superficial layer of the articular cartilage. This leads to erosion and cracking of the articular surface (*chon-

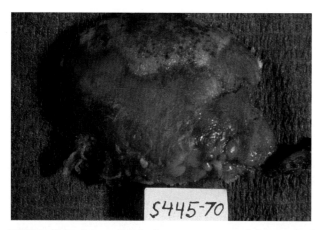

FIGURE 10.2. Osteoarthritis. Gross appearance of degenerated articular surface. (See Color Figure 10.2.)

dromalacia) owing to depletion of proteoglycans, and roughening of the articular surface owing to unmasking and fragmentation of the collagen fibril structure of cartilage (fibrillation). The fibrillated cartilage develops clefts and fissures in the superficial layers that deepen as the cartilage is eroded away from the surface by tangential flaking, pitting, and grooving. Around the erosions, chondrocytes proliferate and synthesize proteoglycans in a failed attempt to repair the lesion. Subchondral trabeculae respond with formation of new bone that becomes lined by granulation tissue. Osteoblastic differentiation increases bone density and the new bone becomes polished or *eburnated* (ivory-like) as a result of friction with the articular surface.[124] Alterations in the bone-cartilage interface lead to fibrocartilage deposition, myxomatous degeneration, subchondral necrosis, and the formation of subchondral cysts that may reach several centimeters in size. It is not clear whether such cysts evolve from synovial fluid forced through defects on the exposed surface of bone or from osteoclastic resorption and remodeling of ischemic sclerotic bone. Bony outgrowths (*osteophytes*, or *spurs*) develop at the margins of the osteoarthritic joint by endochondral ossification. Although generally regarded as a manifestation of the osteoarthritic process, they are also associated with aging in the absence of any other evidence of OA.[125] Osteophytes producing palpable enlargements at the distal interphalangeal joints of the hands are called *Heberden's nodes*, often an early manifestation of OA. The synovial membrane responds with edema, hyperplasia of synovial fronds, and a chronic inflammatory reaction that may be very prominent around detached fragments of subchondral bone (*dendritic synovitis*). This may lead to secondary synovial chondrometaplasia and loose bodies with peripheral concentric rings of hyaline cartilage around the initial nidus. The synovial fluid in OA is usually clear and viscous with normal or slightly increased cellularity.

Spondylitis Deformans (Osteoarthritis of the Spine)

Spondylitis deformans affects vertebral discs and bodies, especially in the lumbar and cervical regions. The pathologic changes are similar to classic OA. Degradation of collagen in the annulus fibrosus leads to disc herniation, predominantly in the anterior aspect of the spine.[126] This produces traction in the bony end plates and osteophyte formation. Osteophytes grow because continuous forces impose on ligaments and tendons that arch and fuse vertebral bodies. The disc may also herniate into the vertebral body (*Schmorl's node*) in a process similar to that seen in osteoporotic spines.[126]

Diffuse Idiopathic Skeletal Hyperostosis (Forestier's Disease)

Diffuse idiopathic skeletal hyperostosis (DISH; Forestier's disease) is characterized by bone proliferation of spinal and extraspinal structures. Frequently, extraspinal manifestations may occur before the involvement of the spine. The patella is one of the most commonly involved sites. Changes are usually symmetrical and involve predominantly the anterosuperior margin of the patella and in the lateral view enthesophytes at the bone attachment of the cruciate ligaments are oriented inside the joint space. In contrast, in osteoarthritis, osteophytes are found on the posterosuperior margin and always oriented toward the outside of the joint. Traction spurs develop in entheses throughout the body in 25% of men and 15% of women older than 50, and 45% of men and 20% of women older than 80. The disease is rare in individuals younger than 45, but is common in some Native American tribes and patients with Paget's disease of the bone and gout. The disease rarely causes symptoms, and it has been associated with obesity, hypervitaminosis A, and adult-onset diabetes, suggesting a pathogenic role of the growth-factorlike activity of insulin.[127,128]

Neuropathic (Charcot's) Joint

Sensory neuropathies can be complicated by neuropathic arthropathy. This complication occurs in 5% to 10% of patients with tabes dorsalis, 14% of patients with leprosy, and 25% of patients with syringomyelia.[129–132] In 30% of the cases there is no evidence of neurologic disease; the distribution of lesions depends on the underlying cause. The synovial fluid may be serous, serosanguinous, or hemorrhagic. The biopsy findings are nonspecific and usually consist of fibrosis, cartilaginous or bony metaplasia, and necrotic debris (dendritic synovitis).[133] Osteoarthritic deformity may result from changes in the shape of the articular surfaces, osteophyte formation, shortening, instability, and subluxation. The pathogenesis probably involves neurotraumatic and neurovascular mechanisms. It is believed that either neural denervation makes the joint insensitive to pain, decreasing its natural adjustment to trauma and microfractures, or that a neural vascular reflex increases vascular flow, leading to osteoclastic activity and osteopenia. In the diabetic patient, the foot is the most common location (tarsometatarsal and metatarsophalangeal joints); it can be confused with osteomyelitis. The disease can present either as severe erosive changes or as massive osteophyte production.[134] One-third of patients, however, may have no demonstrable neurologic deficit. Patients with diabetes, syphilis, syringomyelia, and other neuropathies are particularly prone to developing this joint disease. The diagnosis of Charcot's joints should be considered in anyone who develops what appears to be a severe osteoarthritis or a transverse fracture of the tibia or fibula after minor trauma. Scoliosis with particularly destructive changes on radiography should prompt a search for syringomyelia or syphilis. The most common radiographic abnormalities are those of distension in 3D (dislocation, destruction, and degeneration). An atrophic form with resorption of the proximal humerus, most frequently described in syringomyelia, has been observed in diabetes. Loss of the distal end of the clavicle has not been described before in the neuropathies. These changes, coupled with speckled calcification or shards of bone in the periarticular soft tissue, confirm the diagnosis. Infection and CPPD crystal disease can be difficult to exclude. The joint fluid may be inflammatory and infection may be a complication. The resulting soft-tissue and osseous pathology easily mimics an infective episode.[130–133]

INFLAMMATORY–CONNECTIVE TISSUE DISEASES

In this heterogenous group of diseases, the location and severity of joint involvement depends on the nature of the initial systemic process. Usually, the synovial membrane is affected first and bone and cartilage changes are secondary.[134–136] All forms seem to share a common pathogenic mechanism with an underlying genetic predisposition, an environmental triggering agent, and a cascade of immune events in response to the agent targeted to the synovial membrane. Multiple immunologic and genetic factors are implicated in the pathogenesis.[137,138] Type III immune-complex-mediated mechanisms are involved in the pathogenesis of RA, SLE, and PAN. These complexes are formed by anti-IgG autoantibodies (rheumatoid factors) in RA, antinuclear autoantibodies in SLE, and anti-HBV antibodies in some patients with PAN.[139,140] Autoantibodies to erythrocytes, lymphocytes, platelets, and neuronal cells, and to other cell components, such as phospholipids, appear to have pathogenetic roles in some patients with SLE. There is a significant association between RA or SLE and certain class II (HLA-DR) antigens encoded within the major histocompatability complex (MHC).[141] Because class II genes

can regulate immune responsiveness, such an association may be a reflection of pathogenetic mechanisms underlying the induction of autoimmunity. The *seronegative spondylarthropathies* (SNSA) or *enthesopathies*, previously called "rheumatoid variant diseases," are typically seronegative for rheumatoid factor and involve the entheses (insertion of ligaments and capsules into bones) resulting in sacroiliitis, spondylitis (arthritis of the spine), and other abnormalities. All diseases in this group have a strong association with class I HLA-B27 antigen. This group includes ankylosing spondylitis (AS), psoriatic arthritis, Reiter's syndrome, spondylitis associated with chronic inflammatory bowel disease, and reactive arthritis following enteric bacterial infections such as dysentery.[142–147]

Rheumatoid Arthritis

Rheumatoid arthritis (RA) is a chronic systemic inflammatory disease of unknown etiology characterized by progressive polyarthritis and extraarticular manifestations (rheumatoid nodules, arteritis, pericarditis).[138–140] It affects 0.5% to 1% of the world's population and 3% of Americans between 18 and 79 years of age, with a mean age of onset at 45 years. This incidence is increased fourfold in monozygotic compared to dizygotic twins.[139] Joint involvement is typically polyarticular, bilateral, and symmetric, affecting three or more joints simultaneously, predominantly the metacarpophalangeal, proximal interphalangeal, wrist, elbow, knee, ankle, and metatarsophalangeal joints. The etiology is unknown. However, a predominance in women suggests the influence of reproductive and hormonal factors. Importantly, RA is associated with a specific "shared" epitope in the HLA-DRB1 (Dw4 and Dw14) molecules and, in 80% of cases, anti-IgG autoantibodies against the Fc fragment of human IgG *(rheumatoid factor)* are present in the serum. Rheumatoid factor is not specific for RA and can be detected in other connective-tissue diseases as well as in some infectious and noninfectious diseases. Low titers of rheumatoid factor are found in less than 5% of normal individuals and, although absent in some patients with otherwise typical RA, serum titers in patients with RA correlate with disease severity. Rheumatoid factor complexes polymerize in the absence of antigen and when deposited in synovial membrane, synovial fluid, or cartilage, activate the classical complement pathway, resulting in neutrophils influx, phagocytosis, and release of proteases, collagenases, and prostaglandins, which can degrade the cartilage matrix.[140] In addition to rheumatoid factors, nitric oxide, other autoantibodies, and cytokines such as IL-1 and TNFα, produced by macrophages, lymphocytes, and synovial cells are increased in synovial membrane and fluid. It is unclear if the cellular immune response in RA is directed to autoantigens, exogenous antigens, or both, but the cellular response is polyclonal and antigen presentation capabilities of the synovial membrane are enhanced in RA.[141]

The initial damage to the joint occurs in the synovium as a *diffuse proliferative and exudative synovitis*.[163] The synovial fluid typically shows an inflammatory, nonseptic process with over 5,000 leukocytes/mm^3 with no crystals. The synovial membrane becomes hypertrophic, congested, edematous, and thickened. The synovial villi proliferate over the perichondrial margins of the joint, and synovial cells cover the expanded surface stratifying into four to eight layers. Multinucleated giant cells of possible synovial origin can be found near the synovial surface. After an initial vasculitis the synovial membrane is colonized by B and T (CD4+ more numerous than CD8+) cells, activated cytotoxic T cells, and NK cells. This lymphocyte homing converts the synovial membrane into a secondary immunoorgan where enhanced pathogenic humoral and cellular immune responses are influenced by activated CD4+ cells associated with macrophages via MHC class II molecules. The synovium becomes diffusely infiltrated with macrophages, plasma cells, and lymphocytes that form characteristic lymphoid nodules (Allison-Ghormley nodules) around blood vessels. Fibrin deposition and foci of fibrinoid change and necrosis may be present in the inflamed synovial membrane. The inflammatory exudate eventually organizes into granulation tissue that adheres to the cartilage, forming a *pannus*.[143,144] Under the pannus, the cartilage degrades from the periphery of the joint toward the center. The cartilage matrix is also destroyed from above and below by lytic enzymes (collagenase and proteases) released from synoviocytes and inflammatory cells. The inflamed tissue may penetrate the cortex and extend into the subchondral bone, resulting in cortical erosion at the joint margin. As the cartilage disappears and the pannus is organized, fibrous adhesions are formed and the bone ends are fused by fibrous tissue (fibrous ankylosis) or by osseous metaplasia (bony ankylosis). If the pannus is worn away by motion, the exposed bone becomes the articular surface and secondary osteoarthritic changes may be superimposed. Changes similar to those affecting the synovial membranes may also be seen in tendons and tendon sheaths (rheumatoid tenosynovitis), with fibrous adhesions formed between tendon and sheath. Occasionally the collagen in the tendon undergoes fibrinoid change in a manner similar to rheumatoid nodules in other sites (Fig. 10.3).[144] These firm, nontender, palpable rheumatoid nodules can reach 2 cm in size and may be seen in up to 50% of patients around joints or tendons, commonly over the extensor surface of the proximal ulnar shaft and olecranon process, wrists, Achilles' tendons, and feet. Histologically, the rheumatoid nodule appears as a granulomatous lesion with a central zone of collagen necrosis and fibrinoid change, an intermediate zone of elongated epithelioid cells (modified macrophages) in a palisade arrangement, and an outer zone of granulation tissue infiltrated by lymphocytes, plasma cells, and macrophages. As the disease becomes established, usually over the first year or two, periarticular erosions and loss of joint space may become apparent in affected joints. These erosions are best seen in areas around the margins of the small joints of the hands, wrists, and feet and are often poorly defined with indistinct borders. Changes in larger joints may not be as obvious or characteristic and may not be seen until after years of disease. Erosions are not usually obvious in the elbows, shoulders, hips, knees, and ankles, and the most common finding in these joints is a diffuse symmetric loss of joint space accompanied by periarticular demineralization.[144–147]

Juvenile Rheumatoid Arthritis

The term juvenile arthritis is used to describe approximately 80 clinical entities and syndromes. Juvenile rheumatoid arthritis (JRA, also known as Still's disease), is a chronic systemic polyarthritis of unknown etiology with onset at less than 16 years of age.[148] RA is similar in many respects in both children and adults, but, in JRA, high fever, rash, lymphadenopathy, and monarticular or oligoarticular (four or fewer joints) involvement are more common. Also in JRA, there is little or no joint pain and subcutaneous nodules and rheumatoid factor are uncommon. JRA is classified into three subtypes on the basis of the type of disease onset during the first 6 months: systemic (20% of cases), oligoarticular (35%), or polyarticular (five or more joints) (45%). The synovial changes in JRA are similar to those of adult RA. JRA usually remits by adolescence, but approximately 15% of patients with polyarthritis, systemic onset, or seropositivity for rheumatoid factor have worse outcome.[149,150]

Systemic Lupus Erythematosus

Systemic lupus erythematosus (SLE) is the prototypic immune complex disease. Obvious genetic susceptibility leads to cellular immunity abnormalities, autoantibody formation, and deposits of immune complexes in tissues.

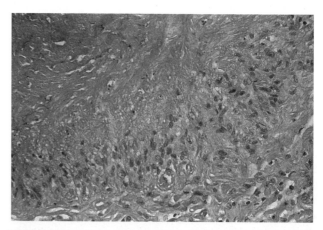

FIGURE 10.3. Rheumatoid arthritis. Palisading nonnecrotizing granuloma. (See Color Figure 10.3.)

Arthralgias and arthritis constitute the most common symptoms in SLE. The acute forms typically involve the small joints of the hands, wrists, and knees in a symmetrical manner and often present with swelling and effusion and nodules similar to those of rheumatoid arthritis. The synovial fluid shows mild inflammatory changes with rare LE cells. Unlike RA, there is no erosion or destruction of the bone. There is, however, synovial thickening of the proximal interphalangeal joints or tendon sheaths.[151]

INFECTIONS

An infection of the joint can be caused directly by Gram-positive or -negative cocci and rods, *Mycobacterium tuberculosis* and atypical mycobacteria, spirochetes, fungi, and viruses (e.g., hepatitis B, rubella). Some microorganisms, especially in genetically predisposed hosts, produce a reactive arthritis mediated by immune reactions to microbial antigens. The arthritis accompanying rheumatic fever, which follows group A hemolytic streptococcus infection, is the prototype reactive arthritis. Other examples are infections caused by *Salmonella, Shigella, Yersinia,* and *Campylobacter.*

Suppurative (Septic) Arthritis

Acute (septic) arthritis is a purulent inflammation of the synovial membrane and synovial fluid produced by pyogenic microorganisms that may reach the joint by several mechanisms: (a) hematogenously from a remote focus (abscess in the skin, teeth infection, respiratory, or urinary tract infection, etc.); (b) in septicemia; (c) directly from a focus of osteomyelitis in metaphysis or epiphysis; (d) via lymphatics from an infection in the vicinity of the joint; (e) by trauma to the joint; or (f) during diagnostic or therapeutic procedures. The synovial membrane is colonized by bacteria that are phagocytosed by synovial cells and neutrophils, resulting in the release of proteolytic enzymes and mediators of cartilage destruction and inflammation. If the infection is untreated, the articular cartilage is destroyed by the purulent exudate, resulting in the exposure of subchondral bone and eventual obliteration of the joint space by fibrous or bony ankylosis. A variety of microorganisms can infect the joint and juxtaarticular tissues (*Brucella, Histoplasma, Blastomyces, Coccidiomycosis, Paracoccidiomycosis, Cryptococcus, Aspergillus, Sporothrix, Protozoa,* and *Helminths*). *Staphylococci* are most commonly involved in very young and elderly persons and in infections of prosthesis where they compete with host cells to colonize the biomaterial. *Hemophilus influenzae* are common in children less than 2 years of age. *Gonococci* produce a migratory polyarthralgia that may resolve spontaneously or evolve into a purulent arthritis. *Tuberculosis* of bone and joints accounts for 10% of extrapulmonary tuberculosis or 2% of the total number of cases. The infection follows hematogenous, lymphatic, or contiguous spread of bacilli from a primary focus of infection (30% in the lung, 20% in the genitourinary tract, and 50% unknown). The process has an insidious onset, affecting a single joint except in malnourished or immunosuppressed individuals. The disease may present as spondylitis (Pott's disease) in 50% of cases, peripheral arthritis in 30% of cases, or as tenosynovitis, bursitis, dactylitis, or aseptic arthritis (Poncet's disease). Pott's disease commonly affects the thoracic and lumbar vertebrae and is usually a combination of osteomyelitis and arthritis of adjacent vertebral bodies and the intervertebral disc leading to vertebral collapse, kyphosis and, in some cases, cord compression or meningitis. Peripheral arthritis often is monarticular, most often involving the hip, knee, or intervertebral joints. The synovial membrane shows epithelioid granulomata containing caseous necrosis and Langhans' multinucleate giant cells. A definitive diagnosis of tuberculous arthritis is made by identifying acid-fast bacilli in the synovial tissue or isolating *M. tuberculosis* in cultures of synovial tissue or synovial fluid (positive in up to 80% of cases). Polymerase chain reaction (PCR) can provide a fast and specific means to diagnose tuberculosis.

Lyme's Disease

Lyme's disease is a systemic inflammatory disease involving skin, joints, heart, and nervous system caused by the spirochete *Borrelia burgdorferi,* a treponemalike organism transmitted by infected deer ticks, primarily *Ixodes scapularis.*[152] The more than 10,000 new annual cases typically present (50% to 75% of cases) as a skin rash at the bite site (erythema chronicum migrans), 3 days to a month after the bite, often accompanied by flulike symptoms.[153] This is followed in weeks to months by an intermediate stage of cardiac (arrhythmia, conduction abnormalities) and/or neurologic involvement (meningitis, encephalitis, cranial nerve palsy).[154] Late stages, occurring months to years after the onset of infection, present as severe neurologic sequelae and a recurrent inflammatory arthritis. Spirochetes have been demonstrated in biopsies of skin and synovial membrane.[153–156] The pathology of the synovium varies and may be indistinguishable from that of active rheumatoid arthritis. A prominent host immune response is characterized by influx of lymphocytes, plasma cells, macrophages, and mast cells and vasculitis. Effusions may be massive (100 mL or more) and a diffuse fibrin deposition beneath the synovial membrane typically is seen. In synovial fluid, the mean white blood cell (WBC) count is 38,000 cells/mm^3 (range, 7,000 to 99,000 cells/mm^3) and neutrophils predominate.

The synovium may have five to six cell layers and may appear as a hypertrophic villous synovitis in which villi show prominent vessels that may mimic a hemangioma. Bone erosion and arthritis occur in 60% of untreated patients. Synovial specimens show perivascular lymphohistiocytic infiltrates, vascular thrombosis, and occasional spirochetes beneath the synovial lining cells and around vessels demonstrated by the Bosma-Steiner silver impregnation method. PCR detection of the organism is a potent tool, and detection of proteoglycans in biological fluids is a way to evaluate the degree of catabolic processes in articular cartilage.[153–156]

Syphilitic Arthritis

Osteoarticular manifestations occur in congenital, secondary, and tertiary syphilis. Bone infection is uncommon in secondary syphilis (5% to 10% of patients). Small joints are affected rarely. The fluid typically contains more than 10,000 WBC/mm^3, predominantly neutrophils. The tissue shows granulomatous inflammation.[157,158]

Rheumatic Fever

Rheumatic fever is an acute or recurrent, inflammatory disease characterized by fever, polyarthritis, and carditis.[159] The inflammatory lesions of rheumatic fever are sterile, develop after a latent period of 2 to 3 weeks following infection, and are attributed to immunologically mediated antibody and cellular immune responses to group A streptococcal pharyngeal infection in genetically predisposed individuals. The response is targeted to streptococcal antigens that cross-react with certain host tissues, such as heart (molecular mimicry). The migratory arthritis of rheumatic fever is usually self-limited and rarely leads to permanent deformity. The synovial fluid in acutely inflamed joints has an average of 26,000 cells/mm^3, predominantly neutrophils and monocytes. Immune complexes are deposited in the joint; subcutaneous nodules similar to rheumatoid nodules with fibroblasts and lymphocytes can also occur.

Seronegative Spondylarthropathies

This heterogeneous group of diseases is characterized by: (a) absence of rheumatoid factor, (b) strong association with the HLA-B27 antigen, and (c) inflammation of synovium and entheses of the sacroiliac joints and small posterior intervertebral (apophyseal) joints and adjacent soft tissues, including intervertebral ligaments and joint capsules. An infectious etiology is likely because germ-free rats transgenic for HLA-B27 do not develop arthritis. Infectious agents capable of inducing this reactive arthritis include various enteric and urogenital bacteria.[160–163]

Ankylosing Spondylitis

Ankylosing spondylitis (AS) is a chronic systemic inflammatory disorder that affects mainly the axial skeleton in approximately 2% of the population, typically during the third decade. Approximately 95% of White and 50% of Black AS patients are HLA-B27 positive (normal frequen-

cies are 8% and 4%, respectively).[164] Patients have a strong predisposition to ligament, tendon, and enthesis inflammation with dactylitis and large joint arthritis. The initial involvement of spinal, sacroiliac, and other joints is similar to that of RA.[165] In advanced disease, however, fibrous and bony ankylosis with bone spurs occur around fused vertebrae (bamboo spine) (Fig. 10.4).[166] The spondylitis starts as an inflammatory erosive process involving the enthesis. This initial inflammation may be focal and brief but it is typically followed by ossification and the formation of a new enthesis above the original cortical surface. Light microscopic studies show surface fibrin, proliferation of synovial lining cells, moderate infiltration with lymphocytes, and sometimes striking numbers of plasma cells. There is also vascular congestion and obliteration, bone and cartilage debris, and a tendency toward fibrosis. In the sacroiliac joints, the cartilage in the iliac surface is much thinner than in the sacral surface and the orientation of the collagen fibers is different in both surfaces. In intervertebral discs, the most common initial feature is an erosive lesion containing lymphocytes and plasma cells and involving the ligament insertion into the anterior or anterolateral attachment of the outer annulus or below the junction of the annulus and the corner of the vertebral body. Ossification of the superficial fibers of the annulus and deeper layer of the anterior longitudinal ligament results in syndesmophyte formation and bone bridging between vertebral bodies throughout the intervertebral disc. Sclerosis of the adjacent cancellous bone and resorption of the limbus result in squaring of the vertebral body.[167] In synarthroses, the inflammation affects the juxtaarticular bone and secondarily destroys the cartilage that is replaced by granulation tissue and eventually ossified. In diarthrodial joints, there may be a villous proliferation of the synovium with pannus formation similar to that seen in RA. Unlike RA, there is extensive bone bridging across the joint, often with preservation of the cartilage and ossifica-

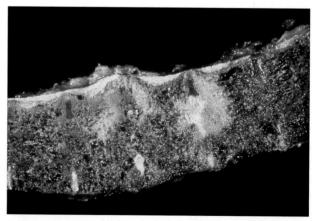

FIGURE 10.4. Ankylosing spondylitis. Fusion of intervertebral joints and spine deformation. (See Color Figure 10.4.)

tion of ligaments and meniscal structures. The synovial fluid contains fewer neutrophils than in RA and Ig and C3 can be demonstrated. In one study WBC varied from 2,200 to 16,500 WBC/mm³, neutrophils from 29% to 93%, and lymphocytes from 0.5% to 32%.

Psoriatic Arthritis

Psoriatic arthritis (PA) occurs in approximately 5% to 8% of patients with psoriasis. It is associated with early onset of psoriasis, extensive skin involvement, and the presence of HLA-B27, -B39, -DR3, -DR4, and -Dqw3 antigens. Several clinical forms are recognized: asymmetric oligoarticular, predominant distal interphalangeal, symmetric polyarthritis, arthritis mutilans, and spondylitis. Psoriatic spondylitis may present, especially in the juvenile form, without evident skin disease. Enthesopathic involvement is responsible for a distribution of skeletal disease similar to that of AS with sacroiliitis, syndesmophyte formation, peripheral synovitis and tendinitis. The pathology of the lesions has net been well studied and it is thought to resemble that of RA.[168]

Reiter's Syndrome

Reiter's syndrome is a reactive arthritis that affects between 30 and 40/100,000 individuals following a clinical or subclinical genitourinary or gastrointestinal tract infection with an arthritogenic strain of bacteria. Males and females are equally affected but the risk is 50-fold in HLA-B27 positive individuals. The genitourinary or endemic form of Reiter's syndrome is most often associated with *Chlamydia trachomatis* urethritis, whereas the gastrointestinal or epidemic form is seen following enteric infections with *Shigella, Salmonella, Yersinia,* or *Campylobacter.*[169] Overall, the prognosis is favorable, but one-third of patients follow a chronic relapsing course with sacroiliitis, often unilateral, and spondylitis with nonmarginal syndesmophytes. Upper extremity joint involvement is somewhat less common. Enthesopathic involvement is even more evident than that seen in ankylosing spondylitis with plantar fasciitis, Achilles' tendinitis, heel pain ("lover's heel"), dactylitis, and inflammation of other tendon and ligament insertion sites being characteristic. Radiographic similarities to ankylosing spondylitis are seen except that sacroiliitis is typically unilateral and syndesmophytes, although less common than in ankylosing spondylitis, are nonmarginal and asymmetric. Periostitis is frequent, reflecting the predisposition to enthesitis. HLA B27 is less strongly associated with Reiter's than with AS, being seen in approximately 80% of the former. Gram stains should rule out septic arthritis. The number of PMN in synovial fluid may be very high in early stages.[170]

Enteropathic Arthropathy in Inflammatory Bowel Disease

Crohn's disease and ulcerative colitis are the two forms of chronic inflammatory bowel disease (IBD) associated with spondylarthropathy. This arthritis shows equal sex distribution, with a prevalence approaching 10% to 20%. HLA-B27 is present in 50% of IBD patients with sacroiliitis and spondylitis but is not related to peripheral arthritis. Axial involvement may be present years before the onset of colitis. The activity of peripheral arthritis, however, seems to correlate with that of the underlying bowel disease. In ulcerative colitis, colectomy can be curative of peripheral joint disease, whereas spondylitic involvement is not influenced. In Crohn's disease, however, colectomy affects neither axial nor appendicular arthritis. Antineutrophilic cytoplasmic antibodies recently have been found with increased prevalence in these disorders.[171-174]

Enterogenic Reactive Arthritis

A variety of gastrointestinal pathogens, which perhaps share an arthritogenic factor, are associated with peripheral arthritis (*Salmonella, Shigella, Yersinia,* and *Campylobacter*). Antigens from bacterial pathogens have been found in the joints, but gastrointestinal symptoms preceding arthritis may be minimal or absent.[175] The arthritis is usually monarticular or pauciarticular and asymmetric and usually involves the lower limbs. Multiple episodes occur in 30% of patients and the arthritis becomes chronic in 5% to 20%. The synovial fluid is sterile and shows mild to moderate inflammation, with 1,000 to 120,000 cells/mm³. PMN predominate and the glucose levels are normal. The prevalence of HLA-B27 varies from 60% to 80%. In Whipple's disease, caused by *Trophermyma whippleii*, peripheral arthritis is observed in 80% of cases and may precede intestinal symptoms by several years. The pattern is polyarticular and symmetric and the synovial fluid contains 4,000 to 100,000 cells/mm³, with PMN constituting almost 100% of this cellularity. Arthritis may also be present in 6% to 50% of patients following intestinal bypass surgery and in patients with celiac disease where an association with HLA-B8 and -DR3 has been reported. It is believed that a molecular mimicry mechanism is responsible for the association of arthritis with gut inflammation.[174-175]

INFILTRATIVE SYSTEMIC DISEASES

Diffuse joint infiltration by proteinaceous materials, metals, or cells can be the manifestation of diseases such as amyloidosis, sarcoidosis, hemochromatosis, sickle cell disease, hemophilia A (factor VIII deficiency) and B (factor IX deficiency), diabetes (neuropathic, Charcot's joint), acromegaly, hyperparathyroidism, hyperlipidemia, cancer, congestive heart disease, lung disorders, chronic infection, or hypertrophic osteoarthropathy.

Sarcoidosis

Approximately 25% of patients with sarcoidosis have joint involvement manifested as either acute or chronic polyarthritis. In the acute form, patients usually present with pain in ankles, knees, elbows, wrists, and hands. In the chronic form, patients have a long history of joint problems, especially in ankles, knees, shoulders, wrists, and small joints of the hands. Biopsy reveals noncaseating granulomata in both forms.[176,177]

Multicentric Reticulohistiocytosis

Multicentric reticulohistiocytosis (MR) is a rare systemic disease of unknown origin that is characterized by a proliferation of histiocytes and multinucleated giant cells in the skin, tendons, and synovial membranes that show villous hyperplasia and may result in a destructive arthritis. The disease is a symmetric erosive arthritis affecting primarily the interphalangeal joints of hands and feet with secondary bone erosion. The diagnosis is confirmed by biopsies of the cutaneous nodules and the synovial tissues of the knee joints. Articular changes are similar to those of RA. Light microscopic examination of the synovial tissue reveals proliferation of histiocytes with large, eosinophilic cytoplasm, numerous multinucleated giant cells, lymphocytes, and plasma cells. Patients may develop diabetes, connective tissue diseases, or neoplasms.[178–181]

TRAUMA

Trauma may interrupt blood supply to bone (osteonecrosis) but it may also damage the articular cartilage, leading to *osteochondritis dissecans*. This entity affects adolescents predominantly in the medial femoral condyle or the dome of the talus, and in one-fourth of cases is bilateral. Detached or partially attached bone and cartilage form a loose osteochondral fragment within the joint. The osteochondral fragment shows viable cartilage and underlying necrotic bone, usually with a fibrous layer on the bony area. Trauma can also produce a group of apophyseal or epiphyseal diseases affecting children and adolescents known as *osteochondroses*, where joint abnormalities are secondary to necrosis of the adjacent bone. Trauma can also produce damage to extraarticular soft tissues, muscles, tendons, ligaments, or bursae leading to tendinitis, bursitis, traumatic arthritis, stress fractures, muscle strains, ligamentous and meniscal tears, and myonecrosis.

DISEASES OF SYNOVIAL MEMBRANE

The synovial membrane can be affected secondarily as part of a systemic disease, typically affecting multiple joints, or primarily usually involving only one joint.

Synovial Chondromatosis (Osteochondromatosis, Synovial Chondrometaplasia)

This progressive, recurrent, and self-limited disease is characterized by nodules of hyaline cartilage within the synovium (Fig. 10.5).[182] The nodules form either secondarily to osteonecrosis or osteoarthritic bone erosion and denudation of the joint surface (*secondary synovial chondromatosis*) or de novo by metaplasia from myofibroblasts (*primary synovial chondromatosis*).[183] Intraarticular disease can coexist with extraarticular involvement. The disease, known as "snowstorm disease," is most likely a different entity, resulting from chondrocyte proliferation in the synovial fluid but with normal synovial membrane. Electron microscopic reveals chondrocytes with abundant rough endoplasmic reticulum, prominent Golgi complexes, and peripheral aggregates of glycogen, the similarity in ultrastructural appearance of chondromatosis, mature hyaline cartilage, and benign cartilaginous tumors.[184–186]

Primary Synovial Chondromatosis

Primary synovial chondromatosis occurs in joints with and without involvement of adjacent tendons and bursae. Early in the disease, the only sign is a focal or diffuse swelling of the synovium best visualized with MRI. Later, the synovium shows an irregular surface with rounded, pedunculated nodules 0.1 to 3 cm in diameter, which arise by metaplasia from myofibroblasts and undergo calcification and peripheral en-

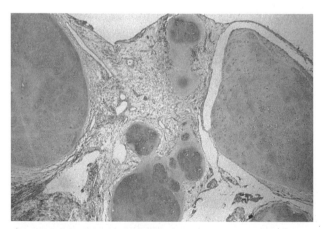

FIGURE 10.5. Synovial chondromatosis. Cartilaginous nodules within the joint. (See Color Figure 10.5.)

chondral ossification, forming well-defined ring-shaped densities.[184] Within the nodules, clusters of chondrocytes are often binucleated and atypical. The nodules detach from the synovial membrane and form hundreds of loose bodies in the articular space where, nourished by synovial fluid, they may coalesce in large osteochondral masses *(massive synovial chondromatosis)*. The extraarticular form, known as *"chondroma of soft parts,"* occurs in tendons of hands and feet, in bursae (biceps, iliopectineal, ischia), or over large osteochondromas *(exostosis bursata)*. The prominent chondrocyte atypia, the large mass if present, and the recurrent character of chondromatosis can be confused with low-grade *chondrosarcomas*, arising either in the periosteum *(periosteal chondrosarcoma)* or the synovial membrane *(synovial chondrosarcoma)*. In chondrosarcoma, however, the cartilaginous component is more mucinous, the atypia is more prominent, and necrosis and invasion of soft tissues are common.

Secondary Synovial Chondromatosis

Fragments of bone and cartilage detach from the synovial membrane and become embedded in the articular space, forming pale, basophilic "nidi" that stimulate cartilage metaplasia and ossification in concentric rings (osteocartilaginous bodies). However, the fragments vary in size and multiple joints are involved.[183–185]

Fibrohistiocytic Proliferations

In a small percentage of the population (two cases per million), the synovial tissues, bursae, and tendon sheaths are involved by local proliferations of fibrohistiocytes that can be grouped prognostically into three separate clinico-pathological entities: (a) pigmented villonodular synovitis (PNS), a diffuse villonodular thickening of large joints; (b) localized nodular synovitis or localized tenosynovial giant cell tumor (L-TGCT), a single lesion or cluster of nodular masses affecting a large joint or tendon sheath; and (c) diffuse tenosynovial giant cell tumor (D-TGCT), an aggressive soft-tissue mass arising from a large joint or bursae.

Pigmented Villonodular Synovitis and Localized Giant Cell Tumor

These lesions are considered to be different manifestations of the same process.[186–189] PNS affects, in decreasing order of frequency, the knee, shoulder, hip, and ankle of adult women in the third or fourth decades. L-TGCT affects a similar patient population but usually involves the volar aspect of finger and toes. They present as monarticular radiolucent processes that can involve the intraarticular and extraarticular synovial membrane in a focal (L-TGCT) (Fig. 10.6) or diffuse manner (PNS).[190] Bone erosion without juxtaarticular osteoporosis is common. In PNS, the synovial membrane is thickened with brownish nodules and fine or coarse villi that may coalesce. In L-TGCT, the tendon sheath and/or the joint show rounded red-brown masses measuring 0.4 to 4 cm and containing bands of fibrous tissue. Histologically, PNS is characterized by various amounts of round to oval mononuclear stromal cells with large nuclei and eosinophilic cytoplasm. These cells, located under the synovial cells, are probably of histiocytic origin and are the diagnostic feature of PNS. Admixed with the mononuclear cells are osteoclastlike multinucleated giant cells, inflammatory cells, foam cells, and hemosiderophages that give the lesion a dark-brown color. Fusion of synovial villi produce empty spaces lined by synovial intima and containing mucopolysaccharides. Fibrinous masses (rice seed bodies) may adhere to the surface or form loose bodies in the articular space and pedunculated lesions may undergo infarction. Mitotic figures are numerous and average 5 per 10 high power fields. In some cases, tumor emboli can be found within local vessels, but this does not predict recurrence or metastasis.[192] The etiology is unclear because lesions are

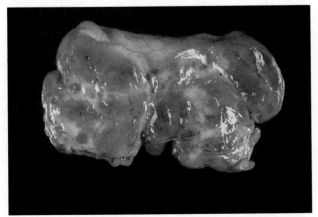
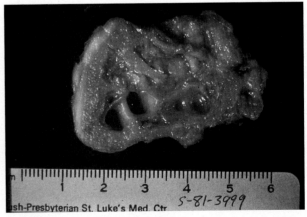

FIGURE 10.6. Pigmented villonodular synovitis. **A:** Gross appearance of hypertrophic synovium. **B:** Inner aspect (specimen bisected). (See Color Figure 10.6.)

diploid in most cases. However, chromosomal abnormalities in mononuclear cells suggest a neoplastic origin.[194] L-TGCT recurs in 10% to 50% of the cases (depending on cellularity) and PNS recurs in one-third of cases.[196–199] Malignant transformation, however, is extremely rare. This diagnosis should be reserved for cases in which the malignant component is seen in association with the benign component, or for cases in which malignant transformation occurs as a recurrence in patients previously diagnosed with benign TGCT in the same location. The differential diagnosis includes: (a) hemosiderotic synovitis secondary to chronic hemarthrosis (the lesion is predominantly subintimal in these cases); (b) giant cell tumor of the bone (PNS involves the bone on both sides of the joint and giant cell tumor of the bone lacks heavy hemosiderin deposition); (c) rheumatoid disease (pigmentation is not typically seen in these lesions); (d) degenerative joint disease; (e) tendinous xanthoma (they are often multiple, composed almost entirely of foamy macrophages, and associated with hyperlipidemia); (f) fibroma of the tendon sheath (this is occasionally seen mixed with L-TGC); and (g) synovial sarcoma (the epithelial component expresses cytokeratin by immunohistochemistry).[195–199]

Diffuse Tenosynovial Giant Cell Tumor

Diffuse tenosynovial giant cell tumor (D-TGCT) is an uncommon lesion, most likely neoplastic, that presents as a large soft-tissue mass in association with a joint or bursa and usually affects the knee, ankle, or foot. The cut surface is white, yellow, or brown and is composed of sheets of polygonal spindle cells, giant cells, and inflammatory cells with scarce cellularity in the periphery of the lesion. Artifactual glandular spaces may be seen, atypia can be minimal, and mitoses and necrosis vary. The main differential diagnosis is with synovial sarcoma.[195,197]

Synovial Tumors

Synovial Hemangioma

Synovial hemangioma is a rare hamartomatous proliferation of blood vessels in the synovial membrane that may affect the joint, tendon sheath, or bursae and is often confused with PNS or other synovial lesions. It usually involves the knee (60%), elbow, or finger joints of children and young adults with a male predominance.[200] The gross appearance varies from a single large nodule to a diffuse villous growth involving the synovial membrane in a focal or diffuse manner. The majority (70%) are discrete nodular lesions 0.8 to 6 cm in size. Microscopically, they resemble hemangiomas in other tissues having cavernous (50%), lobular capillary (25%), or arteriovenous malformation (20%) patterns. Intravascular thrombosis, phleboliths, and hemosiderin deposition are common, and infarction may occur. Large lesions involving the bone, skeletal muscle, and subcutis

should be considered angiomatosis and are likely to recur.[200]

Lipoma and Synovial Lipomatosis (Lipoma Arborescens, Hoffa's Disease)

Lipomas of synovial tissues and tendon sheaths are very rare. They present as rounded masses less than 5 cm in size formed by mature adipose tissue. They may undergo necrosis. A villous subintimal lipomatous proliferation of the synovium known as *lipoma arborescens* is also rare although more common. It is a symptomatic, focal or diffuse villous hyperplasia of the synovial adipose tissue that affects middle-aged men producing slow swelling of knees, wrists, hips, or ankles. It may occur spontaneously but is more commonly found in association with other joint disorders such as a meniscal tear, degenerative disease, chronic synovitis, osteoarthritis, or diabetes mellitus. The entity known as *Hoffa's disease* affects the infrapatellar synovial tissues and is associated with posttraumatic calcification in osseous and chondroid tissues.[201,202]

Synovial Sarcoma

Synovial sarcoma is a rare soft-tissue tumor unrelated to synovium that is often found in the vicinity of the joints and should be considered in the differential diagnosis of joint tumors. Histologically, the epithelial and biphasic types have discernible glandular structures, whereas the spindle type has spindle cells with only immunohistochemical or ultrastructural evidence of epithelial differentiation. Most synovial sarcomas are immunoreactive for cytokeratin, epithelial membrane antigen, and Bcl-2 and negative for CD34, and many express S100 protein and CD99 (MIC2). Nearly all have a specific t(x;18) (p11.2;q11.2) chromosomal abnormality that results in fusion of either of two variants of the SSX gene with the SYT gene.[203]

DISORDERS OF TENDON AND BURSA

Polymyalgia Rheumatica

The synovitis of polymyalgia rheumatica cannot be distinguished histologically or at arthroscopy from mild rheumatoid arthritis. It is not followed, however, by joint deformity or by radiologic erosive changes in the bone ends. Knees are most commonly affected and joint effusions show 300 to 5,700 leukocytes/mm^3, with a mean of 2,900. The synovium shows mild to moderate proliferation with a chronic inflammation that is generally less severe than that of the typical rheumatoid arthritis. Electron microscopy shows microvascular changes and large amounts of vesicular and granular debris in lining cells.[204–208]

ENTHESOPATHY

The enthesis is the site of insertion of a tendon, ligament, or articular capsule into the bone. Histologically, the collagen fibers of the tendon/ligament blend with those of the bone matrix (Sharpey's or perforating fibers), but four continuous zones can be observed: the collagen fibers of the tendon or ligament, the unmineralized fibrocartilage, the mineralized fibrocartilage, and the bone itself. Pathologic alteration of the enthesis is called "enthesopathy"; ossification is known as "enthesophyte." Enthesitis can lead to bone erosion; this may be followed by bone proliferation and progressive ossification at capsular insertions. If the central articular cartilage is replaced by enchondral ossification, a complete ankylosis may develop. These changes can also occur in symphysis pubis and discovertebral and manubriosternal junctions. Enthesopathy can be observed in many disorders: trauma, degenerative diseases (calcaneus, patella, spine), inflammatory diseases (RA, seronegative spondylarthropathies), metabolic diseases (CCPD, hydroxyapatite deposition, alkaptonuria, hypervitaminosis A, chronic fluoride intoxication), and endocrine diseases (acromegaly).

CYSTIC LESIONS

Cysts can occur in the soft tissues in and around the joints as well as in the juxtaarticular bone. Most cysts near joints are in fact myxoid degenerations or *ganglions* or *synovial cysts,* representing bursal sacs or herniations of the articular synovium into surrounding tissues. Juxtaarticular cysts in the subchondral bone *(subchondral bone cyst)* are common in osteoarthrosis. The cysts are filled with fibrous tissue and sometimes cartilaginous metaplasia. Subchondral cysts may contain blood in hemophilia. Juxtaarticular tissues may also respond with cystic changes to the presence of particles of silicone after silicone prosthesis replacement.

Ganglia

Ganglia are cystic spaces surrounded by fibrous tissue with myxoid degeneration and attached to tendon sheaths of the hands and feet. In contrast with bursae, ganglia lack a synovial lining. In some cases, there is a meniscal tear with leakage of synovial fluid. They can involve secondarily the periosteum or the bone. Primary intraosseous ganglia are rare and affect mainly the distal and proximal tibia, proximal femur, and ulna. Histopathologic examination shows that these formations do not originate from articular tissue but from progressive myxoid degeneration of collagen fibers and secondary formation of fluid-filled cavities. Some cysts may coalesce, stimulating fibrosis.[209,210]

Myxoma

Myxomas can be very large and have a tendency to recur. They are composed of spindle or stellate cells in a matrix rich in mucopolysaccharides and they can have cystic spaces surrounded by fibrosis. Atypia is not typical but some lesions can be very cellular. It is important to rule out the myxomatous component of a tumor.[211]

Subchondral Cysts

Subchondral cysts are the end result of prominent granulation tissue with proliferation of bone marrow and myxomatous changes. The histopathological features are similar regardless of specific location and clinical setting. *Osteoarthritic cysts* are a component of the degenerative process of osteoarthritis, but may also be seen in rheumatoid arthritis or crystal arthropathies as large "geodes." They are located adjacent to narrowings of the joint on both sides, predominantly in the hip and knee. They begin as a myxoid degeneration that coalesce to form the cyst. The overlying cortex usually fractures and fragments of bone and cartilage fall into the cyst.[265] In patients with no evidence of osteoarthritis, *intraosseous ganglia* can be seen in the epiphysis under the subchondral plate of middle-aged patients involving the medial malleolus of the distal tibia, the proximal tibia, the carpal bones, and acetabulum. Occasionally, they may develop in the periosteum (periosteal ganglion).[209,210] Subchondral cysts can also develop within several months after trauma to the joint. These *posttraumatic cysts* contain acellular debris and granulation tissue and sometimes bone in the cyst.[212–221]

ARTHROPLASTY

Aseptic loosening of the prosthesis occurs at a rate of 1% per year and is owing to a combination of mechanical and biological factors such as osteoclastic resorption and histiocyte proliferation that degrade the prosthesis material into small debris (particle disease). The components of the prosthesis, polyethylene, methacrylates and metal, are shed into the joint cavity and between prosthesis and bone. Foreign body type giant cells containing engulfed cytoplasmic material accumulate in the area and larger undigested fragments can be seen with polarized light and can also be seen in draining lymph nodes. Methacrylate appears as empty spaces because it is dissolved by xylene during processing. The prominent inflammatory process and the secondary osteolysis may mimic an infection or a tumor (granulomatous pseudotumor) and in very rare occasions can be the setting for malignant transformation.[222–225]

REFERENCES

1. McCarthy EF, Frassica FJ. Diseases of the joints. In McCarthy EF, Frassica FJ, eds. *Pathology of bone and joint disorders with clinical and radiographical correlation.* Philadelphia: WB Saunders, 1998.
2. McCarthy EF, Frassica FJ. Anatomy and physiology of bone. In McCarthy EF, Frassica FJ, eds. *Pathology of bone and joint disorders with clinical and radiographical correlation.* Philadelphia: WB Saunders, 1998.
3. Chanavaz M. Anatomy and histophysiology of the periosteum: quantification of the periosteal blood supply to the adjacent bone with 85Sr and gamma spectrometry. *J Oral Implantol* 1995;21(3):214–219.
4. Aerssens J, Dequeker J, et al. Bone tissue composition: biochemical anatomy of bone. *Clin Rheumatol* 1994;13(Suppl 1):54–62.
5. Mbuyi-Muamba JM, Dequeker J. Biochemical anatomy of human bone: comparative study of compact and spongy bone in femur, rib and iliac crest. *Acta Anat* 1987;128(3):184–187.
6. Biltz RM, Pellegrino ED. The chemical anatomy of bone. I. A comparative study of bone composition in sixteen vertebrates. *J Bone Joint Surg [Am]* 1969;51(3):456–466.
7. Hansen CC, Mazzoni A. Vascular anatomy of the human temporal bone. *Acta Otolaryngol* 1969;(Suppl 263):46–47.
8. Xipell JM, Brown DJ. Histology of normal bone. A computerized study in the iliac crest. *Pathology* 1979;11(2):235–240.
9. Frost HM. Tetracycline bone labeling in anatomy. *Am J Phys Anthropol* 1968;29(2):183–195.
10. Malluche HH, Meyer W, et al. Quantitative bone histology in 84 normal American subjects. Micromorphometric analysis and evaluation of variance in iliac bone. *Calcif Tissue Int* 1982;34(5):449–455.
11. Edger W. Pathological anatomy of osteoporosis with special reference to processes of mineral metabolism in bone tissue. *Verh Dtsch Ges Inn Med* 1965;71:533–568.
12. Sissons HA, O'Connor P. Quantitative histology of osteocyte lacunae in normal human cortical bone. *Calcif Tissue Res* 1977;22:530–533.
13. Garrick R, Doman P, et al. Quantitative histology of bone: the use of a computer program and results in normal subjects. *Clin Sci* 1972;43(6):789–797.
14. Konijn GA, Vardaxis NJ, et al. 4D confocal microscopy for visualisation of bone remodelling. *Pathol Res Pract* 1996;192(6):566–572.
15. Mosekilde L. Consequences of the remodelling process for vertebral trabecular bone structure: a scanning electron microscopy study (uncoupling of unloaded structures). *Bone Miner* 1990;10(1):13–35.
16. Manzke E, Gruber HE, et al. Skeletal remodelling and bone-related hormones in two adults with increased bone mass. *Metabolism* 1982;31(1):25–32.
17. Mosekilde L. Normal age-related changes in bone mass, structure, and strength: consequences of the remodelling process. *Dan Med Bull* 1993;40(1):65–83.
18. Epstein S, Clemens TL, et al. The American Society for Bone and Mineral Research: normal or increased remodelling? [editorial]. *J Bone Miner Res* 1992;7(3):251–252.
19. Agerbaek MO, Eriksen EF, et al. A reconstruction of the remodelling cycle in normal human cortical iliac bone. *Bone Miner* 1991;12(2):1–12.
20. Feik SA, Storey E. Remodelling of bone and bones: growth of normal and transplanted caudal vertebrae. *J Anat* 1983;136(Pt 1):1–14.
21. Cremer MA, Rosloniec EF, et al. The cartilage collagens: a review of their structure, organization, and role in the pathogenesis of experimental arthritis in animals and in human rheumatic disease. *J Mol Med* 1998;76–3(4):275–288.
22. Dijkgraaf LC, de Bont LG, et al. The structure, biochemistry, and metabolism of osteoarthritic cartilage: a review of the literature. *J Oral Maxillofac Surg* 1995;53(10):1182–1192.
23. Dijkgraaf LC, de Bont LG, et al. Normal cartilage structure, biochemistry, and metabolism: a review of the literature. *J Oral Maxillofac Surg* 1995;53(8):924–929.
24. Gardner DL, McGillivray DC. Surface structure of articular cartilage. Historical review. *Ann Rheum Dis* 1971;30(1):10–14.
25. Shay AK, Bliven ML, et al. Effects of exercise on synovium and cartilage from normal and inflamed knees. *Rheumatol Int* 1995;14(5):183–189.
26. Worrall JG, Wilkinson LS, et al. Zonal distribution of chondroitin-4-sulphate/dermatan sulphate and chondroitin-6-sulphate in normal and diseased human synovium. *Ann Rheum Dis* 1994;53(1):35–38.
27. Gulati P, Guc D, et al. Expression of the components and regulatory proteins of the classical pathway of complement in normal and diseased synovium. *Rheumatol Int* 1994;14(1):13–19.
28. Walsh DA, Mapp PI, et al. Neuropeptide degrading enzymes in normal and inflamed human synovium. *Am J Pathol* 1993;142(5):1610–1621.
29. Fairburn K, Kunaver M, et al. Intercellular adhesion molecules in normal synovium. *Br J Rheumatol* 1993;32(4):302–306.
30. Guc D, Gulati P, et al. Expression of the components and regulatory proteins of the alternative complement pathway and the membrane attack complex in normal and diseased synovium. *Rheumatol Int* 1993;13(4):139–146.
31. Wilkinson LS, Edwards JC, et al. Expression of vascular cell adhesion molecule-1 in normal and inflamed synovium. *Lab Invest* 1993;68(1):82–88.
32. Simkin PA. Physiology of normal and abnormal synovium. *Semin Arthritis Rheum* 1991;21(3):179–183.
33. Stevens CR, Blake DR, et al. A comparative study by morphometry of the microvasculature in normal and rheumatoid synovium. *Arthritis Rheum* 1991;34(12):1508–1513.
34. Okada Y, Naka K, et al. Localization of type VI collagen in the lining cell layer of normal and rheumatoid synovium. *Lab Invest* 1990;63(5):647–656.
35. Allard SA, Bayliss MT, et al. The synovium-cartilage junction of the normal human knee. Implications for joint destruction and repair. *Arthritis Rheum* 1990;33(8):1170–1179.
36. Wilkinson LS, Edwards JC. Microvascular distribution in normal human synovium. *J Anat* 1989;167:129–136.
37. Levick JR. Permeability of rheumatoid and normal human synovium to specific plasma proteins. *Arthritis Rheum* 1981;24(12):1550–1560.
38. Wynne-Roberts CR, Anderson CH, et al. Light- and electron-microscopic findings of juvenile rheumatoid arthritis synovium: comparison with normal juvenile synovium. *Semin Arthritis Rheum* 1978;7(4):287–302.
39. Redler I, Zimny ML. Scanning electron microscopy of normal and abnormal articular cartilage and synovium. *J Bone Joint Surg [Am]* 1970;52(7):1395–1404.
40. Teloh HA. Clinical pathology of synovial fluid. *Ann Clin Lab Sci* 1975;5(4):282–287.
41. Schlapbach P, Pfluger D, et al. Identification of crystals in synovial fluid: joint-specific identification rate and correlation with clinical preliminary diagnosis. *Schweiz Med Wochenschr* 1992;122(25):969–974.
42. Freemont AJ. Role of cytological analysis of synovial fluid in diagnosis and research. *Ann Rheum Dis* 1991;50(2):120–123.

43. Von Essen R, Holtta AM. Quality control of the laboratory diagnosis of gout by synovial fluid microscopy. *Scand J Rheumatol* 1990;19(3):232–234.

44. Lakhanpal S, Li CY, et al. Synovial fluid analysis for diagnosis of amyloid arthropathy. *Arthritis Rheum* 1987;30(4):419–423.

45. Kunnamo I, Pelkonen P. Routine analysis of synovial fluid cells is of value in the differential diagnosis of arthritis in children. *J Rheumatol* 1986;13(6):1076–1080.

46. Curtis GD, Newman RJ, et al. Synovial fluid lactate and the diagnosis of septic arthritis. *J Infect* 1983;6(3):239–246.

47. Meier JL. Synovial fluid. Collection, analysis and diagnosis. *Rev Med Suisse Romande* 1988;108(6):535–537.

48. Riordan T, Doyle D, et al. Synovial fluid lactic acid measurement in the diagnosis and management of septic arthritis. *J Clin Pathol* 1982;35(4):390–394.

49. Waytz PH. Synovial fluid analysis. A simple and useful tool in diagnosis. *Minn Med* 1982;61(12):701–703.

50. Blake DR, White T. Synovial fluid analysis. An aid to diagnosis and management in rheumatic diseases. *Practitioner* 1979; 223(1333):101–105.

51. Putz R, Muller-Gerbl M. Anatomy and pathology of tendons. *Orthopade* 1995;24(3):180–186.

52. Ochi T, Iwase R, et al. The pathology of the involved tendons in patients with familial arthropathy and congenital camptodactyly. *Arthritis Rheum* 1983;26(7):896–900.

53. De Santis E, Luppino D, et al. Studies of the pathology of tendons and synovial bursae. IV. Xanthogranuloma of the tendon sheaths and rheumatoid tenosynovitis. *Riv Anat Pathol Oncol* 1969;35:114–135.

54. Thould AK. Arthritis and epidemiology in Europe. *Ann Rheum Dis* 1990;49(3):139–140.

55. Till SH, Amos RS. Neurofibromatosis masquerading as monoarticular juvenile arthritis. *Br J Rheumatol* 1997;36(2): 286–288.

56. McCann PD, Herbert J, et al. Neuropathic arthropathy associated with neurofibromatosis. A case report. *J Bone Joint Surg Am* 1992;74(9):1411–1414.

57. Koblin I, Reil B. Changes of the facial skeleton in cases of neurofibromatosis. *J Maxillofac Surg* 1975;3(1):23–27.

58. Zevin S, Abrahamov A, et al. Adult-type Gaucher disease in children: genetics, clinical features and enzyme replacement therapy. *Q J Med* 1993;86(9):565–573.

59. Bisagni-Faure A, Dupont AM, et al. Magnetic resonance imaging assessment of sacroiliac joint involvement in Gaucher's disease. *J Rheumatol* 1992;19(12):1984–1987.

60. Butora M, Kissling R, et al. Bone changes in Gaucher disease. *Z Rheumatol* 1988;48(6):326–330.

61. Goldblatt J, Sacks S, et al. Total hip arthroplasty in Gaucher's disease. Long-term prognosis. *Clin Orthop* 1988;(228):94–98.

62. Pastakia B, Brower AC, et al. Skeletal manifestations of Gaucher's disease. *Semin Roentgenol* 1986;11(4):264–274.

63. Weizman Z, Tennenbaum A, et al. Interphalangeal joint involvement in Gaucher's disease, type I, resembling juvenile rheumatoid arthritis. *Arthritis Rheum* 1982;25(6):706–707.

64. Siffert RS, Platt A. Gaucher's disease: orthopaedic considerations. *Prog Clin Biol Res* 1982;95:617–624.

65. Aulthouse AL, Alroy J. An in vitro model for abnormal skeletal development in the lysosomal storage diseases. *Virchows Arch* 1995;426(2):135–140.

66. Imaizumi M, Gushi K, et al. Long-term effects of bone marrow transplantation for inborn errors of metabolism: a study of four patients with lysosomal storage diseases. *Acta Paediatr Jpn* 1994; 36(1):30–36.

67. Vogler C, Birkenmeier EH, et al. A murine model of mucopolysaccharidosis VII. Gross and microscopic findings in beta-glucuronidase-deficient mice. *Am J Pathol* 1990;136(1): 207–217.

68. O'Brien JS, Nyhan WL, et al. Clinical and biochemical expression of a unique mucopolysaccharidosis. *Clin Genet* 1996; 9(4):399–411.

69. Erickson RP, Sandman R, et al. A lysosomal storage disease with severe dwarfism, severe joint contractures, mild–moderate mental retardation, corneal opacities and retinal abnormalities. *Birth Defects Orig Artic Ser* 1975;11(6):317–324.

70. Hers HG, Van Hoof F. The genetic pathology of lysosomes. *Prog Liver Dis* 1970;3:185–205.

71. Timsit MA, Bardin T. Metabolic arthropathies. *Curr Opin Rheumatol* 1994;6(4):448–453.

72. Ramsperger R, Lubinu P, et al. Alkaptonuria and ochronotic arthropathy. Arthroscopic and intraoperative findings in implantation of a knee joint surface replacing prosthesis. *Chirurg* 1994;65(11):61–65.

73. Melis M, Onori P, et al. Ochronotic arthropathy: structural and ultrastructural features. *Ultrastruct Pathol* 1994;18(5): 467–471.

74. Lurie DP, Musil G. Knee arthropathy in ochronosis: diagnosis by arthroscopy with ultrastructural features. J Rheumatol 1984; 11(1):101–103.

75. Schumacher HR, Holdsworth DE. Ochronotic arthropathy. I. Clinicopathologic studies. *Semin Arthritis Rheum* 1997;6(3): 207–246.

76. Reginato AJ, Schumacher HR, et al. Ochronotic arthropathy with calcium pyrophosphate crystal deposition. A light and electron microscopic study. *Arthritis Rheum* 1973;16(6):705–714.

77. Kornblum M, Stanitski DF. Spinal manifestations of skeletal dysplasias. *Orthop Clin North Am* 1999;30(3):501–520.

78. Cohen MM. Achondroplasia, hypochondroplasia and thanatophoric dysplasia: clinically related skeletal dysplasias that are also related at the molecular level. *Int J Oral Maxillofac Surg* 1998;27(6):451–455.

79. McKusick VA, Amberger JS, et al. Progress in medical genetics: map-based gene discovery and the molecular pathology of skeletal dysplasias. *Am J Med Genet* 1996;63(1):98–105.

80. Gilbert-Barness E, Opitz JM. Abnormal bone development: histopathology of skeletal dysplasias. *Birth Defects Orig Artic Ser* 1996;30(1):103–156.

81. Cole WG. Osteogenesis imperfecta. *Baillieres Clin Endocrinol Metab* 1988;2(1):243–265.

82. Anderson CE, Sillence DO, et al. Spondylometaepiphyseal dysplasia, Strudwick type. *Am J Med Genet* 1982;13(3):243–256.

83. Rimoin DL, Sillence DO. Chondro-osseous morphology and biochemistry in the skeletal dysplasias. *Birth Defects Orig Artic Ser* 1981;17(1):249–265.

84. Sillence DO, Horton WA, et al. Morphologic studies in the skeletal dysplasias. *Am J Pathol* 1979;96(3):813–870.

85. Schumacher HR. Pathology of the synovial membrane in gout. Light and electron microscopic studies. Interpretation of crystals in electron micrographs. *Arthritis Rheum* 1975;18(6 Suppl): 771–782.

86. Sokoloff L. Pathology of gout. *Arthritis Rheum* 1965;8(5): 707–713.

87. Goldenberg DL, Cohen AS. Synovial membrane histopathology in the differential diagnosis of rheumatoid arthritis, gout, pseudogout, systemic lupus erythematosus, infectious arthritis and degenerative joint disease. *Medicine (Baltimore)* 1978;57(3): 239–252.

88. Smith JR, Phelps P. Septic arthritis, gout, pseudogout and osteoarthritis in the knee of a patient with multiple myeloma. *Arthritis Rheum* 1972;15(1):89–96.

89. Bendersky G. Etiology of hyperuricemia. *Ann Clin Lab Sci* 1975;5(6):456–467.

90. Abraham Z, Gluck Z. Acute gout of the right sacroiliac joint. *J Dermatol* 1989;24(12):781–783.

91. Antommattei O, Schumacher HR, et al. Prospective study of morphology and phagocytosis of synovial fluid monosodium urate crystals in gouty arthritis. *J Rheumatol* 1984;11(6): 741–744.

92. Gordon TP, Bertouch JV, et al. Monosodium urate crystals in asymptomatic knee joints. *J Rheumatol* 1982;(6):967–969.

93. Farebrother DA, Pincott JR, et al. Uric acid crystal-induced nephropathy: evidence for a specific renal lesion in a gouty family. *J Pathol* 1981;135(2):159–168.

94. Canoso JJ, Yood RA. Acute gouty bursitis: report of 15 cases. *Ann Rheum Dis* 1979;38(4):326–328.

95. Agudelo CA, Schumacher HR. The synovitis of acute gouty arthritis. A light and electron microscopic study. *Hum Pathol* 1973;4(2):265–279.

96. Cohen PR, Schmidt WA, et al. Chronic tophaceous gout with severely deforming arthritis: a case report with emphasis on histopathologic considerations. *Cutis* 1991;48(6):445–451.

97. Vargas A, Teruel J, et al. Calcium pyrophosphate dihydrate crystal deposition disease presenting as a pseudotumor of the temporomandibular joint. *Eur Radiol* 1997;7(9):1452–1453.

98. Dijkgraaf LC, Liem RS, et al. Calcium pyrophosphate dihydrate crystal deposition disease: a review of the literature and a light and electron microscopic study of a case of the temporomandibular joint with numerous intracellular crystals in the chondrocytes. *Osteoarthritis Cartilage* 1995;3(1):35–45.

99. Pynn BR, Weinberg S, et al. Calcium pyrophosphate dihydrate deposition disease of the temporomandibular joint. A case report and review of the literature. *Oral Surg Oral Med Oral Pathol Oral Radiol Endod* 1995;79(3):278–284.

100. Huang GS, Bachmann D, et al. Calcium pyrophosphate dihydrate crystal deposition disease and pseudogout of the acromioclavicular joint: radiographic and pathologic features. *J Rheumatol* 1993;20(12):2077–2082.

101. Cooper AM, Hayward C, et al. Calcium pyrophosphate deposition disease—involvement of the acromioclavicular joint with pseudocyst formation. *Br J Rheumatol* 1993;32(3):248–250.

102. Dijkgraaf LC, De Bont LG, et al. Calcium pyrophosphate dihydrate crystal deposition disease of the temporomandibular joint: report of a case. *J Oral Maxillofac Surg* 1992;50(9):1003–1009.

103. Mogi G, Kuga M, et al. Chondrocalcinosis of the temporomandibular joint. Calcium pyrophosphate dihydrate deposition disease. *Arch Otolaryngol Head Neck Surg* 1987;113(10): 1117–1119.

104. Best JA, Shapiro RD, et al. Hydroxyapatite deposition disease of the temporomandibular joint in a patient with renal failure. *J Oral Maxillofac Surg* 1997;55(11):1316–1322.

105. Smith RV, Rinaldi J, et al. Hydroxyapatite deposition disease: an uncommon cause of acute odynophagia. *Otolaryngol Head Neck Surg* 1996;114(2):321–323.

106. Rush PJ, Wilmot D, et al. Hydroxyapatite deposition disease presenting as calcific periarthritis in a 14-year-old girl. *Pediatr Radiol* 1986;16(2):169–170.

107. Bonavita JA, Dalinka MK, et al. Hydroxyapatite deposition disease. *Radiology* 1980;134(3):621–625.

108. Yosipovitch ZH, Glimcher MJ. Articular chondrocalcinosis, hydroxyapatite deposition disease, in adult mature rabbits. *J Bone Joint Surg [Am]* 1972;54(4):841–853.

109. Wiernik PH. Amyloid joint disease. *Medicine (Baltimore)* 1972; 51(6):465–479.

110. Ladefoged C. Amyloid deposits in the knee joint at autopsy. *Ann Rheum Dis* 1986;45(8):668–672.

111. Bird HA. Joint amyloid presenting as 'polymyalgic' rheumatoid arthritis. *Ann Rheum Dis* 1978;37(5):479–480.

112. Sorensen KH, Christensen HE. Local amyloid formation in the hip joint capsule in osteoarthritis. *Acta Orthop Scand* 1983: 44(4):460–466.

113. Athanasou NA, Ayers D, et al. Joint and systemic distribution of dialysis amyloid. *Q J Med* 1991;78(287):205–214.

114. Goodfellow J, Hungerford DS, et al. Patello-femoral joint mechanics and pathology. 2. Chondromalacia patellae. *J Bone Joint Surg [Br]* 1976;58(3):291–299.

115. Al-Rawi Z, Nessan AH. Joint hypermobility in patients with chondromalacia patellae. *Br J Rheumatol* 1997;36(12): 1324–1327.

116. Hvid I, Andersen LI, et al. Chondromalacia patellae. The relation to abnormal patellofemoral joint mechanics. *Acta Orthop Scand* 1981;52(6):661–666.

117. Dandy DJ, Rao NS. Benign synovioma causing internal derangement of the knee. A report of nine cases. *J Bone Joint Surg [Br]* 1990;72(4):641–642.

118. Selesnick FH, Noble HB, et al. Internal derangement of the knee: diagnosis by arthrography, arthroscopy, and arthrotomy. *Clin Orthop* 1985;198:26–30.

119. Tasker T, Waugh W. Articular changes associated with internal derangement of the knee. *J Bone Joint Surg [Br]* 1982;64(4): 486–488.

120. Munzinger U, Ruckstuhl J, et al. Internal derangement of the knee joint due to pathologic synovial folds: the mediopatellar plica syndrome. *Clin Orthop* 1981;155:59–64.

121. Frankel VH, Burstein AH, et al. Biomechanics of internal derangement of the knee. Pathomechanics as determined by analysis of the instant centers of motion. *J Bone Joint Surg [Am]* 1971;53(5):945–962.

122. Aufranc OE, Jones WN, et al. Internal derangement of the knee. *JAMA* 1965;193(13):1116–1117.

123. Ettinger WH Jr. Osteoarthritis II: pathology and pathogenesis. *MD State Med J* 1984;33(10):811–814.

124. Fahmy NR, Williams EA, et al. Meniscal pathology and osteoarthritis of the knee. *J Bone Joint Surg [Br]* 1983;65(1): 24–28.

125. Blanco FJ, Guitian R, et al. Osteoarthritis chondrocytes die by apoptosis. A possible pathway for osteoarthritis pathology. *Arthritis Rheum* 1998;41(2):284–289.

126. Julkunen H, Knekt P, et al. Spondylosis deformans and diffuse idiopathic skeletal hyperostosis (DISH) in Finland. *Scand J Rheumatol* 1981;10(3):193–203.

127. Williamson PK, Reginato AJ. Diffuse idiopathic skeletal hyperostosis of the cervical spine in a patient with ankylosing spondylitis. *Arthritis Rheum* 1984;27(5):570–573.

128. Ono K, Yonenobu K, et al. Pathology of ossification of the posterior longitudinal ligament and ligamentum flavum. *Clin Orthop* 1999;359:18–26.

129. O'Connor BL, Brandt KD. Neurogenic factors in the etiopathogenesis of osteoarthritis. *Rheum Dis Clin North Am* 1993; 19(3):581–605.

130. Xu DY, Cao LB, et al. Neuroarthropathy. Clinico-radiologic analysis of 115 cases. *Chin Med J (Engl)* 1992;105(10): 860–865.

131. Sequeira W. The neuropathic joint. *Clin Exp Rheumatol* 1994; 12(3):325–337.

132. Loudry M, Binazzi R, et al. Total knee arthroplasty in Charcot and Charcot-like joints. *Clin Orthop* 1986;208:199–204.

133. Raju UB, Fine G, et al. Diabetic neuroarthropathy (Charcot's joint). *Arch Pathol Lab Med* 1982;106(7):349–351.

134. Blanford AT, Keane SP, et al. Idiopathic Charcot joint of the elbow. *Arthritis Rheum* 1978;21(6):723–726.

135. Hochberg MC, Spector TD. Epidemiology of rheumatoid arthritis: update. *Epidemiol Rev* 1990;12:247–252.

136. Grassi W, De Angelis R, et al. The clinical features of rheumatoid arthritis. *Eur J Radiol* 1998;27(Suppl 1):S18–24.
137. Glynn LE. Pathology, pathogenesis, and aetiology of rheumatoid arthritis. *Ann Rheum Dis* 1972;31(5):412–420.
138. Van Zeben D, Hazes JM, Zwinderman AH, et al. Association of HLA-DR4 with a more progressive disease course in patients with rheumatoid arthritis: results of a follow-up study. *Arthritis Rheum* 1991;34:822–830.
139. Gonzalez-Lopez L, Gamez-Nava JI, et al. Prognostic factors for the development of rheumatoid arthritis and other connective tissue diseases in patients with palindromic rheumatism. *J Rheumatol* 1999;26(3):540–545.
140. Arnett FC, Edworthy SM, Bloch DA, et al. The American Rheumatism Association 1987 revised criteria for the classification of rheumatoid arthritis. *Arthritis Rheum* 1988;31:315–324.
141. Harris ED Jr. Rheumatoid arthritis: pathophysiology and implications for therapy. *N Engl J Med* 1990;322:1277–1289.
142. Nepom GT, Nepom BS. Prediction of susceptibility to rheumatoid arthritis by human leukocyte antigen genotyping. *Rheum Dis Clin North Am* 1992;18:785–792.
143. Spector TD. Rheumatoid arthritis. *Rheum Dis Clin North Am* 1990;16:513–537.
144. Corson JM. The pathology of rheumatoid arthritis. *Surg Clin North Am* 1969;49(4):733–740.
145. Esser RE, Angelo RA, et al. Cysteine proteinase inhibitors decrease articular cartilage and bone destruction in chronic inflammatory arthritis. *Arthritis Rheum* 1994;37(2):236–247.
146. Glynn LE. Pathology, pathogenesis, and aetiology of rheumatoid arthritis. *Ann Rheum Dis* 1972;31(5):412–420.
147. Macafee AL. Aspects of pathology in rheumatoid arthritis. *Ann Rheum Dis* 1996;31(3):222.
148. Silman AJ. The genetic epidemiology of rheumatoid arthritis. *Clin Exp Rheumatol* 1992;10(3):309–312.
149. Moe N, Rygg M. Epidemiology of juvenile chronic arthritis in northern Norway: a ten-year retrospective study. *Clin Exp Rheumatol* 1998;16(1):99–101.
150. Bywaters EG. Pathologic aspects of juvenile chronic polyarthritis. *Arthritis Rheum* 1977;20(2 Suppl):271–276.
151. Jones JM, Martinez AJ, et al. Systemic lupus erythematosus. *Arch Pathol* 1975;99(3):152–157.
152. Kay J, Eichenfield AH, et al. Synovial fluid eosinophilia in Lyme disease. *Arthritis Rheum* 1988;31(11):1384–1389.
153. Steere AC. Pathogenesis of Lyme arthritis. Implications for rheumatic disease. *Ann NY Acad Sci* 1988;539:87–92.
154. Schned ES. Lyme disease as an etiology of "unexplained" recurrent monoarthritis. *Minn Med* 1984;67(6):325–328.
155. Gross DM, Steere AC, et al. T helper 1 response is dominant and localized to the synovial fluid in patients with Lyme arthritis. *J Immunol* 1998;160(2):1022–1028.
156. Yin Z, Braun J, et al. T cell cytokine pattern in the joints of patients with Lyme arthritis and its regulation by cytokines and anticytokines. *Arthritis Rheum* 1997;40(1):69–79.
157. Keat A. Sexually transmitted arthritis syndromes. *Med Clin North Am* 1990;74(6):1617–1631.
158. Blanch J, Faus S, et al. Syphilitic arthro-osteitis. *Med Clin (Barc)* 1990;94(13):502–504.
159. Paira SO, Roverano S, et al. Joint manifestations of Fabry's disease. *Clin Rheumatol* 1992;11(4):562–565.
160. Burgos-Vargas R. Spondyloarthropathies and psoriatic arthritis in children. *Curr Opin Rheumatol* 1993;5(5):634–643.
161. Cabral DA, Malleson PN, Petty RE. Spondyloarthropathies of childhood. *Ped Clin North Am* 1995;42(5):1051–1070.
162. El-Khoury GY, Kathol MH, Brandser EA. Seronegative spondyloarthropathies. *Radiol Clin North Am* 1996;34(2):343–357.
163. Kettering JM, Towers JD, Rubin DA. The seronegative spondyloarthropathies. *Sem Roentgen* 1996;1(3):220–228.
164. Chang CP, Schumacher HR Jr. Light and electron microscopic observations on the synovitis of ankylosing spondylitis. *Semin Arthritis Rheum* 1992;22(1):54–65.
165. Sampson HW, Davis RW, et al. Spondyloarthropathy in progressive ankylosis mice: ultrastructural features of the intervertebral disk. *Acta Anat* 1991;141(1):36–41.
166. Carrabba M, Chevallard M, et al. Muscle pathology in ankylosing spondylitis. *Clin Exp Rheumatol* 1984;2(2):139–144.
167. Wagner T. The microscopic appearance of synovial membranes in peripheral joints in ankylosing spondylitis. *Rheumatologia* 1970;8(3):209–215.
168. Troughton PR, Morgan AW. Laboratory findings and pathology of psoriatic arthritis. *Baillieres Clin Rheumatol* 1994;(2):439–463.
169. Gonzalez T, Galvan E, et al. Destructive arthritis of the temporomandibular joint in a patient with Reiter's syndrome and human immunodeficiency virus infection. *J Rheumatol* 1991;18(11):1771–1772.
170. Bomalaski JS, Jimenez SA. Erosive arthritis of the temporomandibular joint in Reiter's syndrome. *J Rheumatol* 1984;11(3):400–402.
171. Maher JM, Strosberg JM, et al. Jaccoud's arthropathy and inflammatory bowel disease. *J Rheumatol* 1992;19(10):1637–1639.
172. Enlow RW, Bias WB, et al. The spondylitis of inflammatory bowel disease. Evidence for a non-HLA linked axial arthropathy. *Arthritis Rheum* 1980;23(12):359–365.
173. Queiro Silva R, Ballina Garcia J, et al. Silent axial arthropathy in inflammatory bowel disease. Clinical, radiological and genetic characteristics. *Rev Clin Esp* 1998;198(3):124–128.
174. Mallas EG, Mackintosh P, et al. Histocompatibility antigens in inflammatory bowel disease. Their clinical significance and their association with arthropathy with special reference to HLA–B27 (W27). *Gut* 1976;17(11):906–910.
175. Sieper J, Kingsley GH, et al. Aetiological agents and immune mechanisms in enterogenic reactive arthritis. *Baillieres Clin Rheumatol* 1996;10(1):105–121.
176. Takashita M, Torisu T, et al. Mutilating rheumatoid arthritis associated with sarcoidosis: a case report. *Clin Rheumatol* 1995;14(5):576–579.
177. Kucera RF. A possible association of rheumatoid arthritis and sarcoidosis. *Chest* 1989;95(3):604–606.
178. Kocanaogullari H, Ozsan H, et al. Multicentric reticulohistiocytosis. *Clin Rheumatol* 1996;15(1):62–66.
179. Nakajima Y, Sato K, et al. Severe progressive erosive arthritis in multicentric reticulohistiocytosis: possible involvement of cytokines in synovial proliferation. *J Rheumatol* 1992;19(10):1643–1646.
180. Coupe MO, Whittaker SJ, et al. Multicentric reticulohistiocytosis. *Br J Dermatol* 1987;116(2):245–247.
181. Heathcote JG, Guenther LC, et al. Multicentric reticulohistiocytosis: a report of a case and a review of the pathology. *Pathology* 1985;17(4):601–608.
182. Freemont AJ, Jones CJ, et al. The synovium and synovial fluid in multicentric reticulohistiocytosis. A light microscopic, electron microscopic and cytochemical analysis of one case. *J Clin Pathol* 1983;36(8):860–866.
183. Krey PR, Comerford FR, et al. Multicentric reticulohistiocytosis. Fine structural analysis of the synovium and synovial fluid cells. *Arthritis Rheum* 1974;17(5):615–633.
184. De Bont LG, Liem RS, et al. Synovial chondromatosis of the temporomandibular joint: a light and electron microscopic study. *Oral Surg Oral Med Oral Pathol* 1988;66(5):593–598.

185. Allred CD, Gondos B. Ultrastructure of synovial chondromatosis. *Arch Pathol Lab Med* 1982;106(13):688–690.
186. Moses JJ, Hosaka H. Arthroscopic punch for definitive diagnosis of synovial chondromatosis of the temporomandibular joint. Case report and pathology review. *Oral Surg Oral Med Oral Pathol* 1993;75(1):12–17.
187. Folpe AL, Weiss SW, et al. Tenosynovial giant cell tumors: evidence for a desmin-positive dendritic cell subpopulation. *Mod Pathol* 1998;11(10):939–944.
188. Mancini GB, Lazzeri S, et al. Localized pigmented villonodular synovitis of the knee. *Arthroscopy* 1998;14(5):532–536.
189. Neale SD, Kristelly R, et al. Giant cells in pigmented villonodular synovitis express an osteoclast phenotype. *J Clin Pathol* 1997;50(7):605–608.
190. Darling JM, Goldring SR, et al. Multinucleated cells in pigmented villonodular synovitis and giant cell tumor of tendon sheath express features of osteoclasts. *Am J Pathol* 1997;150(4):1383–1393.
191. Bertoni F, Unni KK, et al. Malignant giant cell tumor of the tendon sheaths and joints (malignant pigmented villonodular synovitis). *Am J Surg Pathol* 1997;21(2):153–163.
192. O'Connell JX, Fanburg JC, et al. Giant cell tumor of tendon sheath and pigmented villonodular synovitis: immunophenotype suggests a synovial cell origin. *Hum Pathol* 1995;26(7):771–775.
193. Darling JM, Glimcher LH, et al. Expression of metalloproteinases in pigmented villonodular synovitis. *Hum Pathol* 1994;25(8):825–830.
194. Palumbo RC, Matthews LS, et al. Localized pigmented villonodular synovitis of the patellar fat pad: a report of two cases. *Arthroscopy* 1994;10(4):400–403.
195. Abdul–Karim FW, el-Naggar AK, et al. Diffuse and localized tenosynovial giant cell tumor and pigmented villonodular synovitis: a clinicopathologic and flow cytometric DNA analysis. *Hum Pathol* 1992;23(7):729–735.
196. Beguin J, Locker B, et al. Pigmented villonodular synovitis of the knee: results from 13 cases. *Arthroscopy* 1989;5(1):62–64.
197. Sciot R, Rosai J, et al. Analysis of 35 cases of localized and diffuse tenosynovial giant cell tumor: a report from the Chromosomes and Morphology (CHAMP) study group. *Mod Pathol* 1999;12(6):576–579.
198. Rowlands CG, Roland B, et al. Diffuse-variant tenosynovial giant cell tumor: a rare and aggressive lesion. *Hum Pathol* 1994;25(4):423–425.
199. Rao AS, Vigorita VJ. Pigmented villonodular synovitis (giant-cell tumor of the tendon sheath and synovial membrane). A review of eighty-one cases. *J Bone Joint Surg [Am]* 1984;66(1):76–94.
200. Wynne-Roberts C, Anderson C, et al. Synovial haemangioma of the knee: light and electron microscopic findings. *J Pathol* 1977;123(4):247–255.
201. Ogilvie-Harris DJ, Giddens J. Hoffa's disease: arthroscopic resection of the infrapatellar fat pad. *Arthroscopy* 1994;10(2)184–187.
202. Des Marchais J, Gagnon PA. Hoffa's disease. Liposynovitis infrapatellaris, inflammation infrapatellar fat-pad. *Union Med Can* 1993;102(6):1313–1315.
203. Dal Cin P, Rao U, et al. Chromosomes in the diagnosis of soft tissue tumors. I. Synovial sarcoma. *Mod Pathol* 1992;5(4):357–362.
204. Salvarani C, Cantini F, et al. Polymyalgia rheumatica: a disorder of extraarticular synovial structures? *J Rheumatol* 1999;26(3):517–521.
205. Chou CT, Schumacher HR Jr. Clinical and pathologic studies of synovitis in polymyalgia rheumatica. *Arthritis Rheum* 1984;27(10):1107–1117.
206. Paice EW, Wright FW, et al. Sternoclavicular erosions in polymyalgia rheumatica. *Ann Rheum Dis* 1983;42(4):379–383.
207. Douglas WA, Martin BA, et al. Polymyalgia rheumatica: an arthroscopic study of the shoulder joint. *Ann Rheum Dis* 1983;42(3):311–316.
208. Miller LD, Stevens MB. Skeletal manifestations of polymyalgia rheumatica. *JAMA* 1978;240(1):27–29.
209. Bauer TW, Dorfman HD. Intraosseous ganglion: a clinicopathologic study of 11 cases. *Am J Surg Pathol* 1982;6(3):207–213.
210. Mainzer F, Minagi H. Intraosseous ganglion. A solitary subchondral lesion of bone. *Radiology* 1980;94(2):387–389.
211. Mosadomi A. Myxoma of the jaw bones. Review of literature and histologic report of 3 cases. *J Natl Med Assoc* 1975;67(3):196–199, 225.
212. Yu JS, Greenway G, et al. Osteochondral defect of the glenoid fossa: cross-sectional imaging features. *Radiology* 1998;206(1):35–40.
213. Taccari E, Spadaro A, et al. Sternoclavicular joint disease in psoriatic arthritis. *Ann Rheum Dis* 1992;51(3):372–374.
214. Galloway MT, Noyes FR. Cystic degeneration of the patella after arthroscopic chondroplasty and subchondral bone perforation. *Arthroscopy* 1992;8(3):366–369.
215. Lemont H, Visalli A. Subchondral bone cysts of the phalanges. *J Am Podiatr Med Assoc* 1990;80(9):479–481.
216. Levine B, Kanat IO. Subchondral bone cysts, osteochondritis dissecans, and Legg–Calve–Perthes disease: a correlation and proposal of their possible common etiology and pathogenesis. *J Foot Surg* 1998;27(1):75–79.
217. Magyar E, Talerman A, et al. The pathogenesis of the subchondral pseudocysts in rheumatoid arthritis. *Clin Orthop* 1974;100:341–344.
218. Schajowicz F, Clavel Sainz M, et al. Juxtaarticular bone cysts (intraosseous ganglia): a clinicopathological study of eighty-eight cases. *J Bone Joint Surg [Br]* 1979;61(1):107–116.
219. Beffa X, Dick W, et al. Subchondral cysts of the iliac acetabulum. *Arch Orthop Trauma Surg* 1978;91(4):259–265.
220. Resnick D, Niwayama G, et al. Subchondral cysts (geodes) in arthritic disorders: pathologic and radiographic appearance of the hip joint. *AJR* 1977;128(5):899–806.
221. Petterson H, Reiland S. Periarticular subchondral "bone cysts" in horses. *Clin Orthop* 1969;62:95–103.
222. Bauer TW, Schils J. The pathology of total joint arthroplasty. II. Mechanisms of implant failure. *Skeletal Radiol* 1999;28(9):483–497.
223. Bauer TW, Schils J. The pathology of total joint arthroplasty. I. Mechanisms of implant fixation. *Skeletal Radiol* 1999;28(8):423–432.
224. Campbell ML, Gregory AM, et al. Collection of surgical specimens in total joint arthroplasty. Is routine pathology cost effective? *J Arthroplasty* 1999;12(1):60–63.
225. Mirra JM, Marder RA, et al. The pathology of failed total joint arthroplasty. *Clin Orthop* 1982;170:175–183.

SURGERY AND ARTHRITIS

G. DOUGLAS LETSON
MICHAEL D. NEEL

Preoperative surgical planning is an essential component of every successful surgery. The surgeon relies heavily on imaging studies and their interpretation to determine surgical approach, implant selection, method of fixation, and even rehabilitation issues. Therefore, in the surgical management of arthritis, a careful radiographic assessment is vitally important. The etiology of the arthritic condition, its resulting bony destruction, and changes in normal anatomy are important issues to be considered when making surgical decisions. Variations in normal anatomy often require custom or specialty implants to be obtained prior to the surgical procedure. Therefore, recognition of these differences is a key ingredient to appropriate x-ray interpretation and subsequent success with surgical procedures.

Working knowledge of basic anatomy about various joints is important for accurate interpretation of imaging studies. The radiologist needs to be aware of normal anatomy, both bone and soft tissue, in order to recognize and make note of variations. Arthritic conditions can result secondary to abnormal anatomy. Conditions such as developmental hip dysplasia can result in severely abnormal anatomy, which becomes important in surgical planning. Arthritic conditions can cause bony erosions, which also result in significant abnormal anatomy. Progressive arthritis can result in or be caused by significant anatomic malalignment from normal alignment. Therefore, it is important to recognize and make note of variations in normal anatomy and alignment.

The determination of the etiology of an arthritic condition is important. Is the etiology of the condition primary osteoarthritis, inflammatory, metabolic, secondary osteonecrosis, or neuropathic? Is there a neoplastic process underlying the condition? Primary osteoarthritis is usually recognized by joint space narrowing with loss of articular height, osteophyte formation, and bone on bone contact with cystic formation. Notation of these should always be made in the interpretation of imaging studies. Inflammatory processes rarely have significant osteophytes or cysts.

Osteopenia with joint space narrowing is usually the only radiographic finding present in an inflammatory process. Osteonecrosis involves only the head of the femur in its early stages. In later stages, it has the appearance of osteoarthritis with collapse of the joint and involvement of both the periacetabular region and the femoral head. Sickle cell disease reveals multiple bony infarctions and progressive joint collapse. Neoplastic conditions and metabolic processes are frequent around the hip and should be considered and ruled out in the appropriate patient population. A periacetabular or femoral lesion can produce collapse and progressive arthritic conditions similar to routine osteoarthritis. Septic arthritis is also a consideration of importance owing to its relative contraindications to total joint surgery. Posttraumatic arthritis often results from acetabular, pelvic, and proximal femoral fractures. Resulting bony deformities, malunions, or nonunions should be noted to aid in preoperative planning.

HIP

The hip joint is a stable ball and socket joint consisting of the femoral head and acetabulum. The femoral head and neck shaft angle is 135 degrees and the femoral neck anteversion is about 15 degrees.[1,2] The head is almost completely covered by the dome of the acetabulum. The head is concentric and spherical within the acetabular socket. The joint space is equal distance between the head and socket circumferentially. The socket itself should be abducted about

45 degrees and anteverted about 15 degrees.[3] The lateral portion of the dome of the acetabulum should almost completely cover the femoral head. There should be a normal medial wall as evidenced by the acetabular teardrop. Ilioischial, iliopectineal, and iliopubic lines should all be present and visualized. The normal center of the femoral head is typically equal to the tip of the greater trochanter. The spherical femoral head should be well centered and seated in the acetabulum. The lesser trochanter is typically located on a line beneath the ischial tuberosity. Often, soft-tissue contractures can be noted based on the inability to fully abduct or adduct the hip for x-ray imaging.

In the evaluation of a patient with hip arthritis, plain AP pelvis and bilateral lateral radiographs are usually sufficient. This allows a thorough review of the proximal femur and acetabulum. Imaging the opposite side is often helpful for preoperative planning in the severely deformed hip. In rare cases, bony destruction is such that oblique views, computed tomography (CT), or magnetic resonance imaging (MRI) is required. These can be helpful in the exact determination of bony defects and alignment.

The indication for proceeding forward with a hip replacement in the elderly patient is pain that interferes with the activities of normal daily living. Patients older than age 65 are candidates for total hip replacement if they have pain that interferes with activities of normal daily living, or pain that is not improved with conservative treatment, including nonsteroidal antiinflammatory drugs (NSAIDs). In patients under the age of 65, you should proceed with conservative care for a trial of 2 years before considering hip replacement. In these younger patients, you must prove that the pain limits their activities and is severe and disabling, often with night pain. Most patients with severe arthritis of the hip are limited in their activities because any ambulation causes increased stress across the hip joint, which results in a significant increase in pain. These patients have significant limitation in normal activities of daily living because of the pressure across the arthritic hip joint. Contraindication for total hip arthroplasty is an active infection, which can be documented by a history and adequate laboratory tests.

When planning a surgical procedure to treat arthritis around the hip, the surgeon needs to be aware of any abnormal anatomy associated with the condition. Excessive varus or valgus alignment around the proximal femur can make soft-tissue balancing and lengthening at the time of surgery difficult. Variations from the "normal" anatomic 135-degree neck shaft angle should be noted. Loss of acetabular bone stock secondary to wear, fracture, or congenital bone abnormalities can make acetabular component selection difficult. Frequently, bone grafts are required to compensate for these defects. Specialty or custom implants may be required owing to extreme varus or valgus anatomy or acetabular insufficiency. Mention of these defects or abnormal anatomic conditions will alert the surgeon that this is not a routine primary hip replacement and that further preoperative planning is required (Fig. 11.1).

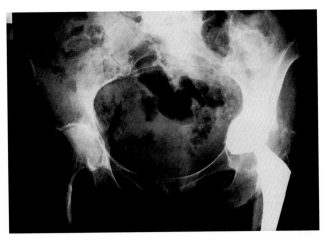

FIGURE 11.1. Rheumatoid arthritis. Hips. There is joint space narrowing and acetabular protrusion of the right hip. There has been a left hip replacement. The cup has eroded bone and is protruding medially.

KNEE

The knee joint is a modified hinge joint consisting of an articulation between the distal femur, proximal tibia, and patella. The patella is a large sesamoid in the extensor mechanism that articulates primarily with the distal femur. The knee joint itself consists of three articulations or compartments: the patellofemoral, medial, and lateral condyles. The distal femur consists of medial and lateral condyles. The medial condyle is usually more distal and has a greater arc of coverage, and thus, is more posterior than the lateral femoral condyle. The condylar coverture is concentric with each of the tibial plateaus. The tibial plateau is gently slanted approximately 10 degrees posteriorly on the lateral view.[4] On the AP projection, the subchondral bone plates in both tibial plateaus are of equal height. On standing films, the joint space between the proximal tibia and distal femurs is of equal thickness throughout. The patellofemoral articulation also has an equally thick joint space. The position of the patella above the tibial tubercle is about 1 to 12 patella lengths from the tubercle to the inferior pole of the patella. The overall alignment of the knee is between 8 and 10 degrees valgus.[5]

In the evaluation of a patient with knee arthritis, plain films are usually sufficient. The particular views required are usually a matter of surgeon preference. However, standing AP, lateral, and Merchant's views, provide a good overall idea of normal anatomy, alignment, and bone stock. Frequently, a leg alignment view from hip to ankle is required. Special imaging techniques such as CT or MRI may be required in rare instances.

Indications for knee replacement are similar to the indications for hip replacement. The patient should be 65 years or older, have failed nonoperative management, have pain associated with activities of normal daily living, and the activities of normal daily living should be altered significantly before considering joint replacement. It is key in considering surgery on arthritic joints that the patient's pain alters activities of normal daily living. There are patients with severe arthritic changes on radiographs who have almost no joint space left; these patients can have normal activities of daily living, but only minor amounts of pain. Other patients with mild to moderate radiographic changes have severe limitations in their activities of normal daily living and severe joint pain; these patients may be candidates for total knee replacements, whereas the patients with unchanged activities of normal daily living, even with severe arthritic radiographic changes, are not candidates for total knee replacement. There are three contraindications to total knee replacement: (a) an active infection, (b) a deficient extensor mechanism, and (c) an asymptomatic solid arthrodesis.

Preoperative radiographic review of the knee raises many of the same issues seen in the hip. When first reviewing images of a patient with knee arthritis, consideration should be given to several areas: etiology, location of arthritis involvement, alignment (hip to knee), degree of bone loss, and abnormal alignment. Causes of the arthritis should be considered and noted. Location, extent, and description of the arthritic process is another area of concern to the surgeon. Is the arthritic condition confined to one compartment or all three (medial, lateral, or patellofemoral)? Is there significant patellofemoral narrowing or osteophyte formation that indicates arthritis? Often, surgical management of arthritis around the knee involves realignment procedures. These involve shifting the weight-bearing axis to an uninvolved compartment. Osteotomies in the distal femur or proximal tibia are utilized. Therefore, information regarding the degree of arthritis (i.e., one, two, or three compartments) helps to determine if the patient is a candidate for such procedures. A diseased patellofemoral joint may be treated with a patellectomy alone if it is the only compartment involved. Alignment, as noted previously, is an important consideration in the planning of a total knee arthroplasty. A significant varus or valgus alignment to the lower extremity can require extensive soft-tissue releases, and possibly specially ordered components. Implant selection is often based on the amount of malalignment present. A severe valgus knee alerts the surgeon to the possibility of the need for complicated soft-tissue balancing as well as peroneal neurapraxia following alignment correction. As always, preoperative consideration prevents or alerts the surgeon to possible postoperative complications and other issues.

Bone destruction is often the result of a severely malaligned knee. Large defects in the proximal tibia and distal femur may result from long-standing varus or valgus malalignment in addition to progressive degenerative cyst formation. These areas may require bulk or particulate bone graft, or special buildups with metallic wedges attached to the prosthesis. Specialty or custom implants may be required to handle large bone defects. Therefore, noting these defects in a radiographic report alerts the surgeon to the potential for a more involved surgical procedure.

Fractures and their treatment can also be important in preoperative planning. Malunited or malaligned fractures can create the same disturbances in normal anatomy that are present in a severe varus or valgus knee. Loss of bone stock can also result from fractures. Additionally, consideration should be given to the presence of retained hardware, which could have an impact on implant selection. Often, specialty implants are required to bridge nonunited fractures or avoid retained hardware.

SHOULDER

The shoulder is the most mobile joint in the human body. Although this is advantageous in that it gives great freedom of motion, it is difficult to maintain joint stability and range of motion when reconstructing the shoulder. The shoulder joint relies mostly on soft-tissue constraint for stability. This is why it is so important to have adequate soft tissue available for reconstructing the shoulder. It is much more important to have adequate soft-tissue constraints to reconstruct the soft tissues for joint replacement in the shoulder than any of the other large joints of the human body. It is also important to realize that range of motion of the shoulder is not limited to just the glenohumeral joint. Much of the motion of the shoulder is also obtained by the sternoclavicular joint and the scapulothoracic motion. The arc of motion of the shoulder joint has been measured to be approximately 150 degrees.[6-8] Two-thirds of this arc of motion is supplied by the glenohumeral joint and one-third is actually supplied by the scapulothoracic motion.[9] When surgeries affect the glenohumeral joint, only approximately two-thirds of the arc of motion of the shoulder is affected; therefore, even if a patient loses motion in the glenohumeral joint, there should be a significant amount of motion still present in the shoulder with the scapulothoracic junction. The articular surface of the humeral head is one-third of the surface of a sphere. This is important because it allows freedom of range of motion. Also, the articular surface is located in 45 degrees of retroversion, which is important not only for the joint replacement, but also in analyzing the glenohumeral joint. Radiographs through this area must be aligned to allow for this 45-degree retroversion so the clinician may obtain an accurate view of the glenohumeral joint.

Imaging of the shoulder is a difficult task because of the anatomy of the shoulder joint. In order to best analyze the glenohumeral surface, a 40-degree posterior oblique radiograph must be obtained. Also, the axillary view can show the extent of cartilage loss, if the patient can get his or her shoulder in position for this radiograph. Arthrograms can be beneficial in joint disease. This is more important in the hypertrophic synovial diseases such as rheumatic arthritis or intraarticular loose bodies. A CT scan is important in looking for bony alterations, especially in patients status post a severe trauma, to help elucidate the bony architecture of the joint.

Indications for joint replacement of the upper extremity are somewhat different from the lower extremity. One important point is that the human body is not forced to ambulate on the upper extremity, allowing patients to tolerate symptoms for longer periods of time prior to having a replacement. This is different from the lower extremity, where most of the pain is associated with activity. One of the most common complaints in shoulder patients is night pain. Patients often remark that their pain is increased at night and that they are often awakened in the middle of the night because of severe shoulder pain. It is more common for these patients to complain of progression of pain while at rest, which indicates a need for some form of surgery, rather than the increase of pain with activity, which is more common with the lower extremity, although patients do usually have a significant increase in pain with activities (especially over-the-head activities). Common complaints that lead to surgery are increased pain at night and increased pain at rest.

Initially, patients' symptoms are relieved with NSAIDs or intraarticular injections. However, these are short-term pain relievers and usually do not address the pathology. Because of the significant role of the soft tissues in the shoulder, many early complaints can be addressed by soft-tissue repair or reconstruction. However, cartilage destruction indicates the need for prosthetic replacement. The progression of pain in areas devoid of cartilage leads to loss of range of motion. Eventually, there is significant loss in the patient's activities of daily living and progression of night pain and rest pain, which eventually lead to joint replacement of the shoulder.

The decision to proceed with a joint replacement of the shoulder is multifactorial. First, there is the failure of the NSAIDs and the intraarticular injections. Then there is progressive loss of motion of the shoulder, progressive loss of the normal activities of daily living, and increase in rest pain. The progressive increase in rest pain is a strong determinant to proceed with a joint replacement.

Implants that are designed for should replacement have to allow for a great amount of motion. Many other joint replacements do not need to allow for such motion; they have their own internal constraints to allow the joint to function. With the shoulder joint, not only must you allow for a significant amount of range of motion, but you also need to be able to reconstruct the soft-tissue constraints, and hook the soft tissues up to the shoulder prosthesis itself. If the shoulder constraints are very poor, you must insert a more constrained prosthesis to allow for stability. This significantly increases the prosthetic loosening and decreases the range of motion of the joint.

There are alternatives to joint replacement of the shoulder, such as arthrodesis and resection arthroplasty, that have varying degrees of success. An arthrodesis is performed more commonly in the younger individual, especially when there is a unilateral pathology. It is often used in the paralytic shoulder, the septic shoulder, and generally with neoplasms that have had a significant bone loss in the shoulder that need to be reconstructed with allografts. The most common problem with this reconstruction is that patients lose a significant amount of function in the shoulder. Patients retain less than one-third the motion of the shoulder in the scapulothoracic area. They lose most of the ability to perform over-the-head activities. They become very dependent on the opposite shoulder. The advantage of an arthrodesis is that this is the only surgical procedure needed. Rarely do these reconstructions fail because of loosening, or become painful.

Resection arthroplasty is another option. Generally, this is performed because of multiple failed replacement surgeries or septic joint replacement. The patient maintains more motion with a resection arthroplasty, but often experiences greater pain.

ELBOW

The elbow joint is very complex. It was originally thought to be just a hinged joint, but it is now well known that it has much more function than a hinge. The elbow has two main functions, flexion and extension, in addition to a function for axial rotation. Flexion and extension of the elbow are the articulation with the ulna and humerus, known as the ulna humeral joint. The axial rotation is with the radius and humerus, better known as the radial humeral joint. The arc of motion of the ulna humeral joint is 0 to 160 degrees.[10] Axial rotation at the radial humeral joint is 75 degrees of pronation and 85 degrees of supination.[10] Normally, a 30- to 130-degree arc of motion of the elbow joint and a minimum of 50 degrees of supination and pronation are required to successfully perform activities of daily living.[11] Patients tend to poorly tolerate the loss of an arc greater than 30 degrees. The elbow joint acts as the link between activities that are done close to and away from the body. With loss of motion in the elbow joint, most of these activities are limited; the patient can only perform activities that are a certain distance from the body. Plain radiographs with a true lateral are essential for evaluating the elbow joint, CT scan is helpful for loose bodies, and MRI is beneficial for hypertrophic synovium.

Patients with RA who are below the age of 50 may require an elbow replacement when disability owing to the disease is present. It is important to note that pain is the main reason to proceed forward with a joint replacement in patients with RA. Most patients with RA do not have significant loss of motion (as do most other patients with elbow problems), and they usually maintain motion throughout the disease. In posttraumatic patients, the reason to proceed with joint replacement is pain relief; however, posttraumatic patients may also have a significant loss of elbow motion. Joint replacement can improve elbow range of motion in posttraumatic patients.[12]

Because of the multiple functions of the elbow joint,

prosthetic replacement design has been poor; there is no consensus on the best design for this joint. Elbow replacements report 80% to 95% relief of pain; however, patients rarely have any significant increase in function. The need for function is not a reason to perform a joint replacement. Following joint replacement of the elbow, patients' only activities are of the sedentary type. Patients may not lift anything greater than 10 pounds. However, it is important to maintain a certain arc of motion, which is believed to be 30 to 130 degrees. Without this arc of motion, even sedentary activities become difficult. Because of the poor longevity of elbow replacements, they are reserved for the elderly population. It is generally felt that a patient should be at least age 50, and usually age 60, before having a joint replacement for traumatic arthritis.

Contraindications for total elbow replacements are infection, soft-tissue contracture, and arthrodesis. Once a person has arthrodesis, it is nearly impossible to perform an adequate reconstruction of the elbow and obtain any motion, although 90% of patients have significant pain relief with a total elbow replacement.[13] One of the major differences between elbow and other joint replacements is that the main indication for elbow replacement is pain relief; this should not be viewed as a surgery to increase function (e.g., so that a patient may be able to return to the work force) as in hip and knee replacements.

Other alternatives to joint replacement are synovectomy, distraction arthroplasty, and elbow arthrodesis. Synovectomy is most commonly performed in patients with RA; this procedure shows significant pain reduction in the earlier forms of rheumatoid disease. Distraction arthroplasty is more common in trauma patients, where there is significant elbow damage, to maintain motion and help decrease pain. A distraction arthroplasty helps to maintain the function of the joint or restore the function of the elbow joint without replacing it. Elbow arthrodesis is rarely performed. It is most commonly performed in unilateral elbow pathology secondary to infection or traumatic arthritis.

The hand and wrist can be treated with joint replacements, resections, and fusion.

CONCLUSION

The accurate, thorough interpretation of imaging studies greatly enhances the ability of the surgeon to achieve a successful outcome. The identification of arthritis around the joint is usually straightforward. However, consideration should be given to etiology, alignment, anatomy, and bone stock. Note of these in the radiologist's report alerts the surgeon to special issues that ensure appropriate preoperative planning. This is vital to the success of any surgical procedure. As the saying goes, "forewarned is forearmed."

REFERENCES

1. Dai KR, An KM, Hein T, et al. Geometric and biomechanical analysis of the femur. *Trans Orthop Res Soc* 1985;10:99.
2. Noble PC, Alexander JW, Lindahl LJ, et al. The anatomic basis of femoral component design. *Clin Orthop* 1988;235:148.
3. Harty M. The anatomy of the hip joint. 45. *Surgery of the hip joint,* 2nd ed. New York: Springer-Verlag, 1984.
4. Ellis MI, Seedhom BD, Amis AA, et al. Forces in the knee joint while rising from normal and motorized chairs. *N Engl J Med* 1979;8:33.
5. Krushell R, Deland J, Miegel RE, et al. A comparison of the mechanical and anatomic axis in arthritic knees. Total arthroplasty of the knee. Proceedings of the Knee Society, 1985–1986. Rockville, MD: Aspen Publishers, 1987.
6. Codman EA. *The shoulder.* Todd, 1934.
7. Dempster WT. Mechanisms of shoulder movement. *Arch Phys Med Rehabil* 1965;46A:49.
8. Steindler A. *Kinesiology of human body under normal pathological conditions.* Springfield, IL: Charles C Thomas, 1955.
9. Walker PS. *Human joints in the artificial replacements.* Springfield, IL: Charles C Thomas, 1977.
10. Boone DC, Azen SP. Normal range of motion of joints in male subjects. *J Bone Joint Surg* 1979;61A:756.
11. Morrey BF, Askew LJ, An KN, et al. A biomechanical study of functional elbow motion. *J Bone Joint Surg* 1981;63A:872.
12. Morrey BF. Treatment of stiff elbow: distraction arthroplasty. *J Bone Joint Surg* 1990;72A:1601.
13. Morrey BF. *Joint replacement arthroplasty.* London: Churchill Livingstone, 1991.

INDEX

Page numbers followed by f indicate figures; those followed by t indicate tables.

Ulnar deviation (*contd.*)
  of fingers, 43*f*
  in Jaccoud's arthritis, 102
  of phalanges, 40–44
  in systemic lupus erythematosus, 99–100
Ulnar notch erosions, 47*f*, 48*f*
Ulnar styloid erosions, 48*f*
Ultrasonography
  in joint disease diagnosis, 1
  in juvenile rheumatoid arthritis, 66–67
  for synovitis, 210
Ultraviolet B light, 88
Uremia, 136–137
  crystal-induced arthritis and, 137
Urethritis, 88, 91
Uric A crystals, intracellular, 124
Uric acid
  in gout, 116, 300
  overproduction of, 301
Uveitis, 94

V
Vacuum sign, 164*f*
  with ankylosing spondylitis, 80–81
  in facet joint osteoarthritis, 35*f*
  with intervetebral disk calcification, 34
Variola, 208
Vascular calcification, 26–27
Vertebrae, aneurysmal bone cyst of, 226
Vertebral bodies
  arthritic changes in, 27–28
  biconcavity of, 30, 31*f*
  changing shape and density of, 30–34
  collapse of, 30, 31*f*, 62

collapse of in septic arthritis, 200
compression fractures of in systemic lupus erythematosus, 101
dense sclerosis of, 33*f*
destructive lesions in, 80–81
diffuse idiopathic skeletal hyperostosis of, 168, 169*f*
flattened, 30–32, 32*f*
forward displacement of, 172–173
fusion of in juvenile rheumatoid arthritis, 69
osteitis of, 76
rheumatoid nodules in, 62
sclerosis of, 76*f*
squaring of, 76*f*, 77*f*, 78*f*
  in psoriatic arthritis of spine, 87
Vertebral joints, 27–28
  pigmented villonodular synovitis of, 210
Vertebral margin, 27–28
Vertebral tuberculosis, 203, 206
Vibration syndrome, 151–152, 153*f*
Villonodular tenosynovitis, 210–213
Viral synovitis, 208
Vitamin D, 297
Volkmann's canals, 297
von Gierke's disease, 301
Von Recklinghausen's disease, 299

W
Weight-bearing joints, chronic neuroarthropathy of, 177
Whipple's disease, 94, 309
Wilson's disease, 140
Wrist

adhesive capsulitis of, 220
chondrocalcinosis in, 129
CPPD in, 128*f*, 129*f*, 130*f*
cyst in distal radius of, 48*f*
deviation of, 46
dialysis arthritis of, 140*f*
erosion of, 270*f*
  in coccidioidomycosis, 10*f*
  patterns in, 40
erosive osteoarthritis of, 150–151, 152*f*
gout in, 118*f*, 120*f*, 120–121
hemochromatosis of, 135
juvenile rheumatoid arthritis of, 13*f*, 67, 68*f*, 73*f*
malposition of, 22*f*
multiple erosions of, 43*f*, 65
neurotrophic arthropathy of, 179, 180*f*
ossification center deformity of, 16*f*
pseudogout in, 129*f*, 130*f*
psoriatic arthritis of, 86
Reiter's disease in, 91
rheumatoid arthritis of, 6*f*, 46*f*, 48*f*, 49*f*, 50*f*, 51*f*, 64*f*, 323*f*
soft-tissue swelling at, 45–46, 47*f*
vibration syndrome involving, 151–152, 153*f*
volar dislocation of, 46

X
Xanthoma, synovial, 210

Y
Yaws osteitis, 208
Yersinia, 307, 309